D1296942

Your
Dry Eye
Mystery
Solved

YALE UNIVERSITY PRESS **HEALTH & WELLNESS**

A Yale University Press Health & Wellness book is an authoritative, accessible source of information on a health-related topic. It may provide guidance to help you lead a healthy life, examine your treatment options for a specific condition or disease, situate a health-care issue in the context of your life as a whole, or address questions or concerns that linger after visits to your health-care provider.

For a complete list of titles in this series, please consult yale books.com.

Your Dry Eye Mystery Solved

Reversing
Meibomian Gland Dysfunction,
Restoring Hope

STEVEN L. MASKIN, MD
with NATALIA A. WARREN, MBA, MHA

YALE UNIVERSITY PRESS/NEW HAVEN & LONDON

Published with assistance from the foundation established in memory of Calvin Chapin of the Class of 1788, Yale College.

The information and suggestions contained in this book are not intended to replace the services of your physician or caregiver. Because each person and each medical situation is unique, you should consult your own physician to get answers to your personal questions, to evaluate any symptoms you may have, and/or to receive suggestions on appropriate treatment.

The authors have attempted to make this book as accurate and up to date as possible, but it may nevertheless contain errors, omissions, or material that is out of date at the time you read it. Neither the authors nor the publisher have any legal responsibility or liability for errors, omissions, out-of-date material, or the reader's application of the medical information or advice contained in this book.

Conflict-of-interest statements: Steven L. Maskin, MD, is the founder and owner of MGDinnovations, Inc., which holds patents on instrumentation and methods for intraductal diagnosis and treatment of Meibomian gland disease as well as jojoba-based topical anesthetics and therapies used in treating MGD. Natalia A. Warren, MBA, MHA, is the chair and cofounder of Not A Dry Eye Foundation.

Yale University Press books may be purchased in quantity for educational, business, or promotional use. For information, please e-mail sales.press@yale .edu (U.S. office) or sales@yaleup.co.uk (U.K. office).

Set in Stone Serif and Stone Sans type by Integrated Publishing Solutions.
Printed in the United States of America.

Library of Congress Control Number: 2021948485
ISBN 978-0-300-25033-6 (paperback : alk. paper)

A catalogue record for this book is available from the British Library.
This paper meets the requirements of ANSI/NISO Z39.48-1992 (Permanence of Paper).

10 9 8 7 6 5 4 3 2 1

Dedicated to patients everywhere suffering with
Meibomian gland dysfunction and Dry Eye

CONTENTS

PREFACE

In late 2018, I was speaking with Jean Thomson Black, my publisher at Yale University Press, about my first book, *Reversing Dry Eye Syndrome*. Sales hadn't slowed; Dry Eye patients were still looking for information on their condition. Having since made significant discoveries about obstructive Meibomian gland dysfunction (MGD), the most common factor in Dry Eye, and its underlying cause, periductal fibrosis, I suggested updating the book. Instead, Jean asked if I might write another book. Although the medical community has known about Meibomian glands for hundreds of years, this would be the first book for lay readers emphasizing the role of these glands in the management of MGD and Dry Eye.

I first encountered periductal fibrosis in the mid-2000s while diagnosing a desperate Dry Eye patient with "mysterious," intractable eye pain. Suspecting the cause was inside his Meibomian glands, I inserted a probe into them. That moment charted the course of my career for the next fifteen years, leading to an expanded practice that includes research on Meibomian glands and MGD, publications in peer-reviewed journals, and a chapter in a textbook for eye doctors treating MGD. I patented the Maskin® Probe and methods for the intraductal diagnosis and treatment of obstructive MGD and started giving presentations on probing and the protocols I follow for successfully managing both straightforward cases and cases of severe and incapacitating MGD. Later I founded MGDinnovations, Inc. (MGDi.com), a biotech translational research company focused on the diagnosis and treatment of MGD.

For this book, I would need a writer and collaborator with in-depth knowledge of Meibomian glands and MGD, preferably someone who could also offer the patient's perspective. I proposed the project to Natalia Warren, one of my patients who had suffered with severe Dry Eye and MGD. She had a journalism background and a master's degree in health administration. She had cofounded Not A Dry Eye Foundation, a nonprofit dedicated to raising awareness of Dry Eye syndrome, and was responsible for content on the organization's website. In November 2018, she agreed to tackle the years-long marathon of writing this book.

Together we conceptualized the book for patients seeking basic information about MGD as well as those interested in learning more. We then curated the salient points from my research and practice and Natalia's experience as a patient and patient advocate. Although our book is not a medical textbook, we delve into important details not typically found in patient-focused Dry Eye literature. We review the science of Meibomian glands and MGD and, based on my research findings, challenge the commonly held view of the proximate cause of this disease. We describe patient symptoms and their impact on daily life and discuss the comorbidities and cofactors that contribute to disease, explaining how successful management of chronic Dry Eye is a process, unlike a quick ten-day course of penicillin for strep throat.

As we were finishing early drafts of two key chapters, 10 and 11, the COVID-19 pandemic surfaced. Once we established safety for our families and I reorganized my practice, patients, and staff, Natalia and I concentrated on the book. Then one day, a new patient from out of state arrived at my practice with eye pain so severe she was suicidal. She had seen over two dozen doctors, some at leading medical institutions in the country. What eluded her doctors, like a "medical mystery," to me was clear. Her other doctors had simply missed occult MGD and other significant comorbid ocular surface diseases. Because they based their diagnoses on incomplete concepts of MGD, their tests and diagnostic techniques didn't discover these diseases. Consequently, they had prescribed insufficient treatments.

The patient initially doubted my advice. Despite having traveled hundreds of miles for treatment, she expected failure and couldn't imagine how her symptoms might improve. Thus, I would have to restore not only the health of her eyes, but also her faith in a future without pain and her trust in at least one doctor.

I started by explaining how the tests and techniques I use to elicit symptoms definitively indicate diseases others can miss. Remaining skeptical, she resisted my diagnosis and treatment plan and consented to treatment only because she believed I was her last hope. Wasting no time, I initiated treatment that day, and her symptoms eased instantly. By the time she left the office, her pain had dropped from a level 10 to a level 3 (with 10 being the worst pain ever, so severe it can lead to suicidal thoughts, and 0 being no pain). Within twenty-four hours, the pain dropped to 1.5. Once we addressed other comorbidities, it dropped below 1.

Unfortunately, this was not an isolated case. Later that week, another new patient came to my office with a similar history. He had seen many doctors and tried many treatments but still suffered with intractable eye pain due to MGD. For these patients, inadequate diagnoses and ineffective treatments were like the random cacophony of an orchestra performing without sheet music. Plus, by not offering Meibomian gland probing, their doctors had acted like orchestra conductors who had sent home entire violin sections.

Although a book is not a substitute for a personal eye doctor, Natalia and I wrote this book for patients just like these two. The views expressed, based on my current thinking and personal research, will equip patients with valuable information about Meibomian glands, MGD, and common ocular surface comorbidities. Our collaboration represents the intersection of a doctor's quest to uncover the mystery surrounding a common but enigmatic eye disease, and his patient's harrowing journey with a painful, incapacitating disease. We hope our joint effort will shift conventional thought about MGD, its diagnosis, and treatment toward a new paradigm based on clinical evidence that reveals the true nature of this disease, and we offer this book as a beacon of hope for patients needlessly suffering with inadequately diagnosed and treated MGD.

ACKNOWLEDGMENTS

A book doesn't materialize out of thin air. First, we acknowledge the important work that preceded ours, from the first descriptions and illustrations of Meibomian glands by Heinrich Meibom, MD, in 1666, to the first mention of periductal fibrosis by Ivan Cher, MD, and the many other researchers in the late 1990s and early 2000s who contributed to our understanding of Meibomian glands and MGD. Their notable contributions created a solid foundation for my research and this book.

Along the way, many other people provided their support and expertise, for which we are grateful.

Steven L. Maskin, MD, offers the following acknowledgments:

First, I am thankful to Natalia A. Warren for her steadfast dedication to this book and many thoughtful contributions. She generously offered her writing talent and a passion for educating those who suffer with a disease that had threatened her own life, and willingly shared this traumatic but ultimately triumphant experience with the world so you, as a patient, may benefit. I fervently pray this book and her story will provide hope and guidance to the countless patients all over the world who are in pain, desperate for help, and suffering with MGD and Dry Eye.

I am thankful for the work of Sreevardhan Alluri, MPH, a graduate student from India who has assisted my research, and Whitney Testa, MBMS, DPT, who made important contributions to my early research.

I thank Katey Mulfinger, operations and marketing specialist at MGDinnovations, for her creativity on illustrations for the text, and Reza Zarif for technical support.

My practice staff continues to care for patients, and I am thankful to them, in particular Maria C. Jaimes, who has worked with me for many years, and Nancy Marte, MHA, who recently joined my practice and has already made a positive impact on patient care.

I thank Shellace James and Ruthie Dibble, PhD, two of my patients who generously shared their stories of being misdiagnosed, losing hope, and finally finding help. Others, understandably, asked that I not use their names, and I appreciate their support and generosity as well.

I am ever grateful for the support of my agent, Linda Konner; my publisher at Yale University Press, Jean E. Thomson Black; as well as Margaret Otzel, senior editor; Kate Davis, copy editor; Maureen Noonan, production manager; Sonia Shannon, book designer; and editorial assistants Elizabeth Sylvia and Amanda Gerstenfeld.

I am grateful to Scheffer C. G. Tseng, MD, PhD, and the experience I gained from 1988 to 1991 as a research fellow in his lab. There, while observing under a microscope, I learned firsthand that Meibomian gland ducts can be held and manipulated without disintegrating. This singular insight led directly to my breakthrough discovery and treatment for an occult, ubiquitous, and sometimes life-altering disease.

Finally, I would like to thank my parents, Sol and Dorothy Maskin, who always provide loving support and who, along with my beautiful children, Benjamin, Jacob, Sarah, and David, have been understanding and patient during the writing of this book.

Natalia A. Warren, MBA, MHA, offers these acknowledgments:

Besides those Dr. Maskin mentioned who contributed generously to this book, I am grateful to my family and friends. You shared your expertise, drove me to appointments, fed me, and gave me support at every step. It takes a village. You were all in mine: Zina D. Hajduczok, MD; Andrew Dmytrijuk, MD; Ceil Warren; John Warren; George Hajduczok, PhD, JD; Lynn Veitch (who clocked the most miles), and Jess Henson, Usha and Mojundar Sridhar, Dede (my BFF) and Curt Rector, Linda Sparn (who clocked the most trips), Nancy Albright, Eithne Clarke, Kim K. Johnson, and so many others who went above and beyond countless times.

For their love and daily encouragement, I thank my parents, Wolodymyr Dmytrijuk and Myroslawa Hayuk Dmytrijuk.

I am eternally grateful to my husband and treasure, Bob, for his loving patience and unwavering support in sickness and in health.

I thank Dr. Maskin, a pioneer and leading expert in his field, for according me the extraordinary honor and privilege of working with him on this book. For me, our countless working sessions were master classes in Meibomian glands and MGD. On behalf of all of his patients, I thank him for his tremendous compassion and dedication to us. Mine is just one of the many lives he has saved.

Finally, I bow my head in gratitude to the One who answered my prayer.

1

Meibomian
Gland Dysfunction

The Most Common Factor in Dry Eye

Maria, a forty-seven-year-old Seattle native, lives in the dark and keeps her blinds closed. She doesn't go out in daylight and never watches TV. The lights cause sharp pains in both eyes. On top of that, her eyes always feel gritty, as if they were full of sand. She's seen a few doctors and tried several treatments, but no one can figure out why she's so sensitive to light or what's causing the gritty feeling. For her, a business analyst who looks at a computer screen all day, work has become unbearable. She's taken long-term leave and might have to apply for Social Security disability. Emotionally distraught and feeling hopeless, Maria now suffers with depression.

Joanne, a seventy-year-old from Illinois who had cataract surgery three months ago, complains that her vision hasn't improved and her eyes are constantly uncomfortable. Despite many visits to the specialist who performed the surgery, her symptoms have been getting worse. Her eyes are red, they always burn, and sometimes they even hurt. Blurred vision makes reading even harder. She wonders why she bothered with the surgery and doesn't trust the doctor anymore.

Bill, a sixty-year-old retired veteran, served in the military for thirty years, during which he was posted overseas and exposed to harsh environments for months on end. The eye pain was tolerable when it started five years ago. Two years ago, on a pain scale of 0 to 10, with 10 being the most severe and incompatible with life, it reached a solid 9 out of 10, sometimes spiking to 10. He struggles every waking moment. His eyes hurt and burn severely, and his vision fluctuates. Light bothers his eyes. They feel very gritty, and his eyelids are always swollen. Bill has seen many doctors and tried many treatments: lubricating drops and ointments, LipiFlow®, warm compresses, lid wipes, punctal plugs, topical antibiotics and steroids, omega-3 fatty acids, and Restasis®. Still, his symptoms haven't improved. The pain is unbearable and unrelenting. He cannot continue living this way much longer.

Patients like Maria, Joanne, and Bill suffer from a wide range of symptoms—burning, sensitivity to light, unbearable pain, and foreign-body sensations, to name just a few. (Except where noted, the names of my patients have been changed for this book.) Sometimes their symptoms creep up, and sometimes they occur suddenly. When one doctor can't get the symptoms under control, the patients seek care from another doctor, then another, then another. Eventually the symptoms take over their lives. They may even measure each day based on how their eyes feel. Is it a "good eye day" or a "bad eye day"? In time, every day becomes a bad eye day.

As an ophthalmologist specializing in Dry Eye for the last thirty-plus years, I've treated thousands of patients just like Maria, Joanne, and Bill. Each of their stories is unique, but most also share one common experience. Their doctors hadn't adequately managed Meibomian (pronounced mī-bō'-mē-an) gland dysfunction. Instead of improving, the disease progressed, triggering comorbidities that exacerbated pain and other debilitating symptoms. (Comorbidities are diseases that occur at the same time.)

There are two primary ways Dry Eye manifests—as aqueous tear deficiency (ATD) and as evaporative Dry Eye. ATD happens when the almond-shaped glands behind the eyelids—the lacrimal glands—don't produce enough moisture. Evaporative Dry Eye is characterized by an abnormal oily layer of the tear film, described in chapter 2, "The Eye." The abnormality allows the watery component of tear film to evaporate too quickly, causing dryness. Meibomian glands inside the eyelids produce this oil, known as meibum.

Meibomian gland dysfunction (MGD), the focus of this book, is a significant factor in Dry Eye. Amazingly, over 35 percent of some segments of the world's populations suffer with Dry Eye. Of those, over 85 percent have MGD. Although ATD and MGD are two distinct conditions, they often coexist as comorbidities.

Contributing to confusion and frustration among patients, the term "Dry Eye" doesn't underscore how serious the condition can be. Because the term sounds benign and inconsequential, many people believe that over-the-counter lubricating eye drops or the anti-inflammatory prescription drops that are widely advertised can cure the condition. But these treatments don't focus on the most common factor underlying most cases of Dry Eye, namely MGD.

As with most complex diseases, to achieve success in treating MGD, it's important to first understand the anatomy and dynamic nature of Meibomian glands. With this understanding we can discern how and why MGD develops and progresses and, applying that knowledge, can innovate targeted and effective treatments.

THE MEIBOMIAN GLAND

Meibomian glands are finger-shaped, oil-secreting glands imbedded in the upper and lower eyelids. Even though most people have never heard of them, Meibomian glands are nearly four times more common than teeth. Most people have about 30 Meibomian glands in their upper eyelids and 25 in their lower eyelids, for a total of 110 glands (compared to just 32 permanent teeth). Not only are these glands key to clear vision and comfortable eyes, but when diseased, they can cause severe pain.

My advanced interest in Meibomian glands started in 1988, when I was a research fellow at the University of Miami, Bascom Palmer Eye Institute, with a grant to study rabbit Meibomian glands in the laboratory. During the next few years I created the world's first laboratory culture system of whole Meibomian glands, as well as cultures of separate ductal and acinar elements, and later clones of Meibomian gland epithelial cells.

While isolating these Meibomian glands and studying them under a specialized phase-contrast microscope, I observed characteristics that appeared interesting but lacked relevance to clinical prac-

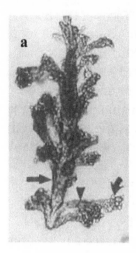
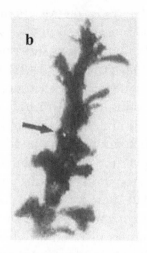
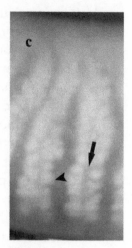

Fig. 1.1. Rabbit and Human Meibomian Glands

a. One of the rabbit Meibomian glands I studied in 1988 (magnified 32 times) after I microsurgically isolated and treated it in an enzyme bath to digest the surrounding connective tissue of the eyelid. Note the central duct (arrow), a ductule (arrowhead), and the cluster of cells that form an acinus (curved arrow). The orifice is at the bottom of the image.

b. The same rabbit Meibomian gland after additional manipulation and staining. Note the reduced numbers of acinar-ductular units around a central duct (arrow) that remains intact.

c. Healthy human Meibomian glands in a lower lid revealed with infrared meibography. The lower lid is fully everted. The two fully-visible vertical glands are generally aligned parallel to each other, and revealed by the acini (arrowhead) that look like small clusters of berries along the length of each central duct (arrow). The orifices of the glands open at the lid margin located at the bottom of the image. The surrounding connective tissue is the darker gray area between the glands.

Source: Steven L. Maskin and Scheffer C. G. Tseng, "Culture of Rabbit Meibomian Gland Using Collagen Gel," *Investigative Ophthalmology & Visual Science* 32 (1991), 214–223. Meibography image courtesy of Steven L. Maskin, MD. Reprinted with permission from the copyright holder, the Association for Research in Vision and Ophthalmology.

tice at that time. Little did I realize this up-close, hands-on study of Meibomian glands early in my career, and my observations that lacked clinical relevance in 1988, would later lead to breakthroughs in understanding and treating MGD. By engaging directly with these glands, I had gained experience, increased my comfort level with them, and developed unique insights into their essential structure. In short, I had journeyed into the uncharted territory of the isolated Meibomian gland.

MEIBOMIAN GLAND DYSFUNCTION

For a variety of reasons that I'll cover in chapter 4, "Meibomian Gland Dysfunction Explored," Meibomian glands can become obstructed and dysfunctional, affecting the production and secretion of meibum and leading to evaporative Dry Eye. For decades, conventional thinking attributed obstructive MGD primarily to thickened meibum and keratinization (skinlike changes to the cells lining the duct wall). My research instead strongly suggests that the scar tissue (periductal fibrosis) that surrounds, constricts, and invades the glands plays an even more important role. These constrictions squeeze the glands, choking them off and preventing the oil they produce from flowing to the tear film. The scar tissue is occult, detectable only with special microscopes or by the tip of a probe inserted into the gland.

A WORLD OF COMPLEXITY: COMORBIDITIES AND COFACTORS

In my previous book, *Reversing Dry Eye Syndrome,* I describe the spiraling events that result when Dry Eye—either ATD or evaporative Dry Eye—develops. One disease exacerbates or leads to other diseases that exacerbate the original disease, triggering a downward spiral. MGD fuels this downward spiral, but a variety of ocular and systemic comorbid diseases and cofactors can fan the flames. The possibilities are vast and unique for each patient (see chapter 5, "Comorbidities and Cofactors").

In the setting of multiple comorbidities, doctors can't administer just one test or prescribe a single treatment to reverse diseases and resolve symptoms. They need to diagnose and treat each distinct comorbidity. Plus, patients may have to examine their lives thoughtfully, just as Maria, Joanne, and Bill would have to, to discover and address the factors contributing to their specific sets of comorbidities and symptoms.

SYMPTOMS: LIFE WITH PAIN

One night in severe pain, Bill drove himself to a local emergency room. But the ER doctor only referred him to a psychiatrist. Bill didn't bother making an appointment. How could a psychiatrist help his eyes? Instead, he visited online forums to find out if anyone else was suffering this way. That's where he learned about Meibomian gland probing and an ophthalmologist in Tampa, Florida.

The three-thousand-mile trip from Southern California to see the specialist was brutal. He could barely keep his eyes open because of the pain. In the terminal, waiting for his flight, with ice on his eyes, he decided this would be his last shot. If Dr. Maskin couldn't help, Bill would end his life.

Maria, Joanne, and Bill are different. They're different ages and genders. They live in different parts of the country and environments. Their jobs and the settings in which they developed symptoms are different. But they each share a common story: undiagnosed and untreated, their symptoms shattered their lives.

Maria had to stop working, lived in the dark, and never left her house. Joanne could hardly see. Bill was so desperate for relief he contemplated suicide. Other diseases can have profound effects on the quality of life, too, but with MGD, even simple, everyday activities like reading, watching TV, or driving can become impossible. That's because the eyes are very sensitive. So even a tiny defect can cause a lot of pain. And when eyes hurt, it's very hard to use them and function normally.

With MGD, patients often feel burning and have tender and sore lids. With ATD, patients often complain of gritty, sandy, or foreign-body sensations. Although these are typical symptoms of MGD and ATD, patients can complain of a variety of painful sensations.

But for some MGD patients, the severity of symptoms doesn't always correlate to the severity of disease. For example, sometimes patients have no symptoms but have signs of MGD. This scenario, described as subclinical (asymptomatic), explains why patients don't always seek help in the early stages of the disease, when it's easier to treat—because they can't always feel it. Conversely, sometimes symptoms are solid 10s even without obvious signs of disease, a reason diagnosis can be difficult.

MGD may aggravate other ocular surface diseases, which themselves produce a wide range of symptoms. These other comorbidities can cause entirely different, overlapping symptoms or might masquerade as MGD by causing similar symptoms that together make accurate diagnosis exceedingly difficult (see chapter 6, "Symptoms:

Living with Pain"). Determining whether it's MGD, ATD, a different comorbidity, or all of these may require some detective work. It's the same with many other diseases. Chest pain can mean a heart attack or GERD or even musculoskeletal inflammation—but which one?

Overlapping and masquerading symptoms often occur near the ocular surface. For example, a sharp, localized pain in the upper inner corner of the eye may indicate any of these:

- One or more blocked Meibomian glands
- A muscle spasm in the eyelid
- Inflammation at the base or root of an eyelash, also called folliculitis
- A traumatic injury to the eyeball or conjunctiva
- A foreign body, like an eyelash or even just a piece of dust, stuck in the eye, in the tear film, or stuck to the eyelid
- Conjunctivochalasis
- Other diseases of the ocular surface or eyelids

With so many possibilities, a symptom alone doesn't necessarily lead to a single, precise diagnosis. Hence, the need for detective work.

Further complicating matters, one very strong symptom can sometimes overlap and mask weaker symptoms. Plus, symptoms are typically felt in a very small area and in parts of the body that touch each other. Determining precisely where the symptom is coming from alone can be difficult. Is it coming from the eyelid, tear film, surface of the eyeball, or referred from somewhere else, like the back of the head? (You will learn how to locate symptoms in chapter 6 (sidebar 6.1) and in chapter 12, "Guidelines for Managing Your Life with Meibomian Gland Dysfunction.")

Because they happen near each other, because they're in such a sensitive part of the body, and because they can wax and wane, symptoms can cause a lot of physical pain and mental frustration. Still, I never tell patients they'll learn to live with their symptoms. Instead, we talk about specific causes, targeted treatments, and ongoing disease management—getting symptoms under control, learning what triggers them, and how to avoid flare-ups.

DIAGNOSIS

During Maria's first exam, I find that her eyes are dry—both her tear meniscus height and Schirmer's tests with topical anesthesia scores are low. (A Schirmer's test checks the tear film volume, with any result under 10 indicating dryness.) When I press on her eyelids, they are very tender, and only a few Meibomian glands express oil. While probing her glands, I find that over 90 percent are constricted by bands of scar tissue choking them off. The bands are firm and fixed in place. Because the constrictions are deep inside the lids, Maria's doctors couldn't see them. Maybe that's why they couldn't tell her why her eyes were so sensitive to light.

While probing Joanne's Meibomian glands, I find that 80 percent are constricted by bands of scar tissue. The glands don't secrete enough oil, a hallmark of MGD. As a result, her tear film is very thin and doesn't lubricate her eyes, causing pain and affecting her ability to focus. Cataract surgery likely exacerbated the disease, triggering her symptoms. But because the MGD wasn't treated adequately before surgery or during her recovery, her symptoms persisted.

Bill had tried many available Dry Eye treatments, but none were specifically targeted for the fixed scar tissue I find during probing, wrapped around almost all of his Meibomian glands, rendering those treatments insufficient. In his left eye, the upper lid has only two functioning (expressible) glands, and his lower lid has only four. In his right eye, the upper lid has three functioning glands, and the lower has just two. Exposure to harsh environments while stationed overseas and friction on his ocular surface from untreated MGD were undoubtedly factors leading to conjunctival wrinkling, known as conjunctivochalasis. On top of that, Bill's watery tears are deficient, scoring 0 mm in his right and only 4 mm in his left eye on Schirmer's tests. Suspecting he may have an underlying systemic condition, I refer him to a local rheumatologist.

When ocular conditions coexist and present with similar symptoms, it can make diagnosis difficult. But difficult or not, it's imperative that doctors identify all existing comorbidities for each patient so they can be treated appropriately. When all comorbidities are not found, there are consequences. Patients' symptoms don't resolve and everyone becomes frustrated, doctors and patients alike. This vicious cycle of symptoms and diseases feeds on itself, continuing until it's finally broken by an accurate diagnosis followed by targeted and effective treatment.

But most people haven't heard of Meibomian glands or MGD. So when patients first learn they have it or common comorbidities, they're surprised. Not helping matters, doctors often use a variety of Dry Eye and MGD-related terms interchangeably. To avoid confusion, here are definitions for several of these terms. They are divided into two categories: the first describes the anatomical location of the disease, and the second describes a functional problem.

Anatomical Location

Blepharitis: Inflammation of the eyelids. (*Blephar* is Greek for "eyelid.") This is a very nonspecific term that is often used as a substitute for the more specific MGD. There are two variants: anterior blepharitis and posterior blepharitis.

- *Anterior blepharitis:* Inflammation of the forward part of the eyelid, in particular the base of the eyelashes. (Anterior means "front.")
- *Posterior blepharitis:* Inflammation of the rear part of the eyelid, including the lid margin and the Meibomian glands. The term is often used instead of MGD.

Functional Problem

Dry Eye or Dry Eye syndrome: The umbrella term that refers to all types of tear dysfunction syndromes, including aqueous tear deficiency and evaporative Dry Eye.

- *Aqueous tear deficiency (ATD):* A disease characterized by decreased production of moisture by the lacrimal glands.
- *Evaporative Dry Eye:* A disease typically characterized by decreased secretion or poor quality of the oil, meibum, which leads to faster than normal evaporation of the tear film. It's usually caused by MGD.
- *Meibomian Gland Dysfunction (MGD):* The disruption of the

normal function of Meibomian glands, a significant factor in over 85 percent of Dry Eye cases.

Sometimes patients aren't accurately diagnosed because tests haven't been administered in a manner that maximizes their ability to detect comorbidities. ATD, for example, may go undetected because of false negative readings in a widely used test for wetness, but it can be easily detected with a simple modification to the test protocol, which I'll explain in chapter 9, "The Diagnosis." Other times it's difficult to interpret patient symptoms because of overlapping or masquerading comorbidities. These can make diagnosis very challenging. But whatever the reason, and especially because there can be many comorbidities, comprehensive and accurate diagnoses are necessary so that the right targeted treatments are prescribed.

TREATMENT

I cauterize Maria's lower tear drainage ducts to increase the volume of tear film and use a probe to release the strictures invading her Meibomian glands, allowing the meibum to flow out. Maria immediately feels better and listens as I carefully explain why it's important to continue practicing good eyelid hygiene. She goes home, turns on the lights, watches TV, and calls her adult children. Maria plans to test out her new eyes for a few days, and then she'll return to work.

I probe Joanne's Meibomian glands. Afterward I instruct her to use topical preservative-free steroid drops for seven days because her glands have been inflamed. When she returns for a follow-up appointment two weeks later, she reports that her symptoms have resolved and that her eye comfort and vision have improved. Joanne is just like the estimated 50 percent of cataract patients with MGD, of which 90 percent have scar tissue invading and constricting their Meibomian glands but who aren't adequately treated before the procedure. Now that she has been effectively treated, Joanne can get on with life and return to the cataract surgeon for a final adjustment of her glasses.

I cauterize Bill's right lower tear duct because that eye is particularly dry, and I probe his Meibomian glands to restore their function. Three weeks after probing, the number of functioning glands has improved. Now, in his right eye, the upper lid has fourteen functioning glands and the

Table 1.1

Bill's Functioning Meibomian Glands Before and After Probing

	Right Eye		Left Eye	
Lid	*Before*	*After*	*Before*	*After*
Upper	3	14	2	17
Lower	2	18	4	11

Courtesy of Steven L. Maskin, MD.

lower lid has eighteen. In his left eye, the upper lid has seventeen functioning glands and the lower lid has eleven. Within three weeks, his pain dropped from a 10 to a 3.

Bill's Schirmer's tests have also improved, scoring up to 6 mm in each eye. But because Bill has conjunctivochalasis, his symptoms are not at 0 and the Schirmer's tests results are still below my preferred target of 10. Bill will need surgery to replace his damaged conjunctiva with amniotic membrane grafts.

Just one week after surgery on his left eye, it surprises Bill how much better that eye feels, and he can't wait to get his right eye done. After I repair both ocular surfaces, Bill's symptoms drop to 0. He can't believe how needlessly close he came to suicide.

Maria, Joanne, and Bill share another common trait. Once MGD

Table 1.2

Bill's Schirmer's Test Results
Before and After Probing All Lids and
Cautery of Lower Tear Duct of the Right Eye

Time Frame	Right Eye	Left Eye
Before	0 mm	4 mm
After	6 mm	6 mm

Courtesy of Steven L. Maskin, MD.

Table 1.3
Bill's Pain Level Before and After Treatment, on a Scale of 0–10 (10 being most severe)

Time Frame	Right Eye	Left Eye
Before treatment	10	10
After probing both lids (left eye)	—	3
After probing both lids and lower punctal cautery (right eye)	3	—
After surgery: AMT for conjunctivochalasis	0	0

Courtesy of Steven L. Maskin, MD.

and other comorbidities were addressed with targeted treatments specific to those conditions, their symptoms subsided dramatically. For example, Maskin® Probing of Meibomian glands dramatically and immediately provided relief for their sore and tender lids and other symptoms, like burning and pain. It released periductal scar tissue, established or confirmed patency (lacking obstruction) of their Meibomian gland ducts, and restored ductal integrity. Together, the relief of symptoms, proof of duct patency, and restoration of ductal integrity create a paradigm shift in the management of MGD.

Many traditional approaches to treating MGD fall short simply because they (1) overlook and fail to release the scar tissue that constricts the glands, (2) overlook and therefore don't treat comorbidities, or (3) prescribe nonspecific treatments that don't target periductal fibrosis or comorbidities.

To bolster their improvements and maintain the renewed level of comfort in their eyes, patients have to be attentive and take care of their Meibomian glands. They should practice good lid hygiene, stay hydrated, get plenty of sleep, eat a healthy diet, and exercise. Bill and Joanne apply warm compresses to their eyes daily. Maria looks away from the computer screen every twenty minutes, rests her eyes, and blinks. (For more tips, see chapter 12.)

In summary, probing to release periductal scar tissue begins the successful management of MGD, while diagnosing and treating co-morbidities and addressing cofactors continue the process.

DO YOU HAVE MGD?: A SELF-TEST

Answer the questions and read the commentary on each. If you answered yes to at least one question, there's a chance you have at least a mild case of MGD.

Question 1: Are your upper eyelids tender if you press very gently on them while looking down, and/or are your lower lids tender if you press very gently on them while looking up?

Lid tenderness can indicate MGD because constricting bands of scar tissue may block Meibomian glands, preventing the flow of meibum. As the meibum builds up behind the constrictions, pressure increases inside the glands, dilating and distorting them. The elevated pressure also causes the lids to become tender. If not properly treated, over time the Meibomian glands will atrophy.

Question 2: Do your eyes burn?

Burning may indicate an allergic reaction as well as an unstable tear film, which can be due to poor quality or abnormal quantity of meibum or other inflammatory factors. A destabilized tear film can expose the nerve endings of the surface tissue of the eye, creating a burning sensation.

Question 3: Are you closing your eyes or squinting more often than usual?

MGD causes evaporative Dry Eye, which often causes an unstable tear film and burning that can be relieved with eye closure. Furthermore, because the tear film is part of the optical system that brings objects into focus, vision may suffer with a tear film destabilized by MGD. To improve vision due to destabilized tear film, you might squint subconsciously. Squinting can help because it concentrates the available tear film into a smaller area, thickening the layer of film over the cornea, thus improving both comfort and vision quality.

MGD-induced destabilized tear film may even cause inaccurate measurements during vision tests routinely used to prescribe glasses and prior to cataract surgery, measurements used to select the strength of the replacement lens.

Question 4: Do you feel something in your eye?

A chronic, localized, foreign-body sensation might indicate MGD. When a Meibomian gland is blocked and swollen, it can feel like a foreign body somewhere in the eye because the swollen part of the lid passes over the eye with each blink. Meibomian glands can also become capped with stagnant meibum. The waxy cap itself, visible on the lid margin at the opening of the gland, can feel like a foreign body in the eye.

Other ocular surface comorbidities, including ATD, conjunctivochalasis, and aberrant eyelashes can all masquerade as foreign bodies in the eye. In addition, a cluster of comorbidities I see often, and which I call *lateral canthal crowding* (discussed in chapter 5, "Comorbidities and Cofactors"), can cause a foreign-body sensation in the outer corner of the eyes.

Question 5: Are your eyes watering a lot?

With MGD, the quality and/or quantity of meibum reaching the tear film declines. This leads to faster evaporation of the tear film. Paradoxically, the eyes may compensate by producing reflex tears, and the result is excessive watering. Conjunctivochalasis, which can channel the tear film flow away from its normal course toward the nose and instead to the lateral (outer) corner of the eye, is another comorbidity often found with MGD. This condition can aggravate watering or lead to moisture collecting on the skin of the lateral corner of the eye. Because the tear film is channeled away, the ocular surface may become dry, leading to reflex tears.

Tear film can build up and overflow not only due to excess reflex tearing, but also if there is something stimulating excess tear secretion, such as a foreign body or infection, or if there is a blockage in the drainage system. A variety of conditions can cause these blockages, including redundant conjunctivochalasis tissue.

Question 6: Do your eyes or eyelids feel heavy?

When meibum builds up behind constricting bands of scar tissue in the eyelids, the lids can become puffy, tender, sore, and feel heavier than normal. There's increased friction on the eye with each blink. The excess weight in the lids contributes to pain, foreign-body sensations, and exacerbates the symptoms of superior (on the upper part of the eyeball) conjunctivochalasis.

Lateral canthal crowding and its different comorbidities, such as inferior conjunctivochalasis, can make the eyelids feel heavy, too. Some people develop dermatochalasis, characterized by loose upper eyelid tissue. The eyelids can look droopy, and the extra weight on the eyeball can feel heavy.

Question 7: Do you spend a lot of time at computer screens, on digital phones, or using tablets?

When you spend a lot of time gazing, performing activities that require visual focus, for example, looking at computer screens, TV screens, digital phones, the road while driving; scanning lists or objects; sewing; knitting; reading books; or even just staring into space while you're on the phone, your blink rate decreases and partial blinks increase.

Your eyes become red and tired because you're not distributing tear film properly across the ocular surface or removing old, dirty tears with each blink. A reduced blink rate can also affect meibum secretion. Lubricating drops can help, but it's also important to remind yourself to blink often—at least every five to seven seconds—and every twenty minutes take breaks from gazing. Look away from what you're doing, stretch your neck, and force yourself to blink purposefully.

EIGHT MYTHS ABOUT MGD

There are many commonly held myths about MGD, and this book covers many of them. Here are eight myths about Dry Eye and MGD and the fundamental facts that refute them. More can be found in the opening of other chapters.

Myth #1

Over-the-counter lubricating eye drops, available at every drugstore, supermarket, and convenience store, are simple and reliable treatments for dry, irritated eyes.

Facts

Lubricating eye drops might make your eyes feel better temporarily, but they will do nothing to reverse the course of obstructive MGD due to diseased Meibomian glands blocked with constricting bands of periductal scar tissue.

Lubricating drops also won't treat allergies or a variety of other ocular surface, eyelid, and eyelash disorders often associated with MGD.

Some eye drops can cause harm, particularly those containing preservatives like benzalkonium chloride (BAK), which can be caustic to the eyes, causing allergic and sensitivity reactions, inflammation, and tissue degeneration. Others may have lubricating properties but can also damage the surface of the eye, like those that constrict blood vessels to reduce eye redness.

Myth #2

Treating inflammation with anti-inflammatory drops is the most important step in treating MGD.

Facts

You've probably seen commercials for anti-inflammatory eye drops that told you to talk to your doctor about Dry Eye. The fact is that inflammation may be a nonspecific result of MGD or its many co-morbidities. For example, inflammation may result from an allergy, ATD, or an infection. To eliminate inflammation caused by these disorders, it's best to treat the specific cause and use the anti-inflammatory drops as adjunctive therapy.

Often there's a mechanical issue that leads to inflammation that anti-inflammatory drops only mask and can't reverse. For example, an anti-inflammatory eye drop won't release the periductal scar tissue, characteristic of MGD, that constricts and invades Meibomian glands, won't tighten the loose tissue of conjunctivochalasis, and won't close the lid of an exposed eye with nocturnal lagophthalmos.

Myth #3

Technology has no impact on eyes. I can look at my phone, TV, or computer screen as much as I want.

Facts

Anytime you use your eyes for gazing activities, as noted previously in question 7 of the MGD self-test, you reduce your blink rate or blink only partially. Playing video games, working at a computer, or bingeing on Netflix can contribute to Dry Eye generally and specifically MGD.

In 2013, the American Academy of Pediatrics reported that the typical eight-year-old spends on average eight hours a day with digital media, and teenagers spend over eleven hours. Right now we can only imagine the long-term impact of these behaviors on ocular health, but at least one recent study already suggests a link between device screen time and Meibomian gland atrophy.

Myth #4

Your environment doesn't cause MGD.

Facts

Every environment can play a role in eye health and comfort. Whether it's helpful or harmful depends on you and the environment. Climates that are dry increase tear film evaporation. In cold climates, forced heat dries the air and destabilizes tear film. (Tip: maintaining humidity levels at around 50–55 percent can help.)

Particulate matter floating in the air reaches the tear film and makes its way to the lid margin and ocular surface, where it can cause inflammation. The air in urban environments tends to be polluted, whereas in suburban and rural areas there may be more allergy-causing pollen. Seashores and lakeshores are more humid but can also harbor molds. Homes with carpeting are more prone to dust on surfaces and in the air. Pets shed hair and dander. Fires produce ash. Fumes from cleaning products, personal hygiene products, cooking, and car exhaust are in the air around us and can lead to lid-margin and ocular surface inflammation with subsequent MGD.

Cavernous spaces are often drafty and full of dust. That includes movie theaters, shopping malls, department stores, and sports arenas, to name just a few. Drafts or turbulent air from heating, ventilation, air-conditioning and ceiling fans in buildings and vehicles, the opening and closing of doors, not to mention the wind in the great outdoors, can all disrupt tear film. Wearing wraparound glasses or goggles can help when wind and drafts are unavoidable. (See chapter 12 for more information on coping with circulating air and dry environments.)

The key is avoiding those environmental factors that cause problems as much as possible, while maintaining good eye and eyelid hygiene. Whenever you can, make lifestyle choices that prevent flare-ups and support Meibomian gland health.

Myth #5

MGD can be easily treated with heat, expression, or massage.

Facts

No amount of heat, massage, or expression can release the periductal scar tissue constricting and invading Meibomian glands. The scar tissue can be released only by internally probing the glands (see chapter 11, "Intraductal Meibomian Gland Probing").

External heat thins meibum secretions, making them more fluid, and is often prescribed as adjunctive therapy to maximize the effectiveness of other treatments. Heat works best if it's applied after the Meibomian glands have been probed to clear fixed obstructions. Otherwise, warm compresses could exacerbate symptoms by increasing blood flow and lid congestion behind the fixed obstructions.

Furthermore, frequently massaging or expressing the glands can increase the intraductal pressure that leads to gland atrophy behind these fixed constrictions. These potentially risky therapies can easily direct meibum away from the opening of the Meibomian gland and, instead, deeper into the gland, the opposite of the intended effect (see chapter 3, "The Meibomian Gland," and chapter 4, "Meibomian Gland Dysfunction Explored").

For this reason, to ensure the released meibum flows outward, expression is best performed after the Meibomian glands have been probed. If you express, always do it lightly to avoid damaging the glands. (For more information about how a doctor should express Meibomian glands, see chapter 11.)

Myth #6

I've already seen several doctors, and none of them helped me. So there's no point in seeing anyone else, because doctors can't do anything for me.

Facts

Eye doctors can help. The key is finding the right one. Look for an eye doctor trained to find and treat MGD, Dry Eye, and comorbidities. You might also need other specialists to treat systemic conditions. (For more information on finding a doctor, see chapter 12.) You could try at-home remedies and simple lifestyle changes, but the fact remains that it is virtually impossible for a patient to accurately and comprehensively self-diagnose these diseases.

Myth #7

You can learn to live with MGD and Dry Eye pain.

Facts

Sadly, sometimes doctors say this. Friends and family members might agree. That's just because they have no way of knowing how dreadful eye pain can be and how much it can affect everything you do.

(Eye pain can be severe. If an eyelash can stop you cold, imagine how a lid full of engorged Meibomian glands feels dragging over dry and wrinkled tissue on the eye's surface every time you blink.)

Your doctor should not be dismissive but instead should consider other diagnoses and treatment options or refer you to a doctor more experienced in treating Dry Eye and MGD.

Myth #8

We produce watery tears when we blink.

Facts

The truth is, we produce normal, nonemotional tears when stimulated corneal nerves signal the brain stem, which then relays signals out to the lacrimal glands and the eyelids. The lacrimal glands receive the signal and produce watery tears while the lids receive the signal to blink. This integrated subconscious system is called the lacrimal functional unit.

The blink itself is a complex function, described in more detail in chapter 2.

2

The Eye

Myth
*As long as your vision is fine,
you don't have to worry about your eyes.*
Fact
*Eyes are complex organs with many highly specialized structures
and tissues. Disease or an abnormality in these can trigger a
cascade of other conditions that can contribute to Dry Eye syndrome
and Meibomian gland dysfunction, even if vision isn't affected.*

To understand Dry Eye, MGD, and other common ocular co-morbidities, it's important to know some basic eye anatomy and become familiar with the external parts of the eye. I've adapted much of the information in this chapter from my previous book, *Reversing Dry Eye Syndrome,* so it may be familiar to you. However, this chapter also contains additional information that will lay a foundation for new concepts discussed in later chapters.

Chapter 2 briefly covers the exterior framework of the eye, the eyeball, glands, tear film, and how healthy tear film is produced and drained. Meibomian glands are mentioned in this chapter and discussed in detail in chapter 3.

EXTERIOR FRAMEWORK

The exterior framework includes the eye socket, eyelids, eyebrows, eyelashes, muscles, and tendons. It houses the eye and protects it from mechanical trauma. Eyelids, the site of Meibomian glands and where MGD arises, are part of this exterior framework.

The Eye Socket

The cavity formed at the juncture of the brow, the cheekbone, and the bridge of the nose anteriorly is known as the eye socket, also called the orbit. It supports and protects the eyeball nestled within. Its bony shell is covered by skin.

The Eyelids

Although thin and seemingly delicate, the eyelid is a complex, powerful apparatus.

Inside the lid are tiny muscles that open and close the eye, blood vessels that nourish the eyelid tissue, nerves that send and receive signals to and from the brain, and Meibomian glands that secrete the oil called meibum.

Anatomically, the lids are divided into two layers, or lamella. The anterior lamella (outer layer) includes the skin, lashes, and orbicularis muscles that close the lids. The posterior lamella (inner layer) includes the tarsal plate (dense connective tissue that forms and supports the lid) and the Meibomian glands. On the side nearest the eyeball, the posterior lamella is covered by a thin layer of pink mucosal tissue called the palpebral conjunctiva, described in more detail in "The Eyeball" section. (*Palpebra* is the Latin word for "eyelid.") The anterior and posterior lamella meet at a junction inside the eyelid called the gray line, which is visible at the lid margin.

The lid margin is the flat edge of the eyelid, between the skin and palpebral conjunctiva. These smooth, flat edges of the upper and lower lids are about 2 millimeters wide (about 1.5 millimeters in children) and meet when you blink.

About three-quarters of the lid margin's width, starting anteriorly at the eyelashes, is covered by keratinized skin. The rest, toward the eyeball, is covered by mucosal tissue. The mucosal tissue of the lid margin, just like all mucosal tissues, is very delicate and permeable.

On the eyelid margin and spanning its length, the keratinized skin and the mucosal tissue meet at a horizontal borderline called

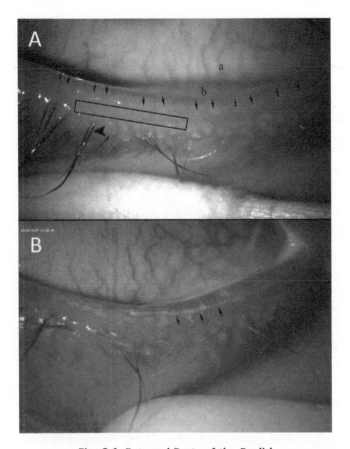

Fig. 2.1. External Parts of the Eyelid

A. An eye with the lower lid margin everted using a white cotton-tipped applicator (bottom of image). The Meibomian gland orifices (small black arrows) are spaced along the lower lid margin. The transparent bulbar conjunctiva (a) covers the sclera, the white of the eye, and the palpebral conjunctiva (b) covers the inner side of the eyelid. Part of the gray line indicating the junction where the anterior and posterior lamella meet inside the eyelid (rectangle) is visible. The arrowhead points to an eyelash.

B. The eye is stained with fluorescein dye revealing the mucocutaneous junction indicated by the light horizontal line (small arrows).

Source: Courtesy of Steven L. Maskin, MD.

the mucocutaneous junction. The mucocutaneous junction line is smooth in younger people and jagged in older people. In healthy eyes the openings, or orifices, of the Meibomian glands are found on the skin side, just anterior to the mucocutaneous junction. Typically, the Meibomian gland orifices lie in a single row across the length of the lid margin, but even in healthy eyes, there can be double rows.

What the Eyelids Do

Eyelids keep the surface of the eye healthy and in working order. They spread tear film, which is constantly being replenished, lubricating and protecting the ocular surface and surrounding tissues.

The upper lid does most of the work during a blink. (The portion of palpebral conjunctiva near the lid margin is sometimes called the lid wiper.) With a normal blink, the eyes close more or less from the temporal (near the temple or outer side of the eye) to the nasal side, distributing fresh tear film over the ocular surface and directing it toward the nose.

When the eyelids open during a blink, negative pressure created in the nose draws old, dirty tear film into the tear drainage system. At the same time, the blinking muscles put pressure on the Meibomian glands, squeezing out droplets of meibum to the eyelid margin.

Blinking can be spontaneous, reflexive, or voluntary. Spontaneous blinking is automatic and unconscious, in the same way that a heartbeat is automatic. It happens constantly every five to seven seconds, although children, and especially infants, blink less often. The rate of spontaneous blinking decreases (you blink less often) when you're gazing—using your eyes for activities that require visual focus, like reading or driving. It can increase slightly during face-to-face conversations to every two to six seconds.

Reflex blinking happens when you get a foreign body in the eye and your eye tries to expel it.

With voluntary blinking, the brain overrides spontaneous blinking, so you can close and open your eyes whenever you choose.

When everything is working as it should and conditions are normal, eyelids operate at a subconscious level, opening and shutting without effort. We don't notice or feel that we're blinking, secreting

---

Sidebar 2.1
Blinking Brings Animated Characters to Life

Did you know that blinking is one way animators give life to their characters? Without blinking, animated characters wouldn't be believable.

Shamus Culhane, the animator who gave life to the seven dwarfs as they marched off to work singing "Heigh-Ho," wrote in *Animation from Script to Screen*, " . . . never have a scene go by without blinks . . . be sure that it happens. A character that does not blink suddenly becomes a lifeless dummy, all the life-quality gone."

Next time you watch an animated film or TV program, pay close attention and you'll notice the characters blinking.

---

the various components of tear film, lubricating our eyes, or channeling old tear film away.

The eyelids also protect the eyes against injury, responding quickly and forcefully when threatened by a foreign object. While we are asleep, the eyelids close over the eyes, shielding and protecting them from desiccating air, airborne foreign bodies, and bedding that might touch and harm our eyes.

Eyebrows and Eyelashes

Eyebrows and eyelashes protect the eyes from all sorts of foreign bodies, including dust and pollen. These hairs catch flying matter before it reaches the surface of the eye. The brows also direct perspiration away from the eyes. Despite seeming very delicate, lashes may be wiry and very sharp. It's normal to lose a few brow and lash strands every day.

As we age, our brows and lashes age, too, and we grow fewer

strands. Sometimes brows grow long or turn gray, and the thickness of individual lashes decreases.

Muscles and Tendons

Tiny muscles in the eyelids control their conscious opening and closing and their subconscious blinking. Protractor muscles close the lids, and retractor muscles open the lids. The orbicularis is the main protractor muscle. The levator is the primary retractor in the upper lid. Lower lid retractors open the lids and hold them in place during a downward gaze.

Tendons that connect muscles to bones are integral to the muscles' function. The canthal tendons, extensions of the orbicularis muscle, are attached to bones of the eye socket near the corners of the eyes. The lateral canthal tendon is the portion attached to the outer corner of the eye. The medial canthal tendon is attached at the inner corner of the eye.

THE EYEBALL

The eyeball is made up of many layers of tissue, each of which plays an important role in vision and eye health.

The Conjunctiva

The conjunctiva (pronounced kŏn-jŭnk-tī'-və) is a smooth, wet, mucosal surface that lines the inner lids and covers the entire white part of the eyeball. It contains goblet epithelial cells that produce a mucuslike substance called mucin, described in "Mucin Layer" under "Components of Tear Film."

There are two main sections of conjunctival tissue: the palpebral conjunctiva, which lines the inner side of the eyelids, and the bulbar conjunctiva, found on the eyeball. They meet at the creases of the eye to form a pouch, or fornix.

The palpebral conjunctiva is about two to five epithelial cell layers deep, variably translucent, and firmly attached. It starts at the inner edge of the eyelid margin and extends to the fornix.

The bulbar conjunctiva is transparent and about six to nine epithelial cell layers deep. It consists of two sections: the limbal conjunctiva, attached to the limbus (where the cornea joins the sclera, the white of the eye); and the scleral conjunctiva, which covers the sclera from the limbus to the fornix. A small fold of bulbar conjunctiva near the caruncle, the small pink ball of flesh at the inner corner of each eye, which contains sweat- and oil-producing sebaceous glands, is the plica semilunaris, or semilunar fold. It helps with tear drainage when the eye moves, and gives the eyeball greater freedom to rotate.

Because it is thin, the conjunctiva would be mostly invisible to the naked eye if not for tiny blood vessels that course through it. These blood vessels nourish all conjunctival epithelial cells and give white blood cells, the universal protector of living tissue, access to the surface of the eye.

The forniceal conjunctiva is loose, relatively deep, and allows the eye to move and rotate freely.

Because the conjunctiva is one continuous piece of tissue, contrary to some popular beliefs, if an eyelash falls into your eye, it won't travel to your brain. It will stay in the front part of your eye, although it might be hidden in the far reaches of the fornix.

Tenon's Capsule, Episclera, and Sclera

The bulbar conjunctiva is attached to an underlying layer of tissue called the Tenon's capsule, which sheathes the eyeball from front to back and separates it from the orbital fat, creating a socket in which the eye moves. The Tenon's capsule is attached to the episclera, a layer of loose fibroelastic tissue. Underneath is the white of the eye, known as the sclera. The episclera, like the conjunctiva, contains blood vessels, but the sclera does not.

As the wall of the eye, the sclera gives the eye its shape by resisting internal and external pressure. Because the tissue is dense and fibrous like cartilage, it protects the structures of the eye essential to vision. Several muscles are attached to the sclera. Their movement is synchronized, so both eyes can move in concert, left, right, up, down, and around.

Although they are attached to the sclera, the bulbar conjunctiva–Tenon's capsule unit can move independently, in the same way that skin can be pushed or pulled without detaching from the body. Closer to the cornea, these tissues have less freedom of movement.

The Cornea

The cornea, at the center of the eye, is divided into three major sections: the epithelium, stroma, and endothelium. The corneal epithelium (outer surface) accounts for about 10 percent of its entire thickness. The stroma, middle layer, accounts for about 90 percent of the cornea's thickness. The endothelium, a single layer of cells lining the inner cornea, keeps the stroma from swelling by pumping excess water into the interior of the eye. A healthy cornea is transparent and is surrounded by the bulbar conjunctiva.

The area where the cornea and conjunctiva connect (where the white part of the eye and the colored part of the eye meet) is the limbus, a zone that is several millimeters wide and includes stem cells that replenish the corneal epithelium. These stem cells on the periphery of the cornea give rise to new cells that continuously replace older degenerated cells of the central cornea. Because this process is continuous and relatively fast, a scratched cornea in an otherwise healthy eye can heal in as little as twenty-four hours. The entire corneal epithelium is replaced about every seven days.

The cornea is among the most innervated parts of the body, having a density of nerve endings at least twenty times that of tooth pulp and four hundred times that of some areas of skin. Because it is highly innervated, the cornea can sense the tiniest defect.

The cornea allows light to enter the eye and, working together with the lens and tear film, permits the eye to focus.

Pupil and Iris

Behind the cornea in the center of the iris is the black dot known as the pupil. The iris is the membrane that gives eyes color: brown, blue, hazel, and so on. The pupil is the aperture that allows light to pass to the back of the eye. The iris acts like the diaphragm of a camera, constricting in bright light and dilating in dim light, thus controlling the diameter of the pupil and the amount of light that passes through.

Anterior Chamber and Aqueous Humor

Between the cornea and the iris lies the anterior (front) chamber. This space is filled with aqueous humor, a transparent fluid that nourishes the cells inside the eye.

Lens

Behind the iris in the posterior chamber is the lens. This clear, colorless, normally elastic tissue is enclosed in a capsule and suspended in the middle of the eye by a net of support fibers. The lens changes shape to focus light rays on the retina. When an object is close, the lens thickens to produce a sharp, close-up image. When the object is farther away, the lens thins out, bringing distant objects into focus.

Retina and Optic Nerve

At the back of the eye is the retina. The retina of the eye is comparable to film in the camera, in that it "processes" the light projected through the cornea and the lens.

The optic nerve takes the electrical impulses recorded by the retina and transmits them to the visual cortex at the back of the brain, where the impulses are interpreted. During an eye exam, your doctor examines your optic nerve for signs of glaucoma, diabetes, and other ocular and systemic diseases.

GLANDS

Glands are groups of cells in the body that produce and secrete chemical substances into the bloodstream (endocrine glands) or through a duct onto an epithelial surface (exocrine glands). The glands that contribute to tear film, the major ones being the lacrimal glands and Meibomian glands, are exocrine glands.

Lacrimal Glands

The lacrimal glands are part of what is known as the lacrimal system or the nasolacrimal apparatus, comprising a complex of glands that produce aqueous (water) tears and of excretory ducts that allow "old" or "dirty" tears to drain from the eyes into the nose.

The large, main, almond-shaped lacrimal gland is found under the upper eyelid, toward the side of the eye near the temple (the temporal side). Smaller accessory lacrimal glands, the glands of Krauss, are mostly situated next to the main lacrimal gland in the conjunctival fornix. Additional accessory lacrimal glands, known as the glands of Wolfring, are found just above the superior border of the superior tarsal conjunctiva.

Meibomian Glands

Meibomian glands are the oil-secreting glands imbedded in the tarsal plate of the upper and lower eyelids. The precise number of glands in each lid varies from person to person, with the upper eyelid typically having approximately thirty individual Meibomian glands, and the lower lids about twenty-five. In both the upper and lower lids, the glands are lined up parallel to each other in a single row perpendicular to the upper and lower eyelid margins.

The glands secrete oil, known as meibum, consisting mostly of liquid wax, cholesterol-related molecules, and other lipids. Released through openings (orifices) at the lid margin, the lids pull meibum onto the eye's surface, where it spreads, joining the aqueous tears produced by the lacrimal glands, and mucins produced by the conjunctiva, to create tear film.

Glands of Zeis and Moll

The glands of Zeis and Moll are found at or near the base of the eyelashes. The glands of Zeis are sebaceous glands that produce an oily substance at the base of the eyelash follicle to keep the lash supple. The glands of Moll are sweat glands found on the eyelid margin near the base of the eyelashes. Although their function is not clear, the presence of enzymes and antibodies that kill bacteria suggest involvement with local immune defense.

TEAR FILM

The tear film, the moist substance that covers the eye all the time, is about 3 microns thick. The portion that covers the cornea is called the precorneal tear film.

Tear film plays a major role in eye health, vision, and comfort in the following ways:

EYE HEALTH

- Tear film acts as a buffer for the eye against harmful foreign bodies or chemical substances.
- Tear film (along with the eyelids) protects the eye from heat and cold, so the eye stays comfortable and doesn't instantly burn or freeze when you open a hot oven or go skiing.

VISION

- Tear film contributes to visual acuity as part of the eye's optical system. The air-tear interface alone contributes two-thirds of the system's refractive power, so if the tear film's thickness changes, visual acuity can change.
- With each blink, the tear film spreads over the eye's surface, smoothing out any irregularities within the epithelium of the corneal surface, supporting visual acuity.

COMFORT

- Tear film provides moisture and lubrication to ocular tissues, making vision, blinking, closing, and opening eyes comfortable.

Components of Tear Film

Tear film consists of three major components: lipid, aqueous, and mucin secretions, which form three layers. The aqueous and mucin secretions combine to make a layer of hydrated mucin gel with increased mucin density nearer the cornea. The lipid secretion, made of liquid meibum, forms a separate and more distinct outer layer.

Lipid Layer

The lipid layer thickness is estimated to be 70–80 nanometers. It performs seven important functions:

- Provides a smooth optical surface for the cornea and air-lipid interface surface
- Reduces the rate of tear film evaporation
- Enhances tear film stability
- Enhances tear film spreading
- Prevents tear film spillover by creating a hydrophobic barrier
- Prevents eye contamination by microbes and undesirable skin oil
- Seals apposing lid margins during sleep

Aqueous Layer

The aqueous layer, secreted by the lacrimal glands and accessory glands, forms the thickest layer of tear film. It nourishes the tissues of the surface of the eye and delivers oxygen and other nutrients to the anterior cornea (which has no blood vessels) to support eye health and promote healing. It also dilutes and helps to clear away irritants.

Aqueous secretions contain a complex collection of proteins, electrolytes, antibodies, and other compounds. These keep the eye healthy and provide immune protection by preventing the growth of bacteria, fungi, or viruses. One of these secretions is lysozyme, a highly effective antibacterial agent. Lysozyme attacks and inactivates bacteria on the surface of the eye in a matter of minutes. Without it and other microbe-fighting secretions, eyes would be prey to disease, and eye infections would be rampant.

Mucin Layer

The mucin layer, attached to the surface of the eye and containing glycoproteins, serves two functions. First, because of its mucousy texture, it adheres the tear film to the corneal epithelium, forming a bridge between the aqueous layer and the corneal surface. Second, together with the aqueous secretions forming the hydrated gel matrix, it allows nutrients from the aqueous layer to moisten and nourish the cornea.

Destabilized Tear Film

When one layer fails at its job, tear film destabilizes faster than it should. The tear breakup time (TBUT)—the time it takes for the tear film to become unstable and the ocular surface to be nonwettable after a blink—decreases. As a result, the cornea and ocular surface become overly exposed. Prolonged or repeated exposure creates symptoms of Dry Eye and may ultimately damage the corneal epithelium. If adequate lubrication is restored, the damaged epithelium will repair itself nicely. If not, the epithelium will continue to break down.

TEAR DRAINAGE

Each eye has a tear drainage system, part of the nasolacrimal apparatus, which originates with an opening portal, or punctum, within the inner corner of the eyelid margin and ends in the nose. The lacrimal caruncle and plica semilunaris assist in directing tear film toward the upper and lower puncta (plural for punctum). The puncta, one in each of the four eyelids, open into the lacrimal canaliculus; the upper punctum into the superior (upper) lacrimal canaliculus; and the lower punctum into the inferior (lower) lacrimal canaliculus. These two canaliculi channel tear film into a single lacrimal sac in the nose. The lacrimal sac then drains tears into the nasolacrimal duct, which finally empties into the nose.

The rate of removal of newly produced tears is called tear clearance.

THE PRODUCTION OF HEALTHY TEARS

With each blink, old tear film containing microbes, chemical substances, and dead cells drains out and new tear film is produced by the lacrimal functional unit. The lacrimal functional unit includes a sensory system, which creates the incoming message; the secretory system, which produces the tear; and the neural communication between the two systems.

The Incoming Message

The brain stem receives messages from stimulated sensory nerves on the surface of the eye. The incoming messages are received every time tear film evaporation exposes nerves, or when a foreign body irritates nerves.

The incoming message can also be activated by emotional stimulation, which is processed differently by the brain but still initiates the tear-producing process.

In healthy eyes that blink normally, the incoming message is often imperceptible. You don't feel it or know it's happening. You just blink involuntarily.

The Outgoing Command

When the brain stem receives the message from the surface of the eye, it processes the information and sends a command to the lacrimal glands to secrete aqueous tears. In addition, the brain sends a message to the eyelid muscles, stimulating the blink mechanism. The blink spreads tear film, helps to deliver meibum to the ocular surface, and draws out old tears.

Closing the Loop

The tear secretion and blinking of the eye in effect close the loop of the lacrimal functional unit. Then the process starts all over again. The tear film begins to evaporate; the exposed nerves send a message to the brain; the brain sends a command to the lacrimal glands and lids. Once again, tears are secreted, the blink distributes them, and the old tear film is drawn out. The process is ongoing because the tears must be continually cleared and replaced to maintain the health of the ocular surface.

EYES DON'T EXIST IN A VACUUM

The eye doesn't exist in a vacuum. It's part of the human body, which includes many systems, all of which interconnect to some degree or another. We are all familiar with many of these systems and how they function. But few of us are aware just how much these systems can impact the health of Meibomian glands. In fact, because of these interconnections, Meibomian glands often serve as barometers of the health of the eye and other parts, or systems, of the body.

How Bodily Systems Affect Meibomian Glands

The immune system helps protect the eyelid margins and Meibomian glands from disease by attacking pathogens (microorganisms that can cause disease) wherever they might be.

The endocrine (glands inside the body) system includes the pituitary gland, the thyroid gland, ovaries, and testicles. It controls many complex bodily systems by exerting influence at the cellular level through chemical messages released into the circulatory system regulating distant target organs, including Meibomian glands.

The metabolic system converts food into energy through a series of complex chemical reactions and is involved in the production of the components of aqueous tear film and the synthesis of meibum.

The nervous system transmits signals involved in the lacrimal functional unit.

The digestive system breaks down food into nutrient molecules the body can absorb, including essential fat soluble vitamins, such as vitamins A and D, important for Dry Eye management and the health of the ocular surface.

The circulatory system delivers nutrients, such as essential fatty acids, and removes waste products.

The muscular system allows the eyelids to blink.

THE HUMAN BODY DOESN'T EXIST IN A VACUUM

The human body itself exists in an endless array of environments that are a normal part of everyday life. Among these are your home, where you work or go to school, the transportation you use, and your habitat. Different times of day and different seasons exert unique stressors on the human body.

Each of these environments can support or detract from the health and comfort of your eyes and Meibomian glands.

3

The Meibomian Gland

Myth
Learning about Meibomian glands isn't important.
Fact
Understanding Meibomian glands will help you take care of them.

Meibomian glands and meibum, the oil they produce, are key to a healthy ocular surface and comfortable eyes. Meibum lubricates the posterior (part closer to the eyeball) eyelid margin and stabilizes the tear film. It prevents tear film from flowing out of the eyes constantly, keeps the wet layer from evaporating when the eyes are open, and creates an airtight seal when the eyes are closed. It also contributes to vision as part of the tear film's refraction system that focuses light on the retina.

Meibomian gland dysfunction (MGD), a disease of the Meibomian glands, is the most common causative factor of Dry Eye, found in over 85 percent of Dry Eye patients. MGD is often the underlying source of chronic discomfort and eye pain.

To understand how MGD develops and how it can be diagnosed and effectively treated, we will first review the anatomy and synthesis of meibum in healthy Meibomian glands.

Sidebar 3.1
Where Does the Word "Meibomian" Come From?

The word "Meibomian" is derived from the name of the German ophthalmologist Heinrich Meibom. Although these glands were discovered decades earlier, he was the first to write about and illustrate them in *De Vasis Palpebrarum Novis Epistola,* a book published in Germany in 1666 (see fig. 3.1).

Interestingly, Dr. Meibom drew only twenty glands in the upper lid, and twenty-five in the lower lid. Today, it is accepted that when healthy, there are more Meibomian glands in the upper lid than the lower lid. Thus, this may be the first graphic representation of atrophic MGD.

MEIBOMIAN GLAND ANATOMY

Meibomian glands are specialized oil-secreting glands classified as *sebaceous holocrine exocrine* glands.

- *Sebaceous* glands produce oil and are found all over the skin.
- *Holocrine* is a mode of secretion. As holocrine cells age within the gland, they synthesize and accumulate oil that is released when the cells degenerate.
- *Exocrine* glands secrete into a duct, or lumen, that leads to the body's surface rather than into the bloodstream. Meibomian gland ducts lead to openings, called orifices, at the lid margin.

Number and Size

There are roughly thirty Meibomian glands in the upper eyelid and twenty-five in the lower lid. Usually the glands form a single row, but some people have more than one row of glands.

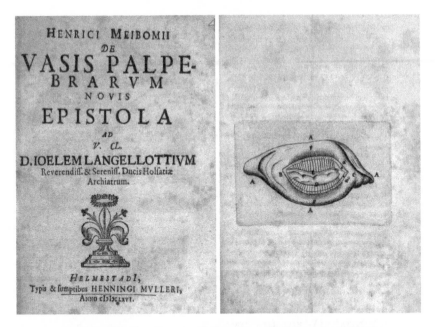

Fig. 3.1. The First Known Illustration of Meibomian Glands

Left: Cover of the book by Dr. Heinrich Meibom, published in 1666. Right: The first known image of the oil-secreting glands that will eventually be called Meibomian glands. The squiggly vertical lines above E represent Meibomian glands in the upper lid. In the lower lid, below D, the glands are less squiggly. The dots in two horizontal curved rows represent orifices at the lid margin. The wispy vertical curved lines above and below these dots are eyelashes.

Source: Heinrich Meibom, *De Vasis Palpebrarum Novis Epistola* (Helmstadt, Germany: Henningi Mulleri, 1666), cover, 17.

In upper lids, Meibomian glands extend more than halfway up the lid corresponding to the dimension of the tarsal plate. At the center of the lid, glands tend to be longer than those on the outer edges, closer to the nose and closer to the ears. The longest glands are about 6.0 millimeters long but can be longer in some cases.

In lower lids, Meibomian glands extend toward the bottom of the lid and are about 2 millimeters long. Glands in the lower lids are usually wider than those in the upper lids.

Meibomian glands are about 400 microns wide, although the width varies.

Generally, the calculated cumulative internal gland volume of upper lids is thought to be at least double that of lower lid glands.

Sidebar 3.2
How Do You Pronounce "Meibomian"?

Most people haven't heard of Meibomian glands or know how to pronounce "Meibomian." Try reading this out loud:

My as in my name is
BOW as in BOW and arrow (the emphasis is on this syllable)
Me as in me and you
An as in an apple a day
my + BOW + me + an = Meibomian (mī-bō′-mē-an)

Meibum, the oil produced by Meibomian glands, is pronounced MY-bum (mī′-bəm).

Location and Flexibility

Meibomian glands are nestled within the tarsal plate, typically parallel to each other. They extend vertically from the lid margin and are lined up across the width of the lid. The tissue between the glands is spongy, allowing for various movements of the eyes and eyelids—opening, closing, looking in different directions, stretching when opening eyes wide, pulling eyelids to lift them up, down, or away, or rubbing the eyes (something you should avoid doing).

The glands themselves are flexible to allow for eye and eyelid movements. They don't distend, or swell like a balloon, unless they're diseased. Because of their flexibility and surrounding spongy tissue, when a probe passes through the central duct of a crooked Meibomian gland, the duct, and with it the entire gland, straightens out. When the gland straightens out, the spongy space between glands evens out (see fig. 3.2).

Table 3.1

Similarities and Differences Between
Meibomian Glands and Other Sebaceous Glands

Feature	Meibomian Glands	Sebaceous Glands
Composition of secretion	Meibum, unique to Meibomian glands: predominantly wax and cholesterol esters	Sebum, similar throughout the body: predominantly triglycerides, squalene, and wax esters
Oil synthesis	Holocrine, produce meibum	Holocrine, produce sebum
Secretion/delivery	Exocrine, secrete directly through the orifice onto the lid margin during blinks. Meibum is then pulled into the tear film during the opening phase of the blink.	Exocrine, secrete into the hair follicle canal. Sebum then reaches the skin surface via a wicking action involving the hair shaft.
Length	Long	Short
Hair follicle	None	One per gland
Regulated by hormones	Yes	Yes
Mode of external regulation	Continuously with blinking	Intermittently
Location	Eyelids only	High concentration on face (nose, chin, forehead). Also found elsewhere: scalp, torso, etc.
Role	Surface lubrication; prevent tear film evaporation and overflow; seal lids when closed; involved with focusing light on retina.	Lubrication to protect against friction; help prevent penetration by moisture.

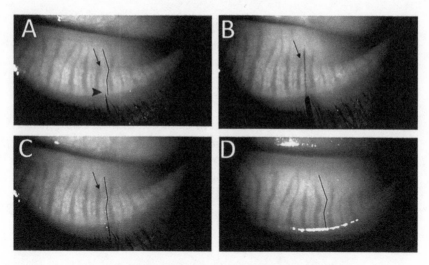

**Fig. 3.2. Straightening of a Mildly Tortuous Duct
and Gland During Intraductal Probing**

A. A 4 millimeter probe (black arrowhead) is about to enter the orifice of the Meibomian gland. The black line that parallels the central duct, placed after the image was taken, indicates the zigzagged shape of a mildly tortuous gland.

B. When the probe advances into the duct, the gland straightens out. The space between the gland and its neighboring gland to the left decreases (arrows in A and B).

C. When the probe is withdrawn, the gland duct is still relatively straight, but some gland tortuosity returns.

D. Two months after probing, the tortuosity returns to preprobing status, suggesting the interglandular (between the glands) tissue is spongy. It compresses and reexpands, allowing duct and gland flexibility.

Source: Reproduced from Steven L. Maskin and Sreevardhan Alluri, "Meibography Guided Intraductal Meibomian Gland Probing Using Real-Time Infrared Video Feed," *British Journal of Ophthalmology* 104, no. 12 (2020), 1676–1682, with permission from BMJ Publishing Group Ltd.

Structure

Each Meibomian gland has a similar structure (see fig. 1.1), which includes:

- Acini
- Ductules
- Central duct

Sidebar 3.3
The Acinar-Ductular Unit

Ductules and the acini connected to them form a unit—
the acinar-ductular unit. More than one acinus can be
connected to a single ductule.

Acini

Along the length of each Meibomian gland central duct are acini
(plural of acinus). An acinus is a cluster of cells that resemble a microscopic raspberry. (*Acinus* is Latin for "berry" or "grape.")

Each Meibomian gland has ten to fifteen rings of multiple acini,
more in longer glands, fewer in shorter glands.

Ductules

Acini are connected to ductules, short tubes that themselves are connected to the central duct of the Meibomian gland. The ductules are
about 150 microns long, 30–50 microns in diameter, and angled
toward the lid margin. A lip of tissue at the juncture of the ductule
and central duct is thought to direct the oil flowing out of the ductule toward the openings at the lid margin. One ductule and the acini
that are connected to it form an acinar-ductular unit.

Central Duct

Each Meibomian gland is arranged around its central duct, which is
about 100–150 microns in diameter.

The ducts are hollow tubes closed off at the end deep inside the
eyelid. Their walls are several epithelial cells thick. The outer layer
of the duct's epithelium attaches to a basement membrane that an-
chors those cells.

Sidebar 3.4
The Continuous Flow of Meibum

The secretion of meibum through the duct and out onto the lid margin makes room for new oil, akin to a car factory's continuous production process. When cars ship out, they make room for new cars. But unlike a factory that can stop production to prevent a buildup of inventory if finished cars can't be hauled away, the Meibomian gland has no known way to stop production if its outflow is blocked. (We explain in chapter 4 what happens to the Meibomian gland when the normal secretion of oil is blocked.)

Secreted meibum pools on the lid margin to supply the lipid layer of tear film during a blink.

Meibum flows into the central duct and seeps out through the orifice onto the lid margin with each blink.

The Excretory Duct

Near the orifice at the lid margin, the central duct narrows, forming the excretory duct. Here, the central duct's skinlike epithelial cells produce keratin. (Keratin is the layer of protein fibers that protects the superficial layer of the skin or epidermis.) The keratinized excretory duct is about 0.55 millimeters long.

In relation to the central duct, the excretory duct looks like the open end of a tube of toothpaste. With plenty of toothpaste in the tube, you can aim toothpaste directly at your toothbrush while squeezing gently. Similarly, the narrowed excretory duct can aim meibum directly at the lid margin with the gentle pressure of a blink.

The Orifice

The orifice is on the posterior quarter of the lid margin on the skin side of the mucocutaneous junction (where the keratinized skin and palpebral mucosal tissue meet). On the other side of the mucocutaneous junction closer to the eyeball, mucosal tissue that is more permeable covers the lid margin. On average a healthy orifice is approximately 100 microns wide, but the width can vary.

Innervation

The Meibomian glands are innervated by sensory and other nerve fibers that transmit nerve impulses which can be interpreted as pain.

SYNTHESIZING AND SECRETING MEIBUM

Meibum is continuously synthesized inside the eyelids, even during sleep. Synthesis begins with stem cells that produce daughter cells known as progenitor cells. These progenitor cells give rise to cells called meibocytes, the cells that break down as they age and transform into meibum. This type of glandular secretion is called holocrine.

Stem Cells

Stem cells are undifferentiated cells that don't yet have specific jobs. They divide slowly and can be pluripotent, meaning they can become almost any type of cell. Stem cells differentiate into daughter cells with specific jobs.

Meibomian gland stem cells are thought to be located along the outer ductal epithelium layer near the junction of the central duct and the acinar-ductular unit, where they give rise to daughter progenitor cells. (Stem cells may also be found near the mucocutaneous junction on the lid margin.)

Research is currently being conducted to determine if there is one stem cell line for both acinar and ductal epithelium or two separate stem cell lines, one for the acinar epithelium and one for the ductal epithelium.

Progenitor Cells

In the case of a single stem cell line, daughter progenitor cells move toward the central duct channel, or lumen, becoming part of its epithelium. Others migrate along the outer ductule wall toward the periphery of the acini, where they divide rapidly and give rise continuously to new meibocytes. The rate of meibocyte production in humans has not been documented, but a study found that in mice, progenitor cells produce new meibocytes every 4.1 days.

Meibocytes

As new meibocytes form on the periphery of the acini, building pressure in the tight space, older meibocytes migrate away from the periphery, toward the center of the acini. Over time, as the meibocytes mature and move toward the ductule, the number and size of organelles inside the meibocytes necessary for lipid production increase. By the time mature meibocytes arrive at the juncture of the acinus and the ductule, the cell membranes and organelles have broken down, transformed into meibum lipid containing remnant cell material. This meibum is pushed through the ductule to the central duct and is secreted through the orifice onto the lid margin.

Meibum synthesis happens continuously because progenitor cells constantly produce new meibocytes.

Regulating the Synthesis and Secretion of Meibum

Hormones, the mechanical force of blinking, and other factors play a role in regulating the synthesis and secretion of meibum and work as a coordinated system.

Synthesis

The same factors that regulate sebum synthesis also regulate meibum synthesis. These factors include corticosteroids, hypothalamic and pituitary hormones, insulin, thyroxine (thyroid hormones), neurotransmitters, and reproductive hormones. Androgens (male sex hormones, such as testosterone) are particularly important and, although less research has been conducted on estrogen, other hormones, and growth factors, they all appear to play a role.

Sidebar 3.5
How Far Do Meibomian Gland Cells Travel?

A single progenitor cell, believed to be the daughter of a stem cell found in the epithelium at the juncture of the central duct and acinar-ductular unit, migrates to a spot along the periphery of the acini more than 100 microns away.

Her daughters—meibocytes—travel much farther. A meibocyte begins life at the periphery of the acini, but as it disintegrates, it's pushed along, out of the acini, into the ductule, through the central duct, through the orifice, and onto the eyelid margin. Then the contents of the cell and remnant material, now part of meibum secretion, flow to the tear film. In mice, it takes about nine days for a Meibomian gland cell to travel the entire distance.

That's quite a distance for a tiny cell to travel in just nine days! How far and how fast human meibocytes travel has not yet been studied.

Sidebar 3.6
Meibomian Glands Can Regrow

A 2019 research presentation at the Association for Research in Vision and Ophthalmology showed that in an animal model, acini can regenerate when the central duct is intact. Consistent with these findings, in an earlier 2018 study, we reported the growth of Meibomian gland tissue after probing glands. Probing, which restores ductal integrity, may have directly led to the growth of Meibomian gland tissue.

Sidebar 3.7
Other Travelers

Daughters of stem cells in the Meibomian glands aren't the only stem cell offspring in the eyes that travel significant distances.

Limbal stem cell offspring—the stem cells on the periphery of the cornea—also travel measurable distances. When there's a need on the cornea—because of an abrasion, for example—these cells travel from the limbus and onto the surface of the cornea, a distance of about 5mm, where they turn into the cells that heal the damaged tissue.

Because of the many stem cells at the limbus, an injured cornea can heal in as little as twenty-four hours.

Peroxisome proliferator-activated receptor gamma (PPAR-γ, a member of the hormone-receptor family within the nucleus of the cell), is also involved with meibum synthesis.

Secretion

Two mechanisms appear to control the secretion of meibum. First, as mentioned previously, pressure builds up in the acini as progenitor cells create new meibocytes, pushing the cells toward the ductule, through the duct and orifice, and out to the lid margin. Second, muscles and tissues in the eyelids squeeze the Meibomian glands during blinks, expressing meibum to the lid margin and clearing space for new meibum.

Some researchers have suggested that the neural signals of the lacrimal functional unit, which stimulate aqueous tear secretion and blinking, may also stimulate Meibomian glands, but this hypothesis has not yet been confirmed.

Amount Secreted

The amount of meibum secreted relates directly to age, sex, time of day, and how the eyes are used.

Young people secrete more meibum than older people. (Fewer than 50 percent of Meibomian glands may function in older adults.) Men, with higher levels of testosterone and with larger Meibomian gland orifices, secrete more meibum than women.

Gazing activities, like reading and driving, reduce the blink rate, so in a given period, the glands secrete less meibum. Gazing can also cause incomplete, partial blinking, where the eye doesn't completely close before opening again, which may reduce the secreted amount.

Upon awakening, eyes may feel great because during sleep meibum accumulates on the lid margins.

THE CHEMISTRY OF MEIBUM

Components of Meibum and Their Synthesis

Meibum consists mostly of molecules of nonpolar cholesterol and long-chain wax esters that promote its stability. (A stable lipid layer is important for the tear film so it can withstand shearing mechanical forces, like blinking and variations in temperature.) The polarity of additional polar lipid molecules within meibum binds the tear film's lipid layer to the aqueous layer.

Flow and Viscosity

When the eyes open after a blink, meibum on the upper and lower lid margins flows to the tear film and spreads. It continues spreading after the eyes stop opening because the speed of a blink is much faster than the spreading of meibum. Then the meibum stops moving until the eyes blink again. When the eyes close, the meibum compresses and either keeps its composition or mixes with more meibum from the lid margins. Each time the eyes open, the process repeats.

Blinking or closing lids applies a shearing force to the ductal contents that helps to lower the viscosity of meibum so it can flow out through the orifice to the lid margin. The narrowed opening of the excretory duct at the lid margin also reduces viscosity, aiding the outflow of meibum.

Melting Point

Eyelid temperature can affect both the liquidity and viscosity of meibum, in the same way that heat affects butter. When melted, butter pours like a liquid. When cold, it can be stiffer than toothpaste. Expert opinion varies widely about the precise temperature at which healthy meibum changes from a solid to an oily liquid, but is thought to range between 20 and 40 degrees Celsius, or 68 and 104 degrees Fahrenheit. This wide range in temperatures may simply indicate that the quality of meibum is subject to diverse individual comorbidity and cofactor profiles.

Thickness

The normal thickness of the meibum layer in the tear film ranges from 70 to 80 nanometers. A thicker layer of meibum slows tear film evaporation more than a thin layer, but if too thick, it can be irritating and reduce vision.

CONCLUSION

Although Meibomian glands are very small, they are complex structures that work continuously, producing meibum to support the health and function of the ocular surface and vision. Their inherent complexity and many internal and external regulatory factors expose them to a variety of risks that can lead to disease. We examine these risk factors, how they can affect Meibomian glands and lead to dysfunction, in the next chapter.

4

Meibomian Gland Dysfunction Explored

Myth
Hyperkeratinization, thick meibum, various environmental stressors, or solutes in the tear film are the proximate causes of Meibomian gland dysfunction.
Fact
Periductal fibrosis is the most common proximate cause of Meibomian gland dysfunction.

To diagnose and treat diseases, experts study their pathophysiologies—how diseases develop and progress. This chapter focuses on the pathophysiology of Meibomian gland dysfunction (MGD), and its proximate cause (the immediate cause that precipitates a condition).

As we explained in chapter 3, Meibomian glands may be small, but they're complex. Because of this complexity, many factors can play a role in the pathophysiology of MGD. Some factors, like age, cold weather, or exposure to low humidity, may be unavoidable. Other factors, like a poor diet or infrequent blinking, which contribute to MGD, are manageable (see chapter 5).

Whether unavoidable or manageable, these underlying factors can trigger anatomic and physiologic changes in Meibomian glands, giving rise to *simple obstructive MGD*, by far the most common subtype of MGD. (When we use the term "MGD" in this book, we are generally referring to simple obstructive MGD.) These changes impair the glands' ability to synthesize and secrete meibum.

HOW MGD PROGRESSES

Most experts agree that simple obstructive MGD progresses following this pattern:

1. Glands become obstructed and unable to secrete meibum at the desired rate.
2. Meibum builds up inside the glands behind the obstruction, increasing intraductal pressure, dilating the acinar-ductular unit and duct, and often increasing glandular inflammation.
3. The buildup of meibum puts pressure on cells in the acini.
4. Because of the pressure on them, meibocytes that are usually square undergo squamous metaplasia (changing shape, characteristics, and function), becoming flat and nonsecretory.
5. Meibum production stops.
6. The production of meibocytes by progenitor cells also stops.
7. Acinar-ductular units atrophy.
8. The whole gland atrophies and disappears.

The disease progresses from stage to stage over time, developing gradually over months and years or, less commonly, it can develop quickly.

PRIOR MODELS OF MGD

Experts generally agree that obstruction plays a role in MGD. But they disagree about the proximate cause of disease and the nature of obstruction and have proposed several models describing how MGD develops. These four models theorized that (1) excessive keratin deposits, (2) thickened meibum, (3) environmental stresses on Meibomian gland stem cells, or (4) infiltration of the Meibomian glands by toxic solutes in the tear film are the proximate causes of MGD.

Sidebar 4.1
Cicatricial MGD, Another Subtype of Disease

Cicatricial MGD, a less common subtype of MGD than simple obstructive MGD, also involves periductal fibrosis (the tissue that invades and constricts gland ducts), which can lead to atrophy. However, with this disease, the location of the gland's orifice changes due to scarring. The scarring develops at the posterior lid margin within the tarsal plate, where it pulls on the terminal gland ducts dragging them to the conjunctival surface of the eyelid margin. As the disease advances, the scarring drags the orifices farther, from the lid margin onto the inner lid's conjunctival surface. Because the orifice location changes, meibum secretes into the aqueous layer of tear film rather than to the outer lipid layer.

Sidebar 4.2
Nonobvious MGD

Nonobvious MGD (NOMGD) is a subtype of MGD without clinical signs other than reduced expressibility of glands. A slit-lamp exam (the mainstay of ophthalmic exams, which uses a microscope to view eyes under magnification, and one you've probably had) shows little or no inflammation, so doctors have to perform diagnostic expression of the Meibomian glands to diagnose it. NOMGD is thought to be a common precursor of inflammatory, atrophic MGD.

Sidebar 4.3
Meibomian Gland Dropout and Whole Gland Atrophy

Meibomian gland *dropout* means one or more of the gland's acinar-ductular units has atrophied and disappeared. Illuminated with infrared meibography, there will be an empty space where an acinar-ductular unit should be. With whole gland atrophy, the entire acinar-ductular population of a single gland will be missing.

Sidebar 4.4
Gland Dropout with an Intact
Orifice = Potential to Regrow Glands

Even with atrophy and a complete loss of acinar-ductular units seen under infrared meibography, as long as an orifice is visible at the lid margin, the gland's central duct essentially remains intact, although compromised. We shared images of this landmark discovery in a poster presented at the American Academy of Optometry conference held in Orlando, Florida, in 2019 and in an article published in the *British Journal of Ophthalmology* in December 2020 and highlighted on the cover of that issue.

This discovery suggests that after duct probing to release fibrosis and restore ductal integrity, glands with total dropout or atrophy may be reprogrammed to initiate acinar regeneration, leading to the growth of gland tissue.

Sidebar 4.5
Is Meibomian Gland Atrophy Reversible?

Periductal fibrosis can compromise the ductal integrity of Meibomian glands, leading to elevated intraductal (inside the duct) pressure and subsequent squamous metaplasia—the metamorphosis of meibocytes from square, secretory cells to flat, nonsecretory cells.

Squamous metaplasia can have a profound effect on Meibomian glands. Most notably, the secretion of meibum stops. Eventually the glands may atrophy.

But is the process reversible?

The answer appears to be yes. After Maskin® Probing, we have seen with meibography imaging the growth of Meibomian gland tissue, and with confocal microscopy, increased duct wall thickness characterized by epithelial proliferation suggestive of stem cell activation. Simultaneously, probing may also decrease the progressive loss of stem cells from periductal fibrotic invasion of the external duct wall (see chapter 11).

The exact physiological process that restores Meibomian gland tissue is not yet known. It may be that relieving the elevated intraductal pressure with probing enables any surviving individual stem cells or acinar epithelial cells that have not yet undergone squamous metaplasia and irreversible atrophy to function normally and proliferate. This may lead to the growth of new acini off a common ductule. Alternatively, the relief of elevated intraductal pressure may reverse early squamous metaplasia, leading to restoration of individual cell function.

Sidebar 4.6
Acinar Epithelial Proliferation Inhibitors

Some cases of MGD can be tied directly to the side effects of systemic treatments of diseases, like acne or cancer, with compounds that directly inhibit proliferation of Meibomian gland acinar epithelial cells. These compounds, for example, the active ingredients in ACCUTANE® (isotretinoin) and various chemotherapy formulations, lead to the loss of gland function and atrophy of acinar-ductular units throughout the gland.

However, we now have evidence of a fifth model, the *periductal fibrosis model* (described after the section on prior models), which shifts the paradigm in our understanding of MGD and its proximate cause.

Four Prior Models of MGD

1. The *hyperkeratinization model* of MGD attributes MGD to an overproduction of keratin (see sidebar 4.7). A thin layer

Sidebar 4.7
Keratin and Hyperkeratinization

Keratin is a protein, naturally found in the form of a mesh within the epidermis, the outer layer of the skin. Keratin is not soluble in water and so, along with sebum oil secreted by skin sebaceous glands, it makes the skin waterproof.
    Hyperkeratinization is an overproduction of keratin.

Sidebar 4.8
How Many People Have Obstructive
Meibomian Gland Dysfunction (O-MGD)?

About 350 million people worldwide are thought to suffer with Dry Eye. Of those, approximately 85 percent, or 297.5 million, are estimated to have MGD.

In one of my published studies among my patients with MGD, probe findings confirmed that 84 percent had obstructed glands. If that ratio holds for everyone with MGD, then about 250 million people worldwide have obstructive MGD.

---

of keratin normally covers the linings of the Meibomian gland's excretory duct and orifice. When there is an overproduction of keratin, known as hyperkeratinization, the theory suggests that keratin blocks the orifice. Some experts claim a host of factors can influence hyperkeratinization of the Meibomian glands, including age, changes in hormone levels, and the toxic effects of medications. Hyperkeratinization has also been attributed to inflammation.

2. The *thick meibum model* attributes MGD to changes in the fluidity of meibum. It becomes thicker and more viscous. This less-fluid meibum stagnates inside the glands, leading to a buildup of pressure inside the acini, eventually leading to their destruction and Meibomian gland atrophy.

3. The *stress model* attributes Meibomian gland atrophy and the degradation of meibum secretions to aging and various environmental stressors that increase demand on Meibomian gland stem cells and meibocytes. According to this model, stressors, such as dry, windy environments, wearing contact lenses, changes in hormone levels, poor diets, allergies, and a reduced blink rate while gazing cause faster tear film evaporation, increasing the need for meibum. This

need speeds up meibocyte production and meibum synthesis, giving cells less time to shed their lipid-producing, protein-rich organelles, increasing meibum's protein-to-lipid ratio. The increased ratio of proteins to lipid in the secreted meibum may increase the meibum's rigidity, making the oil less fluid and affecting tear film stability, leading to evaporative Dry Eye. The increase in gland activity and faster cell turnover also leads to increased desquamated, or sloughed, cells, increasing cell debris in the glands, which causes obstruction. At the same time, acinar stem cells unable to keep up with demand become depleted, leading to acinar atrophy and gland dropout.

4. The *solute gradient model* attributes MGD to solutes (substances dissolved in liquid) in the tear film that constantly wash over the posterior eyelid margin with each blink. Over time, these solutes can cause damage to the delicate mucosal tissue of the eyelid margin and nearby Meibomian gland tissue as follows:

- Dry Eye initiates and intensifies the damage to the eyelid margin caused by solutes, because in reduced volumes of tear film there are even higher concentrations of solutes.
- The damaged mucosal tissue lacks keratin and is more easily penetrated by the hyperosmolar (higher than normal concentration) solutes.
- The mucocutaneous junction moves anteriorly (away from the eyeball), although often irregularly, with more of the lid margin surface exposed as mucosal tissue.
- As the mucocutaneous junction migrates anteriorly, the more permeable mucosal tissue engulfs the site of the Meibomian gland orifices.
- Scarring may pull the orifice posteriorly (toward the eyeball, as in cicatricial MGD), exposing the orifice and excretory ducts to solutes in the tear film.
- Inflammatory peptides and hyperosmolar solutes at the openings of the unprotected Meibomian glands may trigger the development of MGD.

Sidebar 4.9
Understanding Inflammation:
Calor, Dolor, Rubor, and Tumor

First recorded in the first century AD, the terms "calor," "dolor," "rubor," and "tumor" describe the classic signs of inflammation: heat, pain, redness, and swelling, respectively.

When the body senses an attack by microorganisms, pollutants, allergens, chemicals, dust, or countless other irritants, it delivers its own defensive chemicals to the site of the attack. Blood vessels deliver these chemicals—inflammatory mediators—to kill or ward off the attacker. The blood vessels dilate and leak components of the blood that contain the inflammatory mediators, causing the irritated tissue to become warm, painful, red, and swollen.

- The solutes may also stimulate the rapid turnover of the lid margin's epithelial cells with loss of their protective function, leading to further lid margin and distal gland damage.

The *solute hypothesis* may explain why MGD has an age-related component—damage to the eyelid margin tissues happens slowly, over many years and even decades, due to the accumulation of these toxins—and is virtually unavoidable.

Each of these models proposes a plausible theory for the proximate cause of MGD. The *hyperkeratinization model* presents the stagnant protein-containing material sometimes seen accumulated in the orifices of Meibomian glands as the underlying cause of MGD. The *thick meibum model* attributes MGD to changes in the viscosity of meibum. The stressors described in the *stress model* play a significant role in MGD pathophysiology. They may lead to increased ductal cell debris and an altered protein-to-lipid ratio within meibum.

Sidebar 4.10
Harmful and Toxic Solutes in Tear Film

Tear film contains many solutes secreted naturally under normal circumstances. But other more harmful or toxic solutes from fingers, surrounding tissue, or directly from the atmosphere may reach the tear film. Many of these solutes float in the air, independently or as part of larger plumes of particles. Here are just a few:

- Bacteria and their remnants
- Carcasses of demodex mites
- Chemical compounds
- Cooking fumes
- Dust
- Mold
- Pet dander
- Pollens
- Pollutants such as vehicle exhaust
- Scents, both natural and artificial
- Smoke from fires

This is not a complete list of the solutes that might be in your tear film. Imagine *everything* you smell, and add that to the list, too.

The *solute model* elegantly depicts changes to the orifice and lid margin after years of exposure to tear film containing noxious agents with secondary adverse effects on Meibomian glands. The hyperkeratinization, thick meibum, and stress models also delineate the effect of obstruction—increased intraductal pressure as a factor leading to atrophy of the gland tissue. The stress model also raises the possibility of stem cell depletion as an alternative or concurrent path to atrophy.

However, these four models do not explain or account for six unexpected observations I have made while treating patients with MGD. These observations have led me to conclude that periductal fibrosis is the proximate cause of MGD.

THE PERIDUCTAL FIBROSIS MODEL
OF MGD—A NEW PARADIGM

The *periductal fibrosis model* of MGD proposes a specific proximate cause of disease that directly correlates to pathophysiological clinical changes I have observed in Meibomian glands. I discovered this cause inadvertently while treating a patient with advanced obstructive MGD, using a prototype probe I fashioned (described in chapter 11). A popping sound with the release of intraductal resistance, the simultaneous gush of oil trickling down the probe, and the instantaneous relief of symptoms appeared to be related, leading me to believe the probe had encountered and released fibrotic periductal tissue. (Earlier, in 1997, a researcher observed periglandular fibrosis— scar tissue in the area of the gland—using a slit lamp. He also noted dropout at the slit lamp and using an early form of meibography [both devices are described in chapter 9] and wondered if dropout could be related to a strangulation process involving the fibrosis that increased intraductal pressure.)

Success with this patient inspired me to closely observe the Meibomian glands of other patients. Over time my observations coalesced into a model for obstructive MGD that consistently and predictably accounts for clinical findings, patient symptoms, and responses to treatment.

These six key observations, made over the last eighteen years while treating patients with mild to advanced and end-stage cases of MGD, form the basis of this model:

1. Lid Tenderness: A Sign Elicited During an Examination

Lid tenderness, a painful sensation, is a sign I have found to be highly indicative of obstructive MGD and elevated intraductal pressure. I elicit lid tenderness, if present, by applying pressure gently to the lids while evaluating Meibomian glands during the patient's examination.

The majority (approximately 80 percent) of my patients with obstructive MGD have tender eyelids. I reported this observation in my first study describing Meibomian gland probing published in 2010 in the journal *Cornea*. Of the twenty-five patients included in the study, twenty displayed signs of MGD plus lid tenderness. Notably, this was the first time in medical literature that lid tenderness was correlated to MGD, elevated intraductal pressure, and its proximate cause, periductal fibrosis.

Lid tenderness develops in spots over some glands, or it can develop over an entire lid. These patterns of tenderness indicate the location and extent of elevated intraductal pressure and suggest localized constricting periductal fibrosis (see the section "Characteristics of Periductal Fibrosis").

The four prior models of MGD explained earlier do not address lid tenderness and its utility as a marker for elevated intraductal pressure.

2. Lid Tenderness Whether or Not the Gland Shows Expressible Meibum

Eye doctors apply moderate pressure to the eyelids to determine if the Meibomian glands are expressible. If the glands are expressible, doctors usually assume they are unobstructed and healthy, unless the meibum is of poor quality or quantity. Unfortunately, this assumption is wrong.

I have found, and my published studies show, lid tenderness may occur even when glands are expressible, indicating blockage exists deeper within the gland (see "Characteristics of Periductal Fibrosis"). In fact, expressible glands are just as likely to have occult obstruction as nonexpressible glands are to have obvious obstruction.

Again, the four prior models of MGD do not address lid tenderness.

3. Randomly Distributed Atrophic Acinar-Ductular Units Within a Single Gland

Meibography often shows randomly distributed atrophic acinar-ductular units in an otherwise healthy gland. Sometimes there is just one atrophic unit, sometimes more. This pattern of atrophy can only be explained by a selective and disruptive force that targets a single acinar-ductular unit and its stem cells. This force, periductal fibrosis, can preferentially invade the duct at the junction of the duct wall and a single acinar-ductular unit, bypassing other acinar-ductular units in the vicinity.

The four prior models of MGD do not account for this random distribution of acinar-ductular unit atrophy. With hyperkeratinization or thick meibum, the entire population of acinar-ductular units behind the blockage would be atrophic. Similarly, an increased demand on acini to produce meibum would affect all acini, not just one somewhere in the middle of the pack. Also, if solutes at the lid margin caused atrophy, it would likely be found primarily near the orifice, not deeper within the gland.

4. Differing Patterns of Atrophy in Neighboring Glands

Meibography often shows partially atrophied, short, or truncated glands right next to completely atrophied glands (whole gland atrophy) and intact glands. The same invasive force—periductal fibrosis—that selectively attacks acinar-ductular units can selectively attack and encircle different gland ducts at different depths while ignoring neighboring ones.

Because hyperkeratinization, thick meibum, stressors, and solutes equally and diffusely expose Meibomian glands to disease, atrophy patterns in neighboring glands should be homogenous. But they are not. As seen with meibography, the patterns show great variation.

5. Resistance in the Gland Encountered by a Probe

When a 76-micron diameter probe enters a blocked duct, it often encounters fixed resistance. The resistance may ultimately yield, but at first it is firm, fixed, focal, and unyielding, making an audible *pop* sound when released. Often the probe encounters multifocal fixed resistance deep within the gland, not just at the orifice, creating multiple *pops* in quick succession, or a gritty sound, when released.

If a blocked duct contained keratin, if the meibum inside were thick, if its protein-to-lipid ratio were altered, or if the glands were bathed in toxic solutes, as proposed by the four prior models of MGD, a probe would enter and advance through the central duct easily without encountering fixed resistance and without creating an audible *pop* and restoring meibum flow upon its release.

6. Instantaneous Relief of Lid Tenderness When Fixed Resistance in the Gland Is Released and Intraductal Pressure Equalibrates

Passing a probe into the Meibomian gland with MGD has a profound and instantaneous effect on lid tenderness. All twenty patients with lid tenderness in my 2010 study experienced immediate relief after probing. In 2017, doctors at Harvard Medical School's Department of Ophthalmology similarly reported that 91.4 percent of patients with obstructive Meibomian gland dysfunction experienced immediate relief after probing (notably, without complications).

As noted, the four prior models also don't discuss lid tenderness as a hallmark of obstructive MGD. Because inflammation takes time to dissipate, and for these patients relief was instantaneous, inflammation can not be the proximate cause of lid tenderness.

Because of these six observations, in my view, the periductal fibrosis model completes the MGD mosaic, accounting for lid tenderness and atrophy patterns, while *remaining consistent with observations described by the earlier models.*

Characteristics of Periductal Fibrosis

Periductal fibrosis presents with several notable characteristics pertaining to its type, location, and extent within Meibomian glands.

Type of Tissue

Periductal fibrosis is dense scar tissue that may be vascularized (as noted using confocal microscopy), meaning it may contain blood vessels. The presence of blood vessels within this scar tissue may explain why, when a gland is probed and the fibrosis is released, a dot of blood sometimes appears at the orifice or, rarely, within the

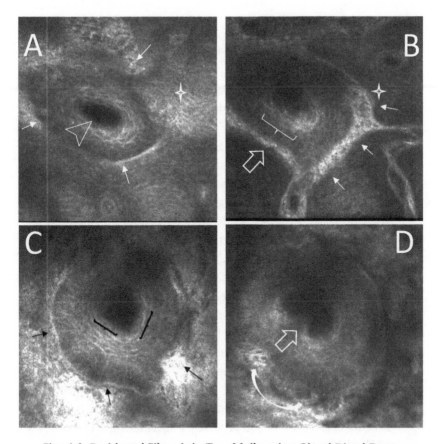

Fig. 4.1. Periductal Fibrosis in Two Meibomian Gland Distal Ducts

Examples of images showing periductal fibrosis seen at different depths in two Meibomian gland distal ducts during examination with confocal microscopy.

Duct 1 (A and B):

A. The oval-shaped lumen (open arrowhead) of the distal duct at a depth of 67 microns, with apparent fibrosis along the perimeter of the external duct wall (arrows), accompanied by a fibrotic sheet (star).

B. The duct at a depth of 112 microns, with fibrosis now appearing as a tight, organized periductal fibrotic band (star and arrows) surrounding, constricting, and invading the external duct wall. The flattened side of the oval lumen (bracket) corresponds to the region with the tightest fibrosis (open arrow).

Duct 2 (C and D):

C. The oval-shaped lumen of the distal duct at a depth of 64 microns, with scalloping and pinching of the external duct wall from apparent invasive fibrosis of the external duct wall basement membrane (arrows). The flattened sides of the oval lumen correspond to regions of fibrosis (brackets).

D. The duct at a depth of 112 microns. A large indentation in the external duct wall (curved arrow) correspond to an indented and strictured lumen (open arrow).

Source: Steven L. Maskin and Sreevardhan Alluri, "Expressible Meibomian Glands Have Occult Fixed Obstructions: Findings from Meibomian Gland Probing to Restore Intraductal Integrity," *Cornea* 38, no. 7 (2019), 880–887, https://journals.lww.com/corneajrnl/Fulltext/2019/07000/Expressible_Meibomian_Glands_Have_Occult_Fixed.16.aspx.

Sidebar 4.11
Detecting Periductal Fibrosis

In 1997, Ivan Cher, MD, an ophthalmologist and re-searcher, first speculated that periglandular fibrotic tissue was a possible cause of Meibomian gland obstruction and atrophy. While studying slit-lamp images of patients with dimples, notches, and other indentations on their lid margins, he observed abnormal duct-gland complexes "beneath each indentation." Dr. Cher explained how fibrosis associated with the abnormalities can tug on the gland orifice to produce the indentations and suggested it may be a cause of atrophic gland "drop-out."

However, without the tactile and auditory (fixed resistance and sounds) insights provided by Meibomian gland probing, and without the confocal microscopy images we have obtained showing periductal fibrosis invading the duct wall, he concluded that the lid margin indentations can occur without fibrosis "breaching the walls of the [duct-gland complex]."

Now, with probing and confocal images, we know fibrosis does invade the duct wall (see fig. 4.1). Exactly to what extent is currently under investigation. Thus far, probe findings suggest, in patients with MGD, fibrosis occurs within 1 millimeter of the orifice in 67 percent of glands, and within 2 millimeters in over 90 percent of glands. (See "Incidence of Periductal Fibrosis" in this chapter, and table 4.1.)

periglandular tissue. The microscopic bleeding is self-limiting (meaning it will stop on its own without the application of pressure), due to the release of fibrovascular tissue (scar tissue that contains blood vessels) and is normal in patients with MGD.

In fact, the appearance of a drop of blood is one way to confirm the existence of periductal fibrosis and its release with probing. It is a sign that duct lumen integrity is restored. *Pops* and gritty findings also confirm the existence of periductal fibrosis and the restored integrity of the duct lumen.

Location and Extent

Periductal fibrosis is occult, or hidden from view, and may occur anywhere along the length of a gland, distally or proximally. Where the fibrosis develops and to what extent determines how it affects the gland. The tissue may occur as one or more circumferential strictures around the duct, like a belt or a python coiling around its prey, elevating intraductal pressure behind the constriction. We also now have evidence of invasion of fibrotic and, at times, fibrovascular tissue into the external duct wall and stem cell zone.

The location and extent of fibrosis are also important factors in diagnosis and the classification of lids with MGD (see chapter 9), and in treatment with Maskin® Probing (see chapter 11).

1. *Distal periductal fibrosis,* which leads to complete constriction and obstruction and develops between the orifice and first acinus, will prevent all meibum from being naturally secreted during blinks or expressed during an exam. Continued meibum synthesis behind this fixed obstruction will lead to increased pressure throughout the gland, causing lid tenderness over the entire obstructed gland. If the fixed periductal fibrosis is not relieved, the entire gland behind the obstruction will undergo atrophy, that is, whole gland atrophy.

2. *Proximal periductal fibrosis,* which leads to complete obstruction deeper within the gland, will cause increased pressure and lid tenderness, but only over the obstructed part of the gland behind the band of fibrosis. The gland will continue to synthesize meibum on both sides of the obstruction. Meibum synthesized in the distal part will secrete and be expressible during exams, whereas meibum in the proximal part will remain sequestered behind the obstruction. If this

proximal fibrosis is not relieved, the segment of the gland behind the fibrosis will atrophy, leading to a short, truncated gland.

Incidence of Periductal Fibrosis

The incidence of periductal fibrosis is remarkably high, underlying most obstructive MGD cases. In one of our studies of nearly twelve thousand glands with MGD that were probed, nearly 67 percent of all glands and 80 percent of obstructed glands had evidence of these fibrotic bands within 1 millimeter below the orifice surface, while over 90 percent of glands had this tissue within 2 millimeters. Table 4.1, "Findings Using a 1-Millimeter Maskin® Probe," summarizes the findings from the study.

Table 4.1
Findings Using a 1-Millimeter Maskin® Probe

Total Number of Patients	108
Male	36
Female	72
Average age	56.4 (±16.8)
Lids probed	404
Glands probed	11,776
Probed glands with no resistance	1,890 (16%)
Probed glands with resistance	9,886 (84%)
Types of resistance	
FFFUR*	7,864 (79.5%)
Not FFFUR	2,022 (20.4%)
Incidence of FFFUR in all glands	67%

*Fixed, firm, focal, and unyielding resistance.
Source: Adapted from Steven L. Maskin and Sreevardhan Alluri, "Expressible Meibomian Glands Have Occult Fixed Obstructions: Findings from Meibomian Gland Probing to Restore Intraductal Integrity," *Cornea* 38, no. 7 (2019), 880–887, https://journals .lww.com/corneajrnl/Fulltext/2019/07000/Expressible_Meibo mian_Glands_Have_Occult_Fixed.16.aspx.

CHANGES TO ANATOMY AND
PHYSIOLOGY OF MEIBOMIAN GLANDS

MGD can cause changes to the anatomy and physiology of Meibomian glands and their secretions.

Changes to Anatomy

MGD can cause several visible and occult changes to the anatomy of the Meibomian glands. Some changes are hidden from view inside the eyelids, although now with meibography and confocal microscopy, these changes are more easily found (see chapter 9).

- The orifice, the excretory duct, or even the entire duct can narrow or close completely, often choked off by *bands of periductal fibrosis.*
- The acini may develop cystic changes and dilate, and the duct and ductules may dilate as they fill with meibum trapped behind the obstruction. (The retention of oil inside Meibomian glands leads to increased pressure and inflammation, altering the composition of meibum.)
- The angle at which the ductule enters the duct may change, from being angled toward the lid margin to becoming horizontal or angled away from the lid margin.
- Acini can atrophy. When they die off, they stop producing meibum and disappear.
- The eyelids can thicken or swell due to inflammation of the Meibomian gland structure and accumulated meibum.
- Because of the effect of inflammation on the nearby lash follicle, eyelashes may grow every which way instead of neatly outward with a curl. They may grow straight out or down, a condition called lash ptosis. With a condition called trichiasis, the eyelashes curl inward and may even scratch against the cornea.
- Inflammation may also cause veining on the eyelid margins, known as telangiectasia.

Changes in Secretions

An important measure of Meibomian gland health is the secretion of meibum. Are the glands producing enough meibum, and is it of good quality?

Quantity

With MGD, the quantity of oil secreted may decline due to the following:

- Closed or blocked Meibomian gland orifices
    - Without an opening, meibum has no exit. If the opening is smaller than normal, less meibum is secreted.
- Dilation of the gland structures (central duct, ductule, and acini)
    - The dilated structures suggest distal duct obstruction, so less oil will be secreted.
    - Reduced pressure within a dilated duct reduces the flow of oil, the same way the flow of water slows through a pipe with a larger diameter, and may not effectively deliver meibum to the tear film.
- Fewer healthy progenitor cells and meibocytes
    - Obstruction causes pressure to build in the acini, causing the cells there to undergo squamous meta-plasia. As a result, fewer progenitor cells give rise to the meibocytes that turn into meibum.
- Atrophy of any part of the Meibomian gland structure
    - If any part of the Meibomian gland structure atro-phies, that part will not synthesize or secrete meibum.
- Cicatricial MGD
    - Meibum secretes into the aqueous layer of the tear film instead of the outer lipid layer.

Sidebar 4.12
Why Glands Become Tortuous

Nobody knows why Meibomian glands sometimes appear bent or curled (see fig. 9.3, C). I have hypothesized that due to inflammation, the tissue in the eyelids surrounding the glands weakens and can no longer hold the glands securely in place. Since glands are secure at the orifice, once gravity takes over, the glands may end up sagging, which may cause them to bend. This may even explain why there is more tortuosity (bending and curling) in the upper lids than the lower lids: the downward force of gravity may naturally cause the unsecured ends of the Meibomian glands near the top of the upper eyelids to bend down.

Quality

When the outflow of meibum is blocked, the stagnant meibum can become a rich environment for bacterial growth and the buildup of undesirable materials, for example, debris from demodex mites (parasites often found at the base of the lashes and in the Meibomian glands), keratin proteins, and inflammatory mediators, to name a few. Although bacteria normally colonize in the glands, an overgrowth of bacteria with an increase in harmful detritus can lead to changes in meibum composition, which affects the stability of meibum and reduces tear breakup time (TBUT). The buildup of undesirable materials can cause inflammation at the cellular level—in stem cells, progenitor cells, meibocytes, and the epithelium of the central ducts—further affecting the synthesis and secretion of meibum.

As a result, the quality of oil secreted may decline, becoming cloudy, full of particulate matter, and no longer clear. The meibum may take on a hue (yellow, pearl, or white, for example) or become thick and pasty, like toothpaste. Its melting point may rise.

IMPACT OF CHANGES

When changes of this magnitude occur (such as reduced and altered Meibomian gland secretions as well as changes to the gland structure with thickening and congestion of lids), other parts of the ocular surface can be affected. That's why MGD rarely occurs in isolation without comorbidities. Then these comorbidities (see chapter 5) may further exacerbate MGD, leading to even more dramatic changes in Meibomian glands, contributing to the spiral of disease. The more common comorbidities are discussed in the next chapter.

5

Comorbidities and Cofactors

Myth
MGD is a simple condition, easily diagnosed and treated.
Fact
Comorbidities often accompany MGD, and
various factors can contribute to this disease.

Many comorbidities can coexist with MGD, and many factors can contribute to this disease. Often MGD and these comorbidities lead to or exacerbate each other.

For example, because periductal fibrosis often blocks the flow of meibum, the eyelid may become congested and thicken. With less secreted meibum and a swollen lid, ocular surface friction during blinking increases. This friction puts additional stress on the Meibomian glands, exacerbating MGD, and may lead to or exacerbate a loosening, stretching, and bunching up of conjunctival tissue, a comorbidity called conjunctivochalasis (a term that combines two words, "conjunctiva" and "chalasis," meaning the conjunctival tissue is relaxed or stretched). Conjunctivochalasis, a very common comorbidity, especially in older patients, can put additional stress on the Meibomian glands by further increasing frictional stresses during blinking. Also, because the Meibomian glands secrete less meibum, tear film evaporation speeds up, exacerbating aqueous tear deficiency (ATD). ATD can worsen ocular discomfort. Because of ocular discomfort, patients sometimes use lubricating eye drops too often. Overuse of eye drops can dilute any nutrients in the ATD-diminished natural tear film or irritate eyes with sensitivities to their ingredients, further exacerbating symptoms. A host of other comorbidities may arise. Thus, the spiral of disease worsens and continues.

For patients, the important takeaway is that resolving MGD may only be the first step in the treatment process. Along with it, various comorbidities and cofactors that can create inherent complexity will also need attention.

COMPLEX PATIENTS

Treating complex patients with multiple comorbidities, like the kind I often see, can pose challenges. However, the challenges need not be insurmountable. It all begins with understanding the underlying cause of MGD—periductal fibrosis—and identifying comorbidities and other factors playing roles in its progression or contributing to symptoms.

These complex patients often want to know what caused their symptoms to spiral out of control. What happened that drove their Meibomian glands and ocular surface into dysfunction and disease, and when?

The fact is, it's often difficult to pinpoint a specific trigger because MGD is a disease that typically progresses over time, with different comorbidities and cofactors influencing that progress. These can be chronic, episodic, or seasonal and may therefore wax and wane. As a result, the disease often progresses in a nonlinear fashion subclinically, without obvious signs or symptoms, delaying diagnosis. Undiagnosed and therefore untreated, MGD worsens, as do other comorbidities.

But an isolated event can cause a mild case of MGD to suddenly spiral out of control. Patients may report they had no pain one day and extreme pain the next, because with that triggering event, the disease finally reached a tipping point and the eyes became symptomatic.

A sculptor suffered with mild, chronic symptoms of MGD for over twenty years. Decades of exposure to ceramic and silica dust finally reached a tipping point, triggering a sudden worsening of symptoms. She saw many doctors but found no relief and eventually became my patient. Meibography revealed significant gland atrophy. I treated her MGD with probing and her other comorbidities as indicated. I also suggested she wear goggles when working to protect her Meibomian glands from the dust swirling in her studio. Today she is symptom free.

Who Has What?

Although my patients often have multiple comorbidities, no patient has every comorbidity, and no two patients are exactly alike. So, although doctors can compare patients to each other, for example, someone with a severe case of MGD versus someone with a mild case of MGD, when it comes to diagnosis and treatment, doctors must approach each patient individually.

I've included an extensive, though not by any means complete, list of comorbidities and cofactors in this chapter, to highlight just how complex MGD and Dry Eye can be.

Clusters of Comorbidities

As unique as everyone is, comorbidities often cluster. Hypertension and diabetes, for example, are often found with obesity. Children with autism spectrum disorders have higher rates of gastrointestinal disorders, seizures, and multisystem disorders than children without. Patients with Sjögren's syndrome often suffer with rheumatoid arthritis, keratoconjunctivitis sicca, and dry mouth. Dental patients with plaque may develop gingivitis. MGD too often clusters with other comorbidities, including aqueous tear deficiency (ATD), conjunctivochalasis, ocular allergies, anterior blepharitis, blepharospasm, and nocturnal lagophthalmos.

Symptoms

Symptoms are the patient's subjective evidence of disease. Virtually all of these comorbidities can cause symptoms of varying degrees. Sometimes the symptoms are severe, extremely debilitating, and even unbearable. The symptoms from comorbidities can mask symptoms from MGD or mimic them, adding to frustration for patients and their doctors.

Sidebar 5.1
The Scourge of Particulate Matter

Exposure to dust and other particulate matter can cause acute or chronic Meibomian gland obstruction with severe pain and lid tenderness. Interestingly, I have seen at least eight patients, besides the sculptor mentioned in the text, with a history of acute obstructive MGD that developed suddenly after exposure to particulate matter: one after exposure to smoke from a volcano in Guatemala; a second to heavy outdoor dust at a renaissance festival; a third to a large dust plume spewed by a vacuum cleaner bag; others to smoke from candles, campfires, and California wildfires; and still others to dust on dairy and deer farms.

Dust may contain a variety of irritants. For example, dust found in the agricultural industry may contain molds, fungi, pesticides, herbicides, animal-derived particles, feed, particles of straw or other bedding, and endotoxins (toxins released by bacteria). Some of my patients who worked in agriculture reported that they had chronic milder symptoms for years, then a sudden onset of severe incapacitating symptoms. These acute symptoms prompted them to seek help, which eventually led them to my practice. (Interestingly, these patients could attribute the onset of acute symptoms to a relatively brief, but specific, incident of exposure to particulate matter.)

Also, eye cosmetics such as foundation, eyeliner, mascara, and eye shadow contain particulate matter that can inflame the lid margins and lead to obstructive MGD.

Adapted from Steven L. Maskin and Sreevardhan Alluri, "Intraductal Meibomian Gland Probing: Background, Patient Selection, Procedure, and Perspectives," *Clinical Ophthalmology*, July 10, 2019, 1203–1223.

Duration

The duration of comorbidities can vary: they can range from being short-lived to being chronic, lasting a lifetime. Duration can depend on the disease, the patient's health and response or adherence to treatment, the diagnostic and therapeutic skills of the physician, environmental and behavioral factors, and more.

It is almost always best to address symptoms as quickly as possible, with the most effective treatment that produces the fewest side effects, to reduce the duration and severity of any disease.

OCULAR SURFACE AND SYSTEMIC COMORBIDITIES

Comorbidities fall into two general categories, those that are related to the surface of the eyes and those that are systemic, affecting many parts of the body but also the eyes and the Meibomian glands.

The tables in this section include the most common ocular surface and systemic comorbidities I have seen in my patients. However, these tables do not include every possible comorbidity. If they did, this book would be unwieldy. Furthermore, an entire chapter could be written about many of these, if not an entire book.

Ocular Surface Comorbidities

Many comorbidities of the ocular surface can play a role in MGD because they exacerbate, or can be exacerbated by, MGD. Because of the vast number of possible comorbidities, it's important to consult a doctor who has experience with diseases of the ocular surface rather than attempt to self-diagnose and self-treat.

Although essentially all types of ocular surface comorbidities lead to inflammation, they can be divided into categories by the underlying manner in which the comorbidity *primarily* impacts Meibomian glands, as follows:

1. Inflammatory comorbidities: comorbidities that primarily induce inflammation, including infections
2. Mechanical comorbidities: problems with the physical properties of ocular tissues, including the continuum of

loose tissue, friction-related disorders, delayed tear clearance, and mechanical lid disorders
3. Tear-related comorbidities: conditions that directly affect tear production
4. Iatrogenic comorbidities: medically induced comorbidities

Arguably, some comorbidities could be included in more than one category. For example, conjunctivochalasis, listed in table 5.2, "Mechanical Comorbidities," may also be associated with tear-related comorbidities because it can channel tears to the outer canthus, leaving the eye dry. Similarly, although the term "filamentary keratitis" indicates both a mechanical problem (*filaments*) and possible inflammation (*itis*), it is only listed in table 5.1, "Inflammatory Comorbidities."

I have included more information about these common comorbidities that often cluster at the end of this chapter:

- Aqueous tear deficiency (ATD)
- Anterior blepharitis
- Friction-related tissue disorders of the ocular surface, including
  - superior limbic keratoconjunctivitis
  - conjunctivochalasis
- Ocular allergies and other sensitivities
- Lateral canthal crowding
- Blepharospasms
- Nocturnal and blink lagophthalmos

Inflammatory Comorbidities

Inflammation occurs when the body senses a noxious stimulus and sends blood filled with white blood cells and other components to fight it off. During this process, the blood vessels dilate, causing the appearance of redness. Inflammation may be a response to a single, acute event or part of the normal healing process. Inflammation can also be chronic, in which case the body constantly senses the noxious stimulus, but for whatever reason, can't win the fight and resolve it. In either case—acute or chronic—ocular inflammation can interrupt the normal function of ocular tissues while causing significant discomfort.

Comorbidities affecting the face and skin, included in table 5.1, can be a factor in MGD when they affect tissues close to the eyes, like the eyelids, area around the eyes, or the forehead. Flakes of dead skin due to these comorbidities can fall into the eyes, causing irritation and inflammation.

Mechanical Comorbidities

Mechanical problems related to the ocular surface (table 5.2) are sometimes overlooked. They can be related to eyelash disorders or elevated ocular surface tissues. They are often due to prolonged friction during blinking or eye movement and are sometimes accompanied by loose conjunctival tissue that causes various symptoms of different severities. The symptoms may be vague, intermittent, or transient and can sometimes be severe and extremely debilitating. Exposure-related comorbidities from mechanical lid disorders occur when the ocular surface is not adequately protected and becomes dry from direct exposure to the atmosphere for prolonged periods.

Tear-Related Comorbidities

Because tear film is an important component in ocular health, comfort, and vision, tear-related comorbidities (table 5.3) can have a profound impact on symptoms. One tear-related comorbidity can exacerbate the other, contributing to a vicious cycle of disease, which can be extremely frustrating for patients and their doctors.

Iatrogenic Comorbidities

Comorbidities due to medical intervention are called iatrogenic, from the Greek *iatros,* meaning "physician" or "medicine." There are many iatrogenic possibilities (table 5.4), including side effects from prescription and over-the-counter eye drops, or surgeries such as LASIK and cataract surgery, among many others. These side effects can contribute to MGD directly or induce new comorbidities that exacerbate MGD. The risks of iatrogenic comorbidities from various treatments vary depending on many factors, including the treatment itself, the patient's specific condition and state of health, the skill of the physician, follow-up care, and so forth.

Table 5.1
Inflammatory Comorbidities
Inflammatory comorbidities affect the ocular surface, lids,
and Meibomian glands leading to periductal fibrosis.

Comorbidity	Description
Allergies (See "Common Ocular Surface Comorbidities" at the end of the chapter.)	Immune system response to an allergen that leads to inflammation of the eyelids, Meibomian glands, conjunctiva, and cornea, with potential for loss of vision and Dry Eye.
Atopic disease	Allergic hypersensitivity accompanied by elevated serum IgE, immunoglobulin E, a marker for atopic disease.
	Often hereditary.
	Can be triggered or exacerbated by many factors, including seasonal allergies, soaps, chemicals, and cold weather, among others.
	Causes ocular surface inflammation with possible fibrosis and symblepharon formation (adhesion of the palpebral and bulbar conjunctiva).
	Associated with chronic inflammation of the skin, such as eczema, a form of anterior blepharitis with inflammation of the skin's upper layer, which can cause itching, redness, blisters, swelling, scaling, or scabbing.
Blepharitis	Inflammation of the eyelids, from the Greek for "eyelid" (*blephara*) and "itis," indicating an inflammatory disease.
	A nonspecific term that is often used in place of a more specific or technical diagnosis.
	Two major types: anterior blepharitis and posterior blepharitis.
• Anterior blepharitis (See "Common Ocular Surface Comorbidities" at the end of the chapter.)	Inflammation of the front part of the eyelids, usually found at the base of the eyelashes.
	Pockets of inflammation can cause small ulcers where the eyelashes meet the lid margin.

Comorbidity	Description
	Often associated with staphylococcus bacteria and much less often herpes simplex virus, which can cause blisters.
	May frequently be due to demodex mites.
	Often characterized by crusting, scaling, flaking, or cylindrical deposits at the base of the eyelashes and lid margin.
	Often associated with allergies.
	Bacteria break down meibum, causing release of irritating free fatty acids and soapy bubbles in the tear film.
• Posterior blepharitis	Inflammation of the posterior eyelids, typically due to MGD.
Conjunctivitis, also called pink eye	Inflammation of the conjunctiva characterized by redness of the tissues. Can be caused by: • Bacterial or viral infections • Allergies (See "Common Ocular Surface Comorbidities" at the end of the chapter.) • Clogged tear drainage duct • ATD • Poor eye or contact lens hygiene • Mechanical disorders such as traumatic injury or conjunctivochalasis • Toxic agent that reaches the surface of the eye, e.g., an ocular medication or makeup. The toxic response may be due to any of the compounds in the formulation including any preservatives. Causes redness of the conjunctival tissues that can cause pain, foreign body and gritty sensations, and even blepharospasm.

(continued)

Table 5.1 *continued*

Comorbidity	Description
Contact dermatitis	Reaction of the skin usually due to direct contact with an allergen or an irritant.
	Allergens can be easily transferred to the eyelids, and even the surface of the eye, when the eyes are touched or rubbed.
Dermatitis (dry skin in the area around the eyes)	Skin that is dry, flaky, and can itch falls into the eyes, creating surface inflammation.
	May have many causes, including thyroid disease and low ambient humidity, as well as excessive cleaning of lid margins.
Filamentary keratitis	Keratitis accompanied by strands (filaments), typically multifocal, of degenerated corneal and conjunctival epithelial cells and mucus adhering to the surface of the cornea.
	Can lead to focal mechanical irritation with accompanying ocular surface inflammation.
	Can be induced and exacerbated by ATD with inadequate blinks.
Folliculitis	Inflammation of the eyelash follicles.
	Produces debris that can disrupt the tear film.
Keratitis	Inflammation of the cornea, among the most sensitive parts of the body, often leading to inflammation of the entire ocular surface.
	Can lead to extremely painful symptoms or reduced corneal sensation in the setting of herpes virus infection or chronic ATD.
Keratoconjunctivitis sicca	Dry (sicca) Eye that includes keratitis and conjunctivitis, painful diseases of the cornea and conjunctiva that are characterized by ATD, inflammation, and sometimes, paradoxically, desensitized corneas.
	May lead to squamous metaplasia of conjunctival and Meibomian gland orifice epithelium, as well as a nonwettable ocular surface.

Comorbidity	Description
	Often exacerbates comorbid friction-induced diseases of the ocular surface.
Rosacea	A chronic skin condition characterized by sebaceous gland inflammation, most recognizable when involving the nose and cheeks with blood vessel dilation.
	Can be associated with surface and Meibomian periglandular inflammation.
	Often accompanied by delayed tear clearance.
	Can lead to blood vessel invasion of the peripheral cornea, often in the setting of delayed tear clearance.
	May be difficult to diagnose in darkly pigmented individuals.
Superior limbic kerato-conjunctivitis (SLK) (See "Common Ocular Surface Comorbidities" at the end of the chapter.)	Inflammation of the tissue at the superior cornea where it meets the conjunctiva, due to mechanical and frictional trauma caused by tight lids without adequate lubrication.
	At times caused by or accompanied by ATD, exacerbated by blinking.

Table 5.2

Mechanical Comorbidities

Mechanical comorbidities create inflammation of the ocular surface, lids, and Meibomian glands, leading to periductal fibrosis.

Comorbidity	Description
Benign essential blepharospasm (See "Common Comorbidities" at the end of the chapter.)	A neuromuscular disorder that often begins with excessive blinking. Causes ocular irritation and ineffective blinks, leading to delayed tear clearance, inflammation, and MGD. The eyelids spasm, close uncontrollably, and may stay closed for variable lengths of time.
Chalazion, chronic	Chronic blockage of Meibomian gland duct with nodule formation, usually without tenderness. Swelling of blocked Meibomian gland can lead to disruption of neighboring glands, causing significant progression of MGD within the lid. Chalazion may develop after hordeolum. Disrupts the normal spreading of tear film. Inflammation, pressure, and swelling can lead to Meibomian gland atrophy.
Computer vision syndrome	Includes a variety of conditions related to computer use, such as eyestrain, irritation, redness, blurred or double vision, and eye fatigue. Environmental factors may also play a role—dry air, positioning of air vents, toxins in office supplies, allergens, dust, height or positioning of computer screen. (See table 5.8, "Behavior and Lifestyle.")
Conjunctival and corneal growths: neoplasia, pinguecula, pterygium, Salzmann's nodular corneal degeneration	Abnormal growths occurring on the cornea and/or conjunctiva. May disrupt the normal spreading of tear film. Associated with increased surface inflammation, ATD, and MGD.

Comorbidity	Description
Conjunctivochalasis (See "Common Ocular Surface Comorbidities" at the end of the chapter.)	Loosening, stretching, and wrinkling of the transparent membrane that covers the white part of the eye.
	The tissue loses elasticity and may become pleated, droop over the lower eyelid margin, or become pinched between the lid and eyeball.
	If chalasis is in the outer corners of the eyes, it alters the normal path of tears, channeling them toward the outer canthus instead of toward the nose, where they flow out through the punctum, leaving the ocular surface dry and inflamed.
	Superior chalasis can cause frictional disease, leading to surface inflammation.
	Can block the tear reservoir behind the lower lid, preventing normal tear film spreading into the precorneal tear film.
	Causes symptoms that may mimic ATD and MGD and that can be difficult for patients to describe, both potentially leading to misdiagnosis.
	To correctly diagnose, symptoms may need to be elicited.
Corneal surface irregularities, such as Cogan's dystrophy, also known as map-dot-fingerprint dystrophy (MDF), and others	Nonsmooth irregular cornea surface (MDF) may lead to painful recurrent corneal erosions (RCE), usually upon awakening.
	Disrupts the normal spreading of tear film.
	RCEs can cause extensive inflammation of the ocular surface and lids.
Delayed tear clearance	Tear film flows out through the tear ducts (lacrimal puncta) into the nose at a slower than normal rate.
	The lacrimal drainage system may be slowed due to narrowing (stenosis) or blockage of the punctum due to infection or swelling from allergies as well as post–punctal occlusion treatment for ATD including thermal cautery and punctal plug. The tissues lining the nasolacrimal duct in the nose may be lax or affected by infection or allergy.

(continued)

Table 5.2 *continued*

Comorbidity	Description
Dermatochalasis	Skin of the brow and particularly the upper eyelids becomes loose and redundant due to age and the effects of gravity.
	The extra weight of the lids on the ocular surface can lead to entropion, trichiasis, and focal-surface microtrauma, and the position of Meibomian gland openings can be altered, affecting normal flow of meibum to the tear film.
	Can lead to protective ptosis if patients close their lids partially for comfort.
Distichiasis	An individual or row of extra eyelashes posteriorly, typically growing from within Meibomian gland orifices.
	Lashes may collide during blinks, preventing the eye from closing completely, leading to dry lid margins and ocular surface, contributing to inflammation.
	Can cause foreign body sensations, mimicking other comorbidities, which may lead to misdiagnosis.
	Lashes may rotate against the eye causing excess tears or trauma.
Ectropion	An outturning of the lower or upper eyelid away from the eyeball.
	Disrupts the normal flow of tear film by causing meibum and tear film to flow out, away from the eyeball, over the lid, and onto the lid skin and cheek.
	Can be due to aging or diseases such as lupus erythematosus or atopic dermatitis, as well as paralysis of the seventh cranial nerve. (See "Paralytic lagophthalmos" in this table.)
Entropion	A turning in of the lower or upper eyelid toward the eyeball.
	The inwardly turned skin of the lid's surface may abrade the surface of the eyeball, causing microtrauma on the eye's surface and lid margin.

Comorbidity	Description
	Lashes rotated inward can scratch the ocular surface, leading to a breakdown of the corneal epithelium with possible infection, loss of vision, and potential permanent loss of the eye.
Floppy eyelid syndrome	Loosening of the upper eyelids that enable them to easily evert when rubbing against an object such as a pillowcase during sleep.
	Exposure of the ocular surface during sleep, causing mechanical trauma to the conjunctiva and ocular surface with inflammation.
	Often associated with obstructive sleep apnea, obesity, keratoconus, and Down syndrome.
Graves' disease	An autoimmune disease involving an overactive thyroid that typically leads to protruding eyes with retracted eyelids, increasing the exposure of the eye's surface.
	Decreases blinking and stretches the tear film.
Hordeolum, acute	Acute blockage of the Meibomian glands, with secondary inflammation, characterized by acute pain and eyelid tenderness.
	Meibum escapes the confines of the Meibomian gland with a severe, typically nodular inflammatory reaction, causing swelling with blurry vision as it exerts pressure on the cornea, changing the cornea's shape (astigmatism).
	Usually sterile (not due to bacteria).
	Can become rather large, encompassing the majority of an eyelid.
	Instead of resolving, sometimes develops into chalazion.
Lagophthalmos	Incomplete closing of the eye when it's supposed to close, such as during a blink or during sleep.
	Leads to dry spots on the ocular surface due to evaporation or insufficient spreading of tear film.

(continued)

Table 5.2 *continued*

Comorbidity	Description
	The lid margins may dry and become desiccated because the lids don't close, leading to orifice squamous metaplasia and gland obstruction.
	Can be associated with recurrent corneal erosion (RCE) and filamentary keratitis.
	There are several variations: blink, iatrogenic, nocturnal, and paralytic.
• Blink lagophthalmos (See "Common Ocular Surface Comorbidities" at the end of the chapter.)	An incomplete closure of the eyelids during a blink.
	Impedes the normal delivery of meibum into the tear film.
	Reduced or incomplete blinking may cause an accumulation of meibum in the glands, which may lead to increased intraductal pressure, which in turn can lead to gland atrophy.
	Often occurs with incomplete or partial blinks during gazing activities, like reading, talking on the phone, screen time, and driving, among many others.
• Iatrogenic lagophthalmos	An incomplete closure of the eyelids caused by medical treatment such as Botox injections around the eyes, eyelid lifts, or blepharoplasty surgery.
• Nocturnal lagophthalmos (See "Common Ocular Surface Comorbidities" at the end of the chapter.)	An incomplete closure of the eyelids during sleep.
	Can happen with the head in any position during sleep.
	A small gap can be seen between the closed eyelids when looking at them from below.
	Often diagnosed when patients describe their symptoms.
• Paralytic lagophthalmos	An incomplete closure of the eyelids caused by paralysis of the seventh cranial nerve, thus preventing the eye from closing.
	May be caused by trauma, tumors, or Bell's palsy and can be accompanied by ectropion.

Comorbidity	Description
Lateral canthal crowding (See "Common Ocular Surface Comorbidities" at the end of the chapter.)	A term I have coined to describe a group of comorbid conditions often affecting the lateral canthus, or outer corner of the eye, including dermatochalasis, entropion, trichiasis, and conjunctivochalasis, leading to altered blink patterns.
	Prevents normal spreading of tear film. Causes local microtrauma and inflammation.
Ocular injuries	Trauma to the surface of the eye, the cornea, the eyelids, the tear drainage system.
	Role in MGD depends on site and extent of trauma, effect of treatments, and other ocular and systemic comorbidities.
	Can disrupt lacrimal functional unit, causing altered tear film production and abnormal spreading of tear film, meibum production, and secretion.
Ptosis	Drooping of the upper lid, which may descend over the pupil, affecting vision.
	May cause decreased blink rate and excursion (the distance the upper lid margin travels from down-gaze to up-gaze), reducing meibum delivery into the tear film.
	May also involve the lower eyelid margin.
	May be congenital (found at birth), due to aging, or caused by diseases including diabetes, stroke, and myasthenia gravis.
	May occur to protect and increase comfort for the eye when the ocular surface is inflamed.
Trichiasis	The follicle of the lash is scarred, altering the direction of lash growth.
	Aberrant lashes may straighten, cross each other, or turn inward toward the eye, scratching the ocular surface, with breakdown of corneal epithelium, ocular surface inflammation, and possible infection.

Table 5.3

Tear-Related Comorbidities

Tear-related comorbidities create unstable tear film,
leading to inflammation of the ocular surface, lids, and
Meibomian glands, in turn leading to periductal fibrosis.

Comorbidity	Description
Aqueous tear deficiency (ATD), also called aqueous deficiency (See "Common Ocular Surface Comorbidities" at the end of the chapter.)	Insufficient production—a poor quantity—of wet tears. Leads to excessive friction during blinking, putting inflammatory stress on the tissues and structures of the ocular surface and inner lining of the eyelids. Associated with delayed tear clearance and poor quality of tear film, leading to blurred vision.
Mucin/goblet cell deficiency	Loss of mucin-producing conjunctival goblet epithelial cells, leading to poor tear quality and rapid breakup times. May be due to thermal or chemical injuries, vitamin A deficiency, or autoimmune conditions such as Stevens-Johnson syndrome, ocular cicatricial pemphigoid, or graft-versus-host disease, causing extensive scarring, inflammation, and atrophy of Meibomian glands.
Seborrheic Meibomian gland disease	Characterized by excess delivery of meibum when the glands are expressed, which can lead to irritation and inflammation of the ocular surface.

Systemic Comorbidities

Systemic comorbidities affect the entire human body. Sometimes they have a larger impact on one organ or one part of the body, but they typically affect the entire body.

As with many diseases, the severity of a systemic comorbidity can change over time, and its effect on the body can vary greatly from person to person. Therefore, individualized diagnosis and

Table 5.4

Iatrogenic Comorbidities
Through a variety of pathways, iatrogenic comorbidities
may each create inflammation of the ocular surface, lids,
and Meibomian glands, leading to periductal fibrosis.

Treatment/Purpose	Adverse Effects
Contact lenses • Soft lenses worn instead of glasses to improve vision, worn temporarily as bandages after surgery or trauma • Rigid gas-permeable cornea and/or scleral lenses, designed to optimize vision in the setting of irregular corneal surfaces • Scleral lenses prescribed for the treatment of Dry Eye	Can alter the chemistry of tear film, increasing inflammatory factors. Increase the risk of ocular surface infections. Alter the normal flow of tear film. Foreign body constantly in the eye may increase inflammation. Some contact lenses may reduce the amount of oxygen reaching the cornea, leading to corneal hypoxia. Can be irritating to Meibomian glands with every blink because of their proximity to lenses (separated only by the thin conjunctival tissue of the inner eyelid and tear film). Can cause old tear film to stagnate on ocular surface, leading to inflammation from decreased tear clearance. Can lead to ocular surface inflammatory diseases such as giant papillary conjunctivitis (GPC). (See "Ocular Allergies and Other Sensitivities" in "Common Ocular Surface Comorbidities" at the end of the chapter.) If masked by a contact lens but left untreated, ocular surface diseases can become more serious. Particles or medications can impregnate into the lens material, leading to a toxic inflammation of the ocular surface, or become lodged in the watery reservoir of the scleral lens, causing irritation and microtrauma.

(continued)

Table 5.4 *continued*

Treatment/Purpose	Adverse Effects	
Lid margin debridement: removing dead cells (exfoliation), debris, and film from the base of the lashes and lid margins with a metal scraper, spinning sponge, or other device	If done excessively, can rough up the delicate tissue of the eyelid margin, making it more permeable to toxic and disease-causing agents in the tear film with adverse effects on distal Meibomian gland tissue. May lead to lid-margin stem cell deficiency, which in turn may lead to increased telangiectasia (abnormal blood-vessel growth) and anterior migration of the mucocutaneous junction with conjunctivalization of the lid margin.	
Lid surgery outcomes, e.g., eyelids don't close properly after ptosis repair (eyelid lifts) or blepharoplasty with removal of redundant skin (See "Iatrogenic lagophthalmos" in table 5.2.)	If surgery is too aggressive, the fissure between the upper and lower lids may become too wide, causing the tear film to thin out. Can prevent proper lid closure, leading to painful ocular surface inflammation. May alter lid contour, adversely affecting the quality of blinks.	
Lubricating eye drops or ointments, i.e., over-the-counter therapies used to soothe and lubricate dry eyes	Some ingredients, such as cellulose, can leave a residue on eyelashes that can cause irritation at the base of the lashes or flake off into the eyes, causing ocular surface irritation.	Irritation causes ocular surface inflammation. Some patients may be sensitive or allergic to ingredients, e.g., lanolin, mineral oils, and petrolatum. May contain preservatives such as benzalkonium chloride (BAC, sometimes BAK), which can be irritating and even toxic, especially if used frequently. Adverse reactions can range from mild irritation or sensitivity to allergy, and may even
Prescription eye drops or ointments used to treat inflammation or infections, glaucoma, and other ocular diseases	Corticosteroids can raise ocular pressure, leading to glaucoma or cataract. Can interact chemically with and disrupt the lipid, aqueous, and mucin layers of tear film.	

Treatment/Purpose	Adverse Effects	
	May induce chronic allergic, toxic, or other type of inflammatory reaction, leading to damaged conjunctival epithelial and goblet cells as well as corneal epithelium.	be worse than symptoms of MGD or Dry Eye. Prolonged use may cause toxic conjunctivitis.
Surgeries (ocular) such as LASIK, PRK, cataract surgery, corneal transplants, etc.	Corneal nerves essential to good quality tear film and cornea health are cut with a blade or lasered, interrupting the lacrimal functional unit. Can decrease blink rate, leading to ocular surface inflammation. Frequent use of eye drops during healing can exacerbate symptoms.	
Therapeutic gland expression; applying pressure to evacuate the contents of Meibomian glands	May feel good afterward in the short term if distal meibum near the gland orifice is expressible, but if done aggressively may cause increased intraductal pressure and inflammation behind any deep, proximal periductal fibrosis. Can be very painful.	
Warm compresses applied to closed eyelids	Usually well tolerated unless the glands are blocked by periductal fibrosis. Can lead to increased inflammation in Meibomian glands. If too warm or if applied for too much time, can irritate and cause warpage of the cornea or scald the eyelids.	

therapy, based on each patient's unique circumstances, are very important.

Systemic comorbidities that play a role in MGD can be categorized as follows:

1. Autoimmune: the immune system mistakenly launches an attack on the body's own tissue

2. Non-autoimmune: comorbidities such as strokes or high blood pressure
3. Iatrogenic: comorbidities due to treatments or medications that cause side effects contributing to MGD

Autoimmune Comorbidities

The body normally protects itself against disease by recognizing foreign agents and attacking them with white blood cells. With autoimmune conditions, the body attacks its own tissue as if the tissue were a foreign agent. It's not always clear what triggers the body to attack itself.

Some autoimmune diseases can cause extreme pain and can profoundly affect quality of life.

Autoimmune conditions often cause chronic inflammation, which can have a significant effect on ocular tissues, including the Meibomian glands.

Table 5.5 lists some common autoimmune diseases that play a role in Dry Eye and MGD, but many other autoimmune diseases that can also play a role in ocular health.

Non-autoimmune Comorbidities

There are many potential systemic non-autoimmune comorbidities. The many possible comorbidities explain why your eye doctor asks for a complete medical history even if you only have dryness or grittiness in your eyes. Your doctor is trying to figure out all the comorbidities that may be contributing to your symptoms. Table 5.6 includes descriptions of commonly found comorbidities.

Iatrogenic Comorbidities: Oral and Intravenous Medications

Some oral and intravenous medications can contribute to MGD because they can affect the Meibomian glands or the lacrimal glands (table 5.7). If the medication is necessary, it may be wise to seek the care of an eye doctor who can help to manage any ocular side effects. Some medications are best avoided if at all possible, especially if they can exacerbate MGD. Others may be taken, but at the lowest dose possible.

Table 5.5

Autoimmune Comorbidities

Comorbidity	Description
Autoimmune thyroid disease	Affects the thyroid gland's production of hormones that play a role in virtually every bodily function, causing a wide range of symptoms, impacting everything from weight and mood to energy levels, and may be associated with chronic Meibomian periglandular inflammation.
• Graves' disease or Graves' ophthalmopathy	Hyperthyroidism, an overactive thyroid. May affect the blink rate and cause eyelid retraction and protruding eyes with exposure and inflammation of the ocular surface. A reduced blink rate also puts stress on the Meibomian glands, leading to dysfunction. Blinks may not be complete and eyes may not close completely. (See "Gazing" in "Behavior and Lifestyle," table 5.8.)
• Hashimoto's hypothyroidism	Hypothyroidism, an underactive thyroid, which in early stages of the disease may be overactive and may be associated with reduced Meibomian and lacrimal gland function.
Diabetes	The pancreas produces insufficient insulin, causing high glucose levels and leading to excessive urination, thirst, and hunger. Leads to decreased corneal sensitivity, disrupting tear production.
Fibromyalgia	A disease characterized by chronic body pain, fatigue, headaches, skin disorders, irritable bowel syndrome, cognitive disorders, problems with coordination, and dizziness, which is associated with Dry Eye and MGD. Can disturb sleep and be psychologically stressful.
Graft-versus-host disease	The bone marrow transplant graft attacks the host tissue with acute and/or chronic symptoms ranging from mild to severe, leading to ocular surface and lid inflammation, fibrosis, and symblepharon.

(continued)

Table 5.5 *continued*

Comorbidity	Description
Irritable bowel syndrome (IBS) and inflammatory bowel disease (IBD), including ulcerative colitis and Crohn's disease	Diseases characterized by chronic inflammation of the digestive tract, which may involve abdominal pain, fatigue, weight loss, and severe diarrhea. Studies have established a correlation between Dry Eye and IBS and IBD treatments.
Lupus (systemic lupus erythematosus)	An autoimmune disease that can affect different systems, tissues, or organs, e.g., lungs, kidneys, heart, joints, muscles, and blood cells, and cause widespread inflammation. Sometimes characterized by a butterfly-shaped rash across the nose and cheeks. Dry eye and MGD are among the most common ocular comorbidities associated with lupus.
Ocular cicatricial pemphigoid	Fibrotic disease that presents in the eye with progressive surface inflammation and loss of fornices, with development of symblepharon and severe MGD.
Sjögren's syndrome	The moisture-producing glands of the body are attacked, including the lacrimal glands, affecting the production of aqueous tears, leading to ocular surface inflammation. Often associated with rheumatoid arthritis, which affects the joints, causing pain, stiffness, swelling, and possibly deformity.
Stevens-Johnson syndrome	An idiosyncratic disease of the skin and mucous membranes, whose onset starts with flulike symptoms with an accompanying red or purple rash that blisters. Eye involvement includes extensive ocular surface and lid-margin inflammation with loss of conjunctival goblet cells, leaving the ocular surface keratinized. May be due to infections, but often a reaction to medications.

Table 5.6
Non-Autoimmune Comorbidities

Comorbidity	Description
Allergy (See "Common Ocular Surface Comorbidities" at the end of the chapter.)	A hypersensitive response by the immune system to foreign substances as if the substances were harmful, leading to systemic inflammation that can interfere with tear production and stabilization, as well as cause inflammation in the tissue of the eyelids. Symptoms can range from mild to life-threatening.
Arthritis: osteoarthritis or degenerative arthritis	Wear and tear on the cartilage of the joints usually due to age or injury. Chronic pain can interfere with sleep, exercise, and food preparation. If it affects the hands or arms, can impede lid hygiene, opening containers, and administering eye drops or other ocular medications, exacerbating ocular symptoms and comorbidities.
High blood pressure, hypertension with atherosclerosis	The force of blood on the narrowed walls of arteries is higher than normal, can lead to heart attacks or strokes, and can cause complications such as kidney disease and possibly dementia. Medications prescribed for high blood pressure are associated with Dry Eye.
High cholesterol, hypercholesterolemia	Levels of unhealthy lipids in the blood that can contribute to hypertension, stroke, and heart disease have been associated with MGD.
Parkinson's disease	A neurological disorder that affects mostly men and causes damage to the brain, often characterized by tremors. May cause a dysfunctional nervous system leading to a reduction in tear secretion. Blink rate and androgen levels may be reduced. Medications may exacerbate symptoms.

(continued)

Table 5.6 *continued*

Comorbidity	Description
	Because it affects hands, may impede lid hygiene, opening of containers, and administration of eye drops or other ocular medications, exacerbating ocular symptoms and comorbidities.
Stroke, also called cerebral vascular accident	The flow of oxygen-bearing blood to the brain is blocked.
	The role in MGD depends on which part of the brain was damaged and to what extent.
	May cause paralysis of eyelids, preventing normal blinking.
	Can lead to desensitized corneas, leading to decreased blink rate.
	Stroke victims sometimes stare into space without blinking.
	If the hands or arms are involved, can impede lid hygiene, opening containers, and administering eye drops or other ocular medications, exacerbating ocular symptoms and comorbidities.

COFACTORS

Besides comorbidities, many factors can contribute to MGD. Some impact the eyes directly, like wearing makeup, and others affect the entire body, including the eyes. These factors fall into four categories:

1. Behavior and lifestyle: activities like our jobs, how much we sleep, read, or drive, among many others
2. Environment: temperature, humidity, pollution, pollens, pets, carpeting, and other aspects of our indoor and outdoor environments
3. Diet: the foods and supplements we consume and how the body processes them
4. Stage of life: age-related health and life circumstances

Table 5.7
Iatrogenic Comorbidities: Oral and Intravenous Medications

Medications	Descriptions
Antiandrogens	Used to treat hair loss and prostate cancers.
	Decreases in androgen levels are associated with Dry Eye and MGD.
Anticholinergics	Can have an anticholinergic effect (blocking of nerve impulses to lacrimal glands) that induces dryness and increases signs and symptoms of Dry Eye and MGD.
• Anticonvulsant	Drugs used for epileptic and other seizures.
• Antidepressants	Medications used to treat depression and often used off-label to treat pain.
• Anti-Parkinson's drugs	Some work to minimize symptoms from the re-duced levels of dopamine found in the brains of people with Parkinson's.
• Antipsychotic	Also called major tranquilizers or neuroleptics, used for managing psychosis, schizophrenia, and bipolar disorder.
Antihistamines	Oral medications used for treating the symptoms of allergies.
	Can dry out the ocular surface while increasing friction during a blink.
Antihypertensives	Medicines that treat high blood pressure.
	May reduce the flow of blood to the ocular surface tissue.
Beta-blockers	Decrease blood flow and consequently blood pressure.
	May reduce the flow of blood to the ocular surface tissue.
	May reduce corneal sensation.
Chemotherapy	Drugs that treat various cancers by reducing cell proliferation.
	Can lead to Meibomian gland atrophy.

(continued)

Table 5.7 *continued*

Medications	Descriptions
Diuretics	Increase excretion of water.
	Can cause dehydration, desiccating the ocular surface, leading to inflammation and friction-related diseases.
Hormone replacement therapy (HRT)	Natural or synthetic estrogen or progesterone prescribed for the symptoms of menopause.
	May suppress Meibomian gland function and production of meibum.
Latisse® and other lash enhancers	Topical treatment that stimulates eyelash growth.
	Can lead to lid margin inflammation.
Pain relievers and anti-anxiety medications	Reduce sensitivity of the surface of the eye, impacting lacrimal functional unit.
• NSAIDs	Nonsteroidal anti-inflammatory drugs.
• Analgesics/ antipyretics	Medications used for reducing pain and fever, e.g., acetaminophen.
• Anxiolytics	Used to relieve anxiety and aid sleep.
Retinoids: isotretinoins (ACCUTANE®), tretinoins (Retin-A®), retinol	Oral medications used in the treatment of severe acne, which can severely damage Meibomian glands, as they suppress the proliferation of meibocytes, the cells that synthesize meibum within acini.

With so many factors affecting Meibomian gland health, it's no wonder MGD can be difficult to diagnose and treat.

Behavior and Lifestyle

Behaviors and lifestyle choices can impact Meibomian gland health (table 5.8). Try to make choices that support the health of your Meibomian glands (see chapter 12).

Table 5.8
Behavior and Lifestyle

Factor	Description
Eyelid tattooing, pigmentation	Tattoos or pigmentation, like permanent eyeliner, that introduce a foreign agent into the tissue near the Meibomian glands.
	Increases risk of periglandular inflammation in the distal segments of the Meibomian gland duct and orifice.
Gazing/ineffective blinking	Activities that involve focusing the eyes for long periods, such as reading, driving, sewing, computer work, gaming, TV binge-watching, and using hand-held devices, or while talking on the phone and staring into space.
	Blinking is less frequent and the eyes may not close completely during blinks.
	Lid margins desiccate, leading to inflammation of the gland orifice and MGD.
	Incomplete blinks interfere with normal spreading of tear film.
	Infrequent blinks lead to ocular surface dryness, inflammation, and decreased tear breakup time (TBUT).
Lifting and/or tinting eyelashes	Chemicals used to lift, curl, or tint eyelashes can be irritating, toxic, or cause allergic reactions.
	Can lead to madarosis (loss of lashes and their protective properties).
	Increases risk of periglandular inflammation in the distal segments of the Meibomian gland duct and orifice.
Not sleeping enough	Sleeping less than the recommended six to eight hours per day in one stretch.
	Meibomian glands don't have enough time to recover; the reserve of meibum that builds during sleep is chronically depleted.

(continued)

Table 5.8 *continued*

Factor	Description
Poor facial hygiene; poor lid hygiene • Not cleansing the the face thoroughly daily • Not cleansing the eyelids or eyelashes daily • Using only water without an effective surfactant to provide lather for removal of excess skin oils and organic material • Cleansing too often, too long, or with too much surfactant • Scrubbing too hard • Not removing surfactant thoroughly	Allergens, bacteria, dead skin, sebum, makeup, pollutants, toxins, and other harmful materials build up around the eyes, in the eyebrows, eyelashes, and on the forehead. Noxious agents can fall onto the ocular surface, involve the eyelids and lid margins, cause irritation and chronic inflammation.
Rubbing eyes	Stretching the eyelids, conjunctiva, lid margin, and Meibomian glands, and potentially exerting pressure on the cornea. Causes an increase in histamine released from mast cells if rubbing is due to an allergy. Can create ocular surface inflammation, which can extend to the lids and periglandular area.
Smoking, vaping	Inhalation and exhalation of smoke or other vapors from tobacco or other products. Toxic particulate matter can settle in the tear film and on the lid margins, causing inflammation.

Factor	Description
Wearing false eye-lashes or extensions	Eyelashes glued to the eyelids or attached with magnets.
	Glue may be irritating or toxic.
	Can cause allergic reactions.
	Can lead to an incomplete blink, impeding secretion of meibum.
	Lashes can harbor harmful bacteria and cause inflammation of the eyelid tissues.
	Can lead to madarosis (loss of lashes and their protective properties).
	Increases risk of periglandular inflammation in the distal segments of the Meibomian gland duct and orifice.
Wearing makeup—eye makeup, foundation, powder, etc.	Applied to the lid and sometimes lid margins, eye makeup can flake, crumble, flow, or, in the case of powders, billow into the eyes or settle on the lashes and lid margins.
	Makeup can cause inflammation of the entire ocular surface, including the tissues of the lid margin and conjunctiva and the periglandular tissue.
	Substances in makeup can be toxic and penetrate the Meibomian glands.
	Applicators harbor bacteria and other microbes that can multiply or spread if shared.
	Makeup can reduce efficacy of topical ocular thera-pies, such as eye drops and ointments, by reducing the availability of the medication to the ocular surface when it contaminates the tear film.
Wearing, using, or exposure to scented products or un-scented products with masking scents	Perfumes, aftershave, hair products, nail polish, soaps, and many other products emit chemicals, as do unscented products with masking scents.
	Can cause toxic, sensitivity, or allergic reactions, causing inflammation of the lids, lid margins, and ocular surface.

Environmental Factors

Both our indoor and outdoor environments play important roles in MGD (table 5.9). Whenever possible, make choices that support the health of your Meibomian glands (see chapter 12).

Dietary Factors

The foods and liquids we consume have a direct impact on the health of Meibomian glands (table 5.10). A healthy diet will support your overall health and the health of your Meibomian glands.

Stages of Life

Although we cannot control the passing of time, we can strive to make choices that support our overall health and Meibomian glands during all stages of life (table 5.11).

COMMON OCULAR SURFACE COMORBIDITIES

Clusters of comorbidities often accompany MGD. Some of the most common comorbidities are ATD, anterior blepharitis, friction-related diseases, ocular allergies and other sensitivities, a condition I call lateral canthal crowding, blepharospasm, nocturnal lagophthalmos, and ineffective blinking (blink lagophthalmos).

Aqueous Tear Deficiency (ATD)

Aqueous tear deficiency describes a condition that affects the lacrimal glands' ability to produce moisture, making the eyes feel dry and gritty.

ATD may lead to cornea desensitization. Desensitized corneas don't sense when the normal tear film is breaking apart. As a result, the corneas don't signal the brain to stimulate the lacrimal glands to produce moisture and trigger the eyelids to blink. Together these factors—desensitized corneas, a reduced blink rate, less moisture production—exacerbate the condition. Gradually, the corneas may become even less sensitized. At the same time, friction from a lack

Table 5.9

Environmental Factors

Environmental factors can cause chronic ocular surface, lid, and Meibomian gland inflammation and irritation that disrupts tear film and the production of meibum.

Factor	Description
Cleaning fluids/household chemicals: aerosol sprays, air fresheners, bleach, detergents, rug cleaners, floor and furniture polish, dishwashing liquids, oven cleaners, etc.	Can emit toxic substances and volatile organic compounds (VOCs). Can cause allergic reactions, contribute to respiratory problems and headaches. Some are thought to cause cancer.
Cooking fumes	Fumes from food, onions, and even fumes from foods that smell good can reach the tear film. When cut, onions release chemicals that turn into a sulfuric compound when it reaches the tear film.
Dusty environments	Dust can settle on the surface of the eyes and lid margins.
Dust mites	Dust mites are a major component of house dust and are present wherever people live, particularly in dark, warm, moist environments, i.e., furniture, bedding, carpeting. They feed on flakes of skin from humans and animals. Their exoskeletons and feces can cause allergic reactions.
Flooring	Carpeting, other flooring, and any protective coatings, especially when they're new, can emit chemical fumes. Fibers can be irritating, and as they disintegrate, particles can float in the air and get into the eyes.
Pets	Some people are allergic to pet dander. Dander and fur can inflame eyes even in people without allergies.

(continued)

Table 5.9 *continued*

Factor	Description
	Even when they are clean and well cared for, pets can carry bacteria that can easily transfer to humans.
Pollution or smoke from fires	Pollutants in the air can contain toxins and particulate matter, as can volcanic ash and smoke from a fireplace, campfire, single candle, controlled burn, or wildfire.
Lawn mowing	Mowing a lawn raises dust and mold and fills the air with particles of grass, dirt, and other plant material.
Moldy environments	Mold in the air can inflame eyes and eyelids.
Ultraviolet (UV) light	UV light, directly from the sun or reflected off snow or water, striking the ocular surface, lens, and retina increases the risk of developing ocular surface diseases, cataracts, and retina damage.
	Can degrade the quality of synthesized meibum by inducing the oxidation of lipids.
	Prolonged exposure to UV light can cause pterygium or pinguecula.
Weather/climate stressors	Increases tear film evaporation and demand on Meibomian glands. (See chapter 4.)
	Causes desiccating stress to the lid margin and ocular surface tissues, leading to inflammation.
• Low humidity	Humidity levels consistently below 50%, whether in the home, at work, or outdoors, increase the rate of tear film evaporation. (Ideal humidity level is 50–55%.)
• Wind, drafts, air currents, and related HVAC	Circulating air passes directly over the eye's surface.
	Slight air currents, e.g., those produced by a closing door, someone walking by, or a loose-fitting mask can be intolerable in the setting of advanced ocular surface disease.

Factor	Description
• Cold: climates, seasons, indoor and outdoor temperatures	Cool temperatures are often accompanied by winds and low humidity.
	Forced-air heating used indoors dries the air.
	Meibum on the ocular surface becomes rigid and spreads less easily.

Table 5.10
Dietary Factors

Factor	Description
Caffeine consumption	Drinking even one cup of coffee or tea a day, consuming chocolate, sodas, and other foods that contain caffeine. (Dark chocolate can contain higher quantities of caffeine than milk chocolate.)
	Because caffeine is a diuretic, it's dehydrating to the ocular tissues.
	As a stimulant, can increase the width of the fissure between the eyelid margins, stretching tear film thin after a blink or when opening eyes, leading to unstable tear film.
	Increases circulating epinephrine and epinephrine in the tear film, possibly increasing pupil diameter, contributing to photophobia and secondary blepharospasm.
	Can contribute to whole-lid or focal blepharospasms with ineffective, incomplete blinks or partial blinks.
	Note: Even after stopping caffeine consumption, effects may linger, because caffeine takes about two weeks to clear the body.

(*continued*)

Table 5.10 *continued*

Factor	Description
Poor ratio of omega-3 to omega-6 fatty acid consumption	A diet low in inflammation-reducing omega-3 fatty acids and high in inflammation-inducing omega-6 fatty acids may lead to a chronic, systemic inflammatory state that also affects the Meibomian glands and meibum production.
Not drinking enough water	Consuming less than approximately eight glasses of water a day and more in dry environments or when exercising.
	It's important to stay hydrated so the lacrimal glands can functional well.
	Note: Healthy eyes produce anywhere from fifteen to thirty gallons of tears each year and need plenty of water to do that.
Poor nutrition	Not consuming adequate quantities of vitamins, in particular A, B's, C, and D, and other nutrients.
	Consuming high quantities of saturated fats, salt, sugar, and cholesterol, as well as binge eating.
	High glucose levels are toxic for Meibomian gland epithelial cells; glands may become dormant, obstructed, and even atrophic.

of moisture on the ocular surface, increased squamous metaplasia of Meibomian gland orifice epithelium, and the reduced blink rate put stress on the Meibomian glands, decrease the meibum secretion rate (although at the same time higher demand is put on the Meibomian glands), and expose the glands to toxic solutes, all leading to surface inflammation, periductal fibrosis, and MGD. Other comorbidities may also arise, such as conjunctivochalasis, or be exacerbated, such as nocturnal lagophthalmos.

About fifteen years ago, a new patient, Elena, came to me seeking relief from extremely tender and painful lids. She was miserable and depressed, and her husband, Jack, distraught. They were retired but unable to enjoy life because of Elena's eye pain. It had taken over their lives.

Upon examination, I found all of Elena's lids showed complete distal obstruction (CDO: tenderness and four or fewer expressible glands). The solution was straightforward. I probed her Meibomian glands, and Elena immediately experienced a dramatic improvement in symptoms. The tenderness and pain resolved, and the number of expressible glands markedly increased. Upon examination after probing, the lids now showed only partial distal obstruction (PDO: five or more expressible glands and no lid tenderness). Elena and Jack left that day thrilled, already making plans to visit friends overseas.

But at her appointment a few weeks later, Elena and Jack expressed concern because the symptoms had partially returned. The pain was only mild, but unmistakable. When examining her, I found that although her lids were not tender, now there were fewer than four expressible glands in each lid (PDO-NF, or nonfunctional) and no comorbidities to explain her exam findings. Her glands appeared to have become dormant. The question was Why?

I started by reviewing Elena's recent medical history and changes in medications and supplements. There were none. Then we discussed her approach to lid hygiene, potential exposure to allergens or toxic fumes, and if there were any changes in her day-to-day life. Nothing she described would have triggered a return of symptoms or caused her glands to become dormant. Then I asked about her diet. Had anything changed?

Elena looked over at Jack, and Jack at Elena. Yes, she admitted, something had changed. She and Jack had been celebrating her pain-free eyes with decadent desserts: a mocha torte, a gallon of mint chocolate-chip ice cream, flaky napoleons, chocolate éclairs, cream puffs, an entire lemon meringue pie, and more in just a few weeks. She had gained weight.

"How much," I asked?

"Ten pounds."

A weight gain of ten pounds in just a few weeks suggests high levels of blood sugar, which could drive Meibomian glands into a state of dormancy. So, rather than probe the glands or administer other treatments, I advised Elena (and Jack) to prevent spikes in blood sugar level by resuming a normal healthy diet and to monitor symptoms.

Two weeks later, Elena reported the symptoms had completely disappeared. When I examined her glands, they were producing adequate meibum, with a good number of expressible glands and no lid tenderness in any lid. Her lids had returned to their PDO status.

Over the years I have seen about a dozen patients with a tempo of disease and recovery similar to Elena's. These patients came to me with tender, painful lids, which I diagnosed as CDO. After probing, the patients experienced dramatic relief immediately, and I reclassified their lids as PDO. But within days, because of bingeing on sweets, the tempo of symptoms returning was quick. At their follow-ups I found nontender lids with nonfunctioning glands, PDO-NF. Once these patients resumed their normal diets, the tempo of recovery was also quick. Within a few weeks, and without added medical interventions, their Meibomian glands began functioning and producing meibum once again.

Table 5.11
Stages of Life

Factor	Description
Aging	Age plays an enormous role in MGD because of the cumulative effects of chronic inflammation, exposure to toxins, and other disease-causing factors over a long period.
	As we age, the body undergoes many hormonal changes that can affect the health of Meibomian glands.
Andropause, sometimes called male menopause	A decrease in testosterone levels, which is associated with Dry Eye and MGD.
Menopause	The cessation of menstrual periods for a year.
	Ovaries decrease production of the reproductive hormones estrogen and progesterone.
	Androgen production also drops and is associated with Dry Eye and MGD.
Perimenopause	The transition into menopause, when the secretions of reproductive hormones estrogen and progesterone by the ovaries begin fluctuating.
	Androgen production drops.
Pregnancy	Changes in hormone levels during pregnancy can cause symptoms of Dry Eye.

There are three types of ATD:

1. Sjögren's-induced ATD
2. Primary acquired lacrimal gland disease, or non-Sjögren's ATD
3. Secondary acquired lacrimal disease, or secondary ATD

Sjögren's syndrome is an autoimmune condition in which the body's immune system attacks moisture producing glands, such as the lacrimal glands and salivary glands, among others, and causes ATD.

Primary acquired lacrimal gland disease (also known as non-Sjögren's aqueous tear deficiency) is the more common form of ATD. Here too the lacrimal glands don't secrete enough moisture, leading to red and irritated eyes, dryness, and vision that fluctuates. Primary ATD is usually age-related because the lacrimal glands aren't functioning as well as they did when they were younger. It may also be linked with the normally lower levels of androgens in older people.

Secondary ATD often occurs when the corneas are desensitized by a comorbidity. A variety of conditions can cause desensitized corneas, including diabetes, stroke, cornea infections with herpes simplex or zoster viruses, chronic ocular inflammation, and others. LASIK, other vision-correcting surgeries, and cataract surgeries can also cause desensitized corneas.

Anterior Blepharitis

There are two types of blepharitis (inflammation of the eyelids), anterior and posterior. Posterior blepharitis develops as a result of abnormal Meibomian gland function, also known as MGD, affecting the side of the eyelid margin closest to the eyeball. Anterior blepharitis refers to inflammation of the anterior (front) eyelid margin and typically develops because of microbes, most commonly bacteria or parasites (often demodex mites) harbored in the lashes and lid margin. Crusting, scaling, other deposits, and inflammation can develop on the lid margin or the base of the eyelashes.

Inflammation of the eyelid margin, if left untreated, can quickly lead to MGD because it can affect the distal Meibomian glands.

Friction-Related Tissue Disorders of the Ocular Surface

Over the course of a lifetime, the surface of the eye is subjected to friction, environmental stresses, and possibly trauma. The tissues of the ocular surface can become inflamed, as seen with superior limbic keratoconjunctivitis (SLK). They may also undergo degenerative changes with loss of elasticity, causing conjunctivochalasis of variable severity. Each of these friction-related disorders requires individualized treatment.

Superior Limbic Keratoconjunctivitis (SLK)

Although tissue may not be excessively loose (the lid may be tight to the globe superiorly), SLK is a condition found on the continuum of friction-related disorders. It is characterized by inflammation of the upper limbus, the tissue where the cornea and conjunctiva meet. The superior bulbar conjunctiva may be inflamed, and there may be filaments (small strands of degenerated epithelial cells and mucus attached to the ocular surface at one end) and erosions on the limbus or on the upper quadrant of the cornea.

Trauma due to mechanical friction is considered the most likely cause.

SLK, usually found in both eyes, is more common in women than men, with onset usually at forty or fifty years of age. About 33 percent of patients with SLK have thyroid disease, and about 25 percent have Dry Eye.

Pseudo SLK, a comorbidity similar in appearance to SLK, with filaments and erosions at the limbus, is caused by ATD. Pseudo SLK can be reversed with successful treatment of ATD.

Like conjunctivochalasis, SLK can cause extreme pain or vague, intermittent symptoms. Doctors sometimes miss it by failing to lift the upper eyelid during exams, or they might misdiagnose it as Dry Eye or blepharitis.

Conjunctivochalasis

Conjunctivochalasis (kŏn-jŭnk-tī′-vō-kal-ā′-sis), sometimes called conjunctival chalasis, is one of those conditions that few patients have heard of, although it is one of the most prevalent MGD comorbidities. In 1908, Anton Elschnig, MD, described the condition as a loose, nonedematous (without swelling) conjunctiva. In 1942, Wendell L. Hughes, MD, a Canadian-born ophthalmologist and pioneer in oculoplastic surgery, coined the term "conjunctivochalasis," a relaxation of the conjunctival tissue.

A 2009 study conducted in Tokyo, Japan, showed that nearly everyone develops this condition as they age: 71.4 percent of thirty-one- to forty-year-olds, 90.2 percent of forty-one- to fifty-year-olds, 94.2 percent of fifty-one- to sixty-year-olds, and 98 percent of sixty-one- to seventy-year-olds were diagnosed with conjunctivochalasis. It is found more frequently in patients with thyroid eye disease, among contact lens wearers, and after lid tightening procedures. Unfortunately, though conjunctivochalasis is common, doctors often miss or misdiagnose it when patients have signs and symptoms of comorbid MGD or Dry Eye.

The specific cause of conjunctivochalasis is not well understood, and inflammation is not usually considered a primary cause, although it may play a role. Instead, mechanical friction, trauma or injury to the eye, exposure to UV light, and delayed tear clearance may be underlying factors, as is aging.

Conjunctivochalasis develops when the conjunctiva, the transparent membrane that covers the white part of the eyeball, loses its elasticity and detaches from the Tenon's capsule. Some believe the Tenon's capsule thins out, losing its adherence to the globe, and can bunch up, presenting itself as a mass in the superior temporal quadrant. The conjunctival tissue can stretch and wrinkle (chalasis), changing the topography of the normally smooth surface of the eye. The peaks of the bunched-up or wrinkled tissue can rise above the level of the tear film, thus obliterating it and exposing the delicate tissue to desiccating air and toxins. Instead of spreading over the entire eye's surface, misdirected tear film channels into the folds of the wrinkled conjunctiva. Unevenly distributed tear film increases friction during blinks, exacerbating drag on the already-stretched conjunctival tissue.

Conjunctivochalasis can occur in any part of the conjunctival tissue, in a small focal area, or it can cover a large part of the eye's surface. It is often found on the superior part of the bulbar conjunctiva, where there is more friction during blinks and eye movements up, down, left, and right. Sometimes it is accompanied by prolapsed orbital fat into the subconjunctival space. Inferiorly, the bulbar conjunctiva can prolapse over the lid margin. When the prolapsed chalasis is temporal, it can channel tears to the outer corner of the eye, where it can dampen the skin in that area. The prolapse can also extend from the lateral canthus to the nasal canthal area, or it can cover the plica semilunaris, extending over the punctum, causing epiphora (the overflowing of tears). Again, the extent and exact site of prolapse varies from person to person, as does general wrinkling, requiring individualized and targeted treatment.

Even small sections of bulbar conjunctivochalasis can cause irritation, and severe chalasis can cause extremely debilitating symptoms.

Like many diseases that rarely cause obvious symptoms early on, for example, high blood pressure or many types of cancer, conjunctivochalasis may cause no obvious, specific symptoms. Even when it causes symptoms, it's not widely recognized. A simple test to elicit symptoms of conjunctivochalasis is also not widely known (see chapter 9).

Adding to frustration, conjunctivochalasis can mimic symptoms of Dry Eye and MGD. Because of this mimicry it can be easy to miss. Doctors may not even consider conjunctivochalasis because they think they've already found the cause of symptoms when they diagnose Dry Eye or MGD. Or patients may report symptoms that are vague and not easily diagnosed, or find it difficult to describe their symptoms. When patients can't describe their symptoms precisely, doctors may not know what to look for. Undiagnosed and untreated, symptomatic conjunctivochalasis, particularly in tandem with ATD and occult MGD, can cause severe pain, leading patients to lose hope and even become suicidal (see chapter 6).

Ocular Allergies and Other Sensitivities

About 20 percent of the population has ocular allergies. These can affect the cornea and eyelid, but most commonly affect the conjunctiva. Ocular allergies are often mistaken for Dry Eye because their symptoms are similar. Often patients have both conditions, Dry Eye and ocular allergies (see sidebar 5.3).

There are six types of ocular allergies:

1. Seasonal conjunctivitis: the allergic response occurs at certain times of the year, especially when there is a lot of pollen or mold in the air.
2. Perennial conjunctivitis: the allergic response occurs

Sidebar 5.3
Allergies, ATD, and MGD: A Vicious Cycle

Allergies, ATD, and MGD, can play an important role in the onset and development of each other, leading to a vicious cycle of disease.

Allergies can lead to ATD and MGD or contribute to their progression.

Allergy medications can exacerbate ATD and MGD.

ATD can exacerbate MGD and increase the toxic effects of allergens.

MGD can exacerbate symptoms of allergies and ATD.

Thus, this causal relationship between allergies, Dry Eye, and MGD can create a vicious cycle of ever-increasing, debilitating symptoms.

---

year-round because allergens are always present. Some common allergens are dust, pet dander, indoor molds, pesticides, cotton, and feathers (in pillows).

3. Contact conjunctivitis: the allergic response occurs after an allergen, such as an eye drop or makeup, touches the eye.

4. Giant papillary conjunctivitis (GPC): the allergic response, bumps of inflamed mucosal tissue on the superior palpebral conjunctiva, is usually found in people who wear contact lenses.

5. Atopic keratoconjunctivitis: the allergic response may affect the cornea, limbus, bulbar and palpebral conjunctiva, as well as Meibomian glands and may lead to severe scarring of the ocular surface. If the impact on the cornea is severe, it can lead to blindness.

6. Vernal keratoconjunctivitis: the allergic response is seen in boys under age ten, in dry, hot climates or areas with high

pollution. It stabilizes by adulthood or advances to atopic keratoconjunctivitis.

Several other systemic allergies are closely associated with ocular allergies, including dermatitis (skin allergies), rhinitis (nasal allergies), and asthma (allergies of the breathing airway, often associated with atopic keratoconjunctivitis).

Allergies can exacerbate Dry Eye or even cause it or MGD because the allergic reaction causes a release of inflammatory mediators that disrupt the tear film, alter its quality, and shorten tear breakup time. If the inflammation is chronic, the lids can swell and fibrosis can grow around, as well as invade, the Meibomian gland duct wall. The chronic inflammation can also numb the cornea, thus disrupting the lacrimal functional unit and exacerbating Dry Eye.

Medications can compound the problem. Oral medications that contain antihistamines for treating allergies reduce aqueous tear secretions from the lacrimal gland. Ingredients in eye drops can themselves be irritating, cause allergic reactions, or even be toxic to the ocular tissues. Vasoconstrictors (medications that shrink or constrict small blood vessels in the eyes to reduce redness) can mask symptoms or reduce blood flow to the tear glands and ocular surface tissues. When the medication's effect wears off, the blood vessels relax and then dilate, allowing even more blood to flow back quickly, exacerbating redness. Chronic use can also lead to very large, abnormal blood vessels on the surface of the eye.

Lateral Canthal Crowding

Lateral canthal crowding is a term I use referring to a cluster of comorbidities that often occur simultaneously in the outer corners of the eyes (the lateral canthus) and includes dermatochalasis of the brow or upper eyelid, entropion, trichiasis, and conjunctivochalasis. Patients with lateral canthal crowding often squint, keeping their eyes partially closed.

The weight of the drooping upper eyelid or brow causes an inturning of the upper lid, and with it, the inturning and misdirection of the eyelashes. The lashes at the outer corners of the eyes frequently collide, which can cause squinting. At the same time, drooping and inward rotation of the lid puts pressure from the lid margin onto the eye. Skin can rotate against the eye, increasing friction against the bulbar conjunctival tissue. Lateral conjunctivochalasis is often associated with these other findings.

Sometimes just by removing lashes in the lateral canthal area, the eye can more easily open up, restoring comfort and a good quality blink.

Blepharospasms: Benign Essential Blepharospasm and Secondary Blepharospasm

Blepharospasm is a spasm of the eyelid. Benign (not life threatening) essential (of unknown cause) blepharospasm (BEB), once thought to be a psychiatric disorder, is now recognized as a neuromuscular disorder.

The lids may blink too fast and appear to flutter, or the eyes may stay closed for extended periods. Over time, BEB may intensify and occur more frequently, leaving the sufferer functionally blind at times.

BEB is often associated with other comorbid neurodegenerative disorders, such as Parkinson's disease and multiple sclerosis. Medications used in treating these diseases may exacerbate symptoms of Dry Eye.

Another type of blepharospasm, secondary blepharospasm, is caused by tear or ocular surface problems, including ATD, MGD, allergy, conjunctivochalasis, and distichiasis (an extra row of lashes sometimes emanating from a Meibomian gland orifice) or trichiasis. It may also be caused by dehydration, stimulants such as caffeine, or an electrolyte imbalance.

Often blepharospasm is mixed; BEB and secondary blepharospasm occur simultaneously.

Nocturnal and Blink Lagophthalmos

There are several types of lagophthalmos, a condition in which the eyelids don't close properly or completely. Of these, nocturnal and blink lagophthalmos are very common comorbidities.

Sidebar 5.4
Orbicularis Muscle Spasm

The orbicularis muscle that closes the eyelid can spasm, resulting in general or focal pain. The pain of an orbicularis spasm can mimic many conditions, including conjunctivochalasis, MGD, ATD, mechanical trauma to the eye, folliculitis, or trichiasis, among others. Because of symptom mimicry and when there are no other signs, an orbicularis spasm can be very difficult to diagnose and may be one of those causes of phantom eye pain sometimes diagnosed as ocular neuropathic pain (see chapter 9).

Usually, the condition is easily treated with nothing more than using a clean finger to massage the lid very gently where there is pain or applying warm compresses.

With nocturnal lagophthalmos, the eyelids don't close completely during sleep, leaving a gap that exposes the ocular surface. Those exposed spots can become dry and painful when the eyes open fully upon awakening.

Blink lagophthalmos refers to partial or incomplete blinks. The eyelid margins don't meet when the eyes close. This can happen during gazing activities, such as reading or driving. Eyelashes may collide and prevent the eyelids from closing. Entropion or ectropion can leave a gap between the eyelids during a blink. With blink lagophthalmos there is the risk of chronic inflammation, which can lead to desensitized and exposed corneas, ATD, and obstructive MGD.

CONCLUSION

Many medical specialties strive to establish standards of care for an endless variety of diseases to ensure that patients receive timely, effective care. The goal is zeroing in on a diagnosis and treating the condition quickly and effectively because patients need their symptoms and diseases resolved to minimize their suffering.

The first challenge with an occult disease like MGD is making the right diagnosis, that is, not missing the presence and extent of a hidden disease or its impact on a patient.

The second challenge with MGD is accurate diagnosis and treatment of other comorbidities, like the ones discussed in this and other chapters, so all symptoms resolve. There is no set rule about which factors may play a role in disease or which comorbidities each patient might have, although there are clusters of common comorbidities that doctors should look for. Ultimately, patient symptoms, discussed in the next chapter, and clinical signs should guide both diagnosis and treatment.

6

Symptoms

Living with Pain

Melissa, a doctor of internal medicine, had dedicated her life to serving patients at a clinic in rural Ohio. Then one morning she woke with a sore, dry mouth and stabbing pain in her eyes. She called in sick and saw an ophthalmologist. He examined her eyes, diagnosed Dry Eye, and told her to use lubricating drops. She used them for a few days, but they didn't help. When she returned one week later, he dismissed her pain.

"You'll learn to live with it," he said.

"With what?" Melissa wondered. "I feel like I have screwdrivers in my eyes."

In extreme pain but undeterred, Melissa searched through troves of medical information. Could Sjögren's syndrome strike overnight? Melissa realized she would need to see a specialist, but the pain in her eyes and the dryness in her mouth were winning. Surely there were ophthalmologists and rheumatologists who could help. But who and where?

The life Melissa knew ceased to exist. Instead of ministering to patients, Melissa became the patient. Not only were twelve years of medical school, some funded by taxpayer dollars, and years of experience wasted, but an underserved community lost a badly needed doctor. Colleagues took over her patient load, and her partner took leave from work. Someone had to care for Melissa and drive her to appointments.

Melissa's excruciating pain eclipsed even the psychological and financial burdens of the mysterious disease. The doctors she had seen offered no hope, so she planned her suicide. The pain would not stop, but committing suicide meant going against everything she had strived for as a physician.

Somehow Melissa endured, eventually finding her way to my practice in Florida to begin her journey back to a normal, productive life.

AN EYE WITH MGD

Imagine your eye with MGD. The constricted Meibomian glands secrete little meibum, so the aqueous layer of tear film evaporates too quickly.

With only a thin layer of tear film, your cornea is overexposed to the environment. Your lids feel like sandpaper with each scratchy blink. Bright light causes pain because when it's too thin, tear film can't protect your exposed corneal nerves from noxious stimulus. Your vision blurs and fills with glare because inadequate tears can't smooth out imperfections in the cornea's surface. While sleeping, your eyelids stick to your eyeballs, and when the eyes open the congested eyelids rip tissue from the sensitive corneas. As Melissa said, it's like waking with a screwdriver in the eye.

You might avoid looking—never mind reading—because just looking seems to exacerbate your eye pain. You seek out doctors, and at each of their offices you're forced to fill out forms, even though looking at the forms exacerbates your pain. When one doctor doesn't help, you find another, then another. But their treatments don't help, either. You might lose faith in these doctors, maybe even in the entire medical profession. Though desperate for help, you might retreat completely from your daily life. You may suffer from depression. In extreme cases, completely without hope and believing there's no chance you'll ever get better or be free of the extreme pain, you may have suicidal thoughts. Tragically, and avoidably, some of you may give in to these thoughts and end your lives.

Why the Eyes Are So Sensitive

Because of a high density of nerves in the cornea, the eyes are extremely sensitive. A speck of dust, let alone an eyelash, can feel enormous.

Besides the nerves of the cornea, the rest of the eye is also very sensitive. Mucosal tissue of the palpebral and bulbar conjunctiva and the eyelid margin contribute to this sensitivity. This tissue lacks the protective layer of keratin protein found in the skin, making it vulnerable to the environment and its irritants in ways that skin is not.

Because of densely innervated corneas and highly sensitive mucosal tissues, and because humans are visual beings, the symptoms caused by MGD and comorbidities can impact day-to-day life tremendously.

Small Footprint—Where Does It Hurt?

Complicating matters are size and location. Meibomian glands are tiny, about the width of a hair. They're just several millimeters long and often less than 1 millimeter apart. The excretory duct is only about 0.5 millimeter long. Plus, there's minimal space between the eyelid and the surface of the eyeball. Tear film less than 5 microns thick is the only thing that separates them. Bulbar conjunctival tissue is about 100–200 microns thick, palpebral conjunctival tissue is only about 33 microns thick, and both become thinner with age. The Meibomian glands secrete meibum to the lid margin, a very thin strip of tissue. And eyelashes, which can be sharp like tiny wires, are about 1 millimeter away.

Because MGD occurs in a microscopic space, and because pain can linger even after the pain stimulus is gone, it's often difficult to identify the exact location of pain.

Is it in the eye? In the eyelid? In the eyelashes? In the Meibomian glands? On the skin? On the lid margin?

Even if the pain feels like it's in the eyeball, it may be referred from somewhere else, sometimes making diagnosis, and treatment, tricky (see sidebar 6.1).

Sidebar 6.1
Where's the Pain?

Because the eyes are highly sensitive, when there's pain or a foreign-body sensation in the eye it's sometimes difficult to figure out the source of pain.

Is it something on the eyeball?

Is it in the tear film?

Is it on the palpebral conjunctiva (lining the eyelid closest to the eyeball)?

Here's a quick test that can help you figure out where the pain is. With a clean finger, very gently pull the eyelid away from the eye in the area of pain. Don't pull hard or lift the eyelid very far, just far enough so the eyelid isn't touching the eye.

- If the pain remains in the same spot, it's probably coming from the eyeball.
- If the pain persists but moves around, there's probably something in the tear film.
- If there's no pain, then it probably came from the lid rubbing the eye. There may be an abnormality of the lid (for example, thickening, an abnormal eyelash) that rubs uncomfortably against a healthy eye surface. Or the lid may be healthy, but with each blink it rubs against an already irritated eye (for example, in the setting of a corneal abrasion).

DIFFERENT TYPES OF PAINFUL OCULAR SENSATIONS

Ocular pain due to MGD or comorbidities can take many forms, causing distinct sensations that can vary in degree. (For information on the diseases indicated by the different types of pain, sensations, signs, and symptoms, see chapter 9.) The pain can range from

Some experts have suggested that chronic ocular surface pain without an obvious cause may be neuropathic,
rather than nociceptive due to corneal nerve damage resulting from a variety of causes, such as chronic Dry Eye
and LASIK.

Nociceptive pain is caused by mechanical, thermal, or
chemical injury. You feel nociceptive pain when you stub
your toe, burn your finger, or splash soap in your eye.
The nociceptive pain sensation may be delayed. When
you burn your finger or stub your toe, there might be a
momentary delay before you feel the pain.

Neuropathic pain is generated by altered or damaged
nerves. Ocular neuropathic pain is believed to be either
peripheral, emanating from nerves on the surface, or central, emanating from within the brain. Although the patient experiences ocular symptoms, there is no detectable
external stimulus causing the pain.

In fact, a long-term nociceptive stimulus may drive the
pain threshold of highly sensitive ocular surface tissue
even lower. This lower threshold can cause exaggerated
pain from a stimulus known to cause pain (hyperalgesia)
or from a stimulus that does not normally provoke pain
(allodynia) such as exposure to light or a puff of air.

This exaggerated pain is not the same as neuropathic
pain. If your burned finger touches a warm surface, it
might feel like it's burning even more. If you just tap your
stubbed toe, it might hurt more. A bright light or a puff
of air can make an irritated eye feel worse, too.

Although a patient may suffer with neuropathic pain,
I believe the condition is overdiagnosed (see chapter 9).
A 2015 study found nerve endings around the ducts and
acini of Meibomian glands which may give rise to incor-

rectly diagnosed neuropathic pain symptoms in patients with MGD. In my three decades of experience, the hundreds of desperate and suicidal patients who came to me in extreme pain, diagnosed with ocular neuropathic pain (sometimes called corneal neuropathic pain) by other doctors, were actually suffering with severe nociceptive pain due to advanced MGD and Dry Eye. Because of occult gland obstruction, these patients had developed lid tenderness and soreness. Because of a lack of meibum in the tear film, they had developed painful, burning irritation, photophobia, and other symptoms. Comorbidities of the ocular surface also contributed symptoms. As long as the pain stimuli went untreated, their pain persisted.

traumatic mechanical pain, like when you stub your toe, to burning, itching, or soreness. Patients may experience a variety of intermittent foreign-body sensations: scratchy, grainy, sandy, gravelly, or a feeling that there's always something in the eye. The eyes might feel heavy or tired, or patients might say their eyes are "exposed," as if without protection (see sidebar 6.3).

The truth is, patients with MGD or comorbidities can experience a variety of uncomfortable sensations in many spots on the eyelids or ocular surface, and to different degrees.

Patients sometimes struggle to accurately depict how their eyes feel and may need coaching from their doctors to help them find the right words.

OTHER VISIBLE SIGNS AND SYMPTOMS

In addition to pain, patients may notice a wide range of other bothersome signs and symptoms associated with MGD. These may impact vision, make the eyes look unhealthy, or cause embarrassment. When eyes are chronically red and inflamed, patients sometimes

Sidebar 6.3
Different Ways Patients Describe
Symptoms of MGD and Comorbidities

MGD and comorbidities often cause distinct sensations. Patients have used these terms or phrases to describe their symptoms:

- Acid
- Burning
- Crawling on eyelashes
- Crushed glass in the eyes
- Difficulty opening eyes
- Dry eyes
- Exposed; eyes have no protection
- Eyes feel like open wounds
- Foreign-body sensation
- Gasoline
- Grainy
- Gravelly
- Gritty
- Heaviness
- Heavy eyelids
- Heavy eyes
- Inflammation
- Itching
- Lid puffiness
- Light causes pain
- Menthol
- Raw
- Sandy
- Scratchy
- Screwdriver in the eye
- Sensitive to drafts, wind, or any air movement
- Sensitive to fumes
- Sensitive to perfumes

- Sensitive to temperature
- Sharp; sharp pain
- Skin around the eyes is tender
- Soapy
- Something in the eye
- Sore
- Stabbing; stabbing pain
- Stinging
- Tearing
- Tender eyelids
- Tickling
- Tissue paper under eyelids
- Twitching eyelids
- Watery; wetness; wet eyes

worry it looks like they're abusing drugs or alcohol even when they aren't. Some other visible signs and symptoms of MGD are the following:

- Blurred vision
- Crusty eyes, lashes, and lids
- Debris in the eyes
- Frequent blinking
- Frothy tears (saponification), which can feel like soap in the eyes
- Lid puffiness
- Lids sticking to the eyes, especially at waking
- Misdirected lashes inward, outward, or sideways
- Mucus discharge in the corners of the eyes
- Redness on the surface of the eye, at the eyelid margins, and on the eyelids
- Swelling of the eyelids

- Twitching eyelids
- Veining on the sclera, lids, and lid margin (telangiectasia)
- Watery eyes, constant tearing, and overflowing tears (epiphora)

SEVERITY AND PERSISTENCE OF SYMPTOMS

In many cases, symptoms can be merely annoying. My patients sometimes say it feels like they have an eyelash in their eye all the time, or they might say their lids feel puffy or tender. Their eyes might be heavy, tired, red, or itchy. When they blink they feel dragging. Their eyes might sting or burn. But in time, that annoyance can turn into a major problem, impacting lives, careers, and families.

20 out of 10!

Health-care providers often ask how bad the pain is on a scale of 0 to 10, with 0 being no pain, and 10 being the worst pain you've ever felt, the kind incompatible with life.

By most measures, the pain of childbirth is considered among the worst, 10 out of 10. Others say pain caused by kidney stones, notably the kind that persists without momentarily abating, can be even worse than childbirth. Some of my patients say that eye pain can be even worse than either of these, rating their eye pain 11, or even 20, out of 10! No wonder MGD and Dry Eye patients without hope of finding relief might consider suicide.

Fine One Day, and Then . . .

Some of my patients, like Melissa, say their symptoms occurred suddenly. As discussed in chapter 5, eyes might feel fine one day, and the next there's unbearable pain. This can happen when an asymptomatic disease reaches a tipping point and, when triggered, suddenly causes symptoms.

For example, exposure to something benign, like an eyelash in the eye, may cause this seemingly sudden onset of acute symptoms. A new oral medication might cause dryness, triggering a cascade of symptoms. An allergic reaction can also trigger sudden symptoms. Cofactors and comorbidities like these can themselves increase symptoms or exacerbate the symptoms of MGD. Or the pain may be due to acute exacerbation of subclinical chronic MGD or other comorbid diseases.

If the symptoms occur upon awakening, it's usually due to either nocturnal lagophthalmos (incomplete closing of the lids during sleep), recurrent corneal erosion exacerbated by nocturnal lagophthalmos, floppy eyelid, or MGD.

One Eye or Both?

Pain in one eye, even extreme pain, is barely manageable. But you can use the other eye for seeing, and the brain can focus away from the pain to some extent. But when extreme pain is in both eyes, the brain has nowhere else to focus. The pain can stop you cold, making it virtually impossible to function well, if at all.

Often when the eyes experience extreme pain, they close automatically, or you close them deliberately. They may feel better or protected when closed. However, you can't close both your eyes and drive, read, see a sunset or your children's faces. Life stops. Simple daily tasks—getting dressed, preparing a meal, walking to the bathroom—can be impossible.

Constant, Intermittent, or Ever-Changing?

Some patients report having the same symptoms constantly and for years. They have them from the moment they wake up in the morning till the moment they go to sleep. Sometimes these patients don't want to get out of bed in the morning because they know they will suffer all day.

Other patients report having intermittent pain. It's gone after a few hours, or it's there one day and gone the next. They never know when the pain will start or stop, and they hope it won't last long.

Still other patients report having pain that constantly changes. This ever-changing pain baffles patients. They wonder why they suffer with a variety of symptoms or why the symptoms can change quickly.

Intermittent or constantly changing pain may occur because a variety of factors affect the onset of MGD and its progress (see chapter 5). These factors themselves often fluctuate, for example, with weather and temperature, sleeping habits and work assignments, prescription medications, the onset of comorbidities, exposure to triggers, and so forth. The waxing and waning of these factors can impact the seasonal or episodic nature of both symptom onset and severity.

Sometimes the symptom of one comorbidity eclipses symptoms of other comorbidities. The more prominent symptom masks the others, the way a pebble in a shoe might mask a headache. Once the more prominent symptom resolves, the masked symptoms come into focus, sometimes with as much severity as the treated symptom.

Typical symptoms of Dry Eye pain may even be masked by pain from other parts of the body, for example, facial pain, neck pain, or by pain referred to the eyes from other parts of the body (see the section "Other Causes of Eye Pain Masquerading as Dry Eye or MGD"). Once these nonocular conditions receive treatment, the symptoms they cause abate. Then the patient may experience the more typical symptoms of comorbid Dry Eye or MGD, like dryness and burning.

What Each Symptom Means

Symptoms indicate something is happening in the body. For example, severe chest pain or tightness that radiates down the left arm usually indicates a heart attack. Dizziness and nausea can be symptoms of food poisoning, stroke, disorders of the inner ear, pregnancy, side effects of medications, chemotherapy, and so forth. WebMD lists no less than eighty-seven conditions associated with lightheadedness, dizziness, vomiting, and nausea.

Clayton Christensen, the Harvard Business School professor whose 1997 book, *The Innovator's Dilemma,* introduced "disruptive innovation"—how cheaper or simpler products and services can blindside established companies—described the body's limited vocabulary in a 2009 book, *The Innovator's Prescription.* Diseases vastly outnumber symptoms. So any symptom, or even group of symptoms, might indicate various diseases. For doctors, the challenge is correlating the symptoms to the right diseases.

During diagnosis your doctor will ask a variety of questions. What is your chief complaint? Where does it hurt? How often? Does anything trigger the pain or make it feel better? Your answers to these and other questions will help your doctor pinpoint your co-morbidities, formulate a diagnosis, and prescribe treatments.

Medications That Hide Symptoms

Because symptoms give clues used in diagnosis, drugs that reduce or alter the symptoms without addressing the cause of those symptoms may hide the disease. Gabapentin, an antiepileptic and anticonvulsant medication, or LYRICA®, prescribed for diabetic nerve pain, fibromyalgia pain, pain caused by the shingles virus, or injuries of the spinal cord, are sometimes prescribed off-label for a working diagnosis of ocular neuropathic pain. When prescribed to patients suffering with nociceptive ocular pain, these drugs may reduce that pain. But the underlying conditions causing the pain will go untreated and may advance. If the patient stops taking the nerve-altering medication, symptoms may return and be even worse.

Plus, if the body is completely or partially silenced—nerve-altering drugs restrict its already limited vocabulary—it won't have the ability to express itself through symptoms. The absence of symptoms will challenge doctors to make any diagnosis or accurately evaluate the effectiveness of any treatment.

OTHER CAUSES OF EYE PAIN
MASQUERADING AS DRY EYE OR MGD

Not all eye pain is due to MGD, Dry Eye, or other common ocular surface comorbidities. Many conditions can cause eye pain, including these:

- Glaucoma (when intraocular pressure is significantly elevated)
- Corneal ulcer
- Heterophoria, the latent misalignment of eyes
- Ametropia, needing glasses
- Uveitis, inflammation of the pigmented layer of the eye

- Endophthalmitis, infection of the inner part of the eye
- Hypotony, low intraocular pressure
- Orbital diseases

Still other comorbidities cause eye pain even though the pain does not emanate directly from eyes. We call this referred pain because it is felt in the eyes but is referred from somewhere else. One such comorbidity is occipital neuralgia, a painful condition due to muscular tension around the occiput (the part of the skull at the back of the head above the neck). This muscle squeezes the nerves that course through it, leading to pain referred to the eyes. Tension in the trapezius muscle of the upper back or in facial muscles as well as sinusitis and migraines can also cause referred eye pain.

Some experts attribute eye pain with no visible signs to ocular neuropathic pain, sometimes called corneal neuropathy or neuralgia. Unfortunately, a popular test often administered to diagnose neuropathic pain is not definitive and can lead to misdiagnosis (see sidebars 6.2 and 9.14).

Sometimes comorbidities masquerade as MGD, mimicking its symptoms, which can lead to misdiagnosis. Sometimes other symptoms mask MGD symptoms altogether, also leading to a missed diagnosis. These masquerading and masking conditions can mislead doctors into prescribing ineffective or incomplete treatments.

IMPACT ON DAY-TO-DAY LIFE

During my career I have seen the lives of countless patients impacted by chronic, debilitating eye pain. It upended their lives and the lives of their loved ones.

Prior to consulting with me, a few of my patients had delayed weddings because of MGD symptoms. Others had quit working, retired early, or gone on disability. Some had delayed or quit going to college, ending promising careers before they even started. Too many had considered suicide, though even one case of suicidal ideation would be too many. During a nearly thirty-year career I have had hundreds of patients admit that before seeing me they had suicidal thoughts because of their intractable eye pain. Some had attempted suicide, some were hospitalized for suicidal ideation, and some had detailed plans for ending their lives. Each had seen many doctors, including some at the world's leading ophthalmic institutions. At their first visits with me, these patients shared that I was literally their last hope and if I couldn't help them, they would commit suicide. (In her volunteer work as a patient advocate since 2015, Natalia, my co-writer and collaborator, has spoken with dozens of people diagnosed with Dry Eye and MGD who had suicidal thoughts.)

Assessment Tools

To objectively measure the impact diseases like Dry Eye and MGD have on individuals and society as a whole, experts use a variety of assessment tools. Sometimes doctors also use surveys and questionnaires to aid in the diagnosis of Dry Eye and assess its impact on, or severity in, individual patients.

Utility Measures

Utility in economics is a measure of usefulness, satisfaction, or happiness. In health care, utility measures physical and mental well-being, how much a disease impacts patients, or if a specific treatment is worth the potential side effects to patients. Utility measures are based on patient responses to common questions, such as:

- Are you comfortable? How comfortable are you?
- Are you able to work?
- Is your day-to-day life impacted? How much?
- Is your family's life impacted? How much?
- Does someone take time off to take care of you?

By comparing the answers to these questions, experts can assess a disease's personal, social, and economic impact.

Dry Eye Utility Assessments

In a 2006 utility study of Dry Eye patients, those who had moderate and severe symptoms rated their utility on a par with patients

Sidebar 6.4
Suicide Measured Objectively

Health-care economists have developed various utility assessments to quantify a disease's personal, social, and economic impact, namely Time Trade-Off (TTO), Standard Gamble, Rating Scale, and Quality of Life (QOL).

TTO asks how many years of life a patient would give up to be disease-free. For example, an October 2019 TTO study of adults in the United Kingdom concluded that people would be willing to give up 6.4 years of life to keep perfect vision for just 10 years. (The study also concluded that people valued vision more than other senses.)

Standard Gamble asks how much risk of immediate but painless death a patient would accept to be disease-free. Rating Scale measures how well a patient is doing on a scale of 0 to 100, with zero being death and 100 being in perfect health. QOL, usually considered a less objective measure because one person's "feeling great" might be another person's "just OK," asks how a patient would rate their quality of life.

Applied to MGD and Dry Eye patients who consider or attempt suicide, the Time Trade-Off scale would say they are willing to give up their entire lives to be disease-free. Standard Gamble would score them at 100 percent. The Rating Scale would score them at 0. QOL would be null. These numbers reveal a stark reality. Patients who gave up their jobs or retreated from society would score only slightly better.

I never think of my patients in these objective terms. They are individuals with rich lives. But their brushes with suicide illustrate how much suffering and despair undiagnosed and untreated MGD can cause.

Sidebar 6.5
The Economic Impact of Dry Eye

The economic impact of Dry Eye on society is significant. A 2011 study estimated the annual cost of managing the disease for a patient was $11,302, and $55.4 billion for the United States overall. The burden on the U.S. health-care system was estimated at $3.84 billion.

---

requiring kidney dialysis in hospitals, those with severe angina, or those who had a disabling hip fracture. The study showed that the utility of patients with moderate and severe Dry Eye—MGD being a leading cause—was seriously impacted and that as the severity of Dry Eye increased, utility decreased. Furthermore, the study reported that diagnostic tests for Dry Eye don't always capture how much of an impact the disease can have on the quality of life (QOL). This may be another reason for the "at least you don't have cancer" comments by some doctors. They don't seem to appreciate the impact eye pain can have on daily life.

Commonly Used Dry Eye Surveys

Sometimes doctors use questionnaires or surveys with their patients to help determine if symptoms are due to Dry Eye. A survey gives doctors an objective measure of the patient's symptoms by scoring patient answers to several questions. The score indicates if the patient has Dry Eye and, if yes, its severity, whether it is mild, moderate, or severe.

Several dozen Dry Eye surveys have been developed over the years. Three commonly used ones are the Ocular Surface Disease Index© (OSDI©), Standard Patient Evaluation of Eye Dryness (SPEED™) and System Assessment iN Dry Eye (SANDE).

The OSDI questionnaire was developed in 1995 by Allergan, the pharmaceutical company known for Restasis®—the prescription eye drop for Dry Eye released in the 2000s and widely advertised on TV for many years. This questionnaire focuses on the frequency, not severity, of symptoms, asking if they happen all, most, half, some, or none of the time. Therefore, the survey has several limitations. For example, clinicians using OSDI may not learn that their patients are intermittently in severe pain or suicidal. OSDI asks about the general symptoms of Dry Eye, such as light sensitivity, grittiness, pain, soreness, and blurred vision, but does not ask about common symptoms of MGD, such as burning; itching; heavy, tired, or fatigued eyes; redness; or about symptoms at waking. Consequently, patient responses will not always indicate if they have MGD, the most common factor in Dry Eye.

SPEED was developed by TearScience, the maker of LipiFlow®—a device that heats and massages the eyelids, now sold by Johnson & Johnson Vision. SPEED asks about the severity (unlike OSDI) and frequency of dryness, grittiness, or scratchiness; soreness or irritation; burning or watering; and eye fatigue. But it too has limitations because it doesn't ask about itching, redness, symptoms upon waking, and suicidal thoughts. Without these questions, although directed more toward MGD than OSDI, the survey may still miss some cases of MGD and conceal MGD's full impact on patient lives.

SANDE was developed at Harvard Medical School in 2007 and asks only about the frequency and severity of symptoms on a 100-point visual analog scale (VAS). Because it doesn't ask specifically which symptoms the patient is experiencing, a clinician evaluating a patient won't know without further evaluation which specific comorbidities a patient suffers with.

Improving the Surveys

As indicated earlier, surveys might better serve patients if they included questions common to MGD, for example, about itching, heavy or tired eyes, redness, or about any symptoms at waking.

Surveys should also ask patients to rate the impact of symptoms on their lives on a scale of 0 to 10, with 10 being suicidal ideation.

This prompt might help patients communicate the severity of their pain and its impact on their lives, and doctors will know if they are treating a high-risk patient.

Surveys in My Practice

I have not relied on surveys in my practice because I believe they are restrictive and too narrow in scope, not reporting everything a patient might be experiencing. Instead, for me, asking questions and having a patient respond in their own words, explaining what they feel or how much their symptoms affect their lives, is a better way to approach the diagnostic process. Furthermore, in my practice I often see patients who tell me I am their last hope, so I need specific and actionable information, the kind that emerges during my open and unscripted dialogue with patients.

Living with Pain

Eye pain often forces patients to change how they live their everyday lives. These dramatic changes, in line with the Dry Eye utility studies conducted in 2006, suggest that the psychosocial impact of MGD and Dry Eye can be significant, impacting every aspect of life.

Work can become intolerable. Teachers, truck drivers, students, writers, editors, engineers, programmers, web designers, analysts, nurses, surgeons, and many, many others use their eyes for gazing activities constantly. Butchers might work in freezing environments that make the meibum on the ocular surface brittle, so it breaks up too quickly. Bakers work with billowing flour. Farmworkers are exposed to chemicals, animals, and masses of particulate matter. Are there any professions that don't pose risks to Meibomian glands?

Beyond work and school, MGD can limit participation in other everyday activities. Some patients stop getting their hair cut or avoid it for as long as they can. They fear irritating scents, getting a hair or splash of shampoo in their eyes, and the cascade of severe symptoms that ensue.

Women stop wearing makeup, which can be very difficult because people often identify with the image they present. Animal

---

Sidebar 6.6
Does Depression Cause Dry Eye?

Although clinical depression and symptoms of Dry Eye are associated, and patients whose lives were upended by Dry Eye may develop psychosocial conditions such as anxiety, stress, and depression, in my practice, I have not found evidence that depression alone causes Dry Eye. However, if patients are depressed, they may not take good care of their eyes, increasing the risk of developing MGD. Also, treatment with antidepressant medications can cause or exacerbate Dry Eye. Adjusting dosage can minimize side effects.

---

lovers may have to give up their beloved pets if a pet allergy causes debilitating Dry Eye symptoms.

Patients with red eyes often forgo social activities to avoid embarrassment.

Sometimes it hurts to keep the eyes open, so people stay home with their eyes closed. Natalia kept her eyes closed for seven months. That's no way to live.

People with severe MGD often avoid incense, fumes, odors, cooking smells (raw onions can be particularly irritating), dust, smoke, exhaust fumes, and everything else out in the world that might irritate eyes. They don't go shopping or to the movies. They don't go to restaurants. They don't visit friends. They stop attending their places of worship where candles or incense burn.

In short, MGD can impact virtually every aspect of life.

Skeptics and Supporters

Sometimes skeptics don't believe patients have MGD-induced pain. Friends, family members, acquaintances, and even strangers may see nothing wrong, so they doubt the pain exists. Doctors may mistakenly diagnose the pain as psychosomatic ("it's all in your head") or neuropathic ("it's a problem with your nerves") because they can't find the specific cause of a patient's discomfort. The doctor's misdiagnosis then reinforces the skeptics' disbelief.

The lack of correlation between patient reported symptoms and clinician assessment was underscored in a 2013 National Health and Wellness Survey revealing that as many as six million people reported not having their symptoms of Dry Eye diagnosed. When patients are diagnosed with Dry Eye, providers often underestimate the severity of symptoms. In one 2010 study, as many as 43 percent of women and 54 percent of patients over sixty-five had the severity of their Dry Eye symptoms underestimated by their health-care provider. A 2005 study reported that providers graded the severity of Dry Eye one level lower than 41 percent of patients in self-assessments.

On the other end of the spectrum are the supporters—family members and friends who sometimes put their own lives on hold to help their loved one suffering with MGD. They take extended vacations from work or school, travel long distances, arrange for someone to look after things at home, and do whatever it takes to help. Even as a trained surgeon, it's difficult for me to watch someone suffering with advanced MGD. But sometimes it's just as hard to watch the person who loves the one who is suffering. They feel helpless. They don't understand what's happening and don't know what to do. When they do something, they worry if it's the right thing. Because of their sacrifices and sentiments, I always thank those who support my patients for doing whatever they can to help.

MGD in Eight-Year-Olds

Although considered a disease of older adults, MGD has been diagnosed in children as young as eight. The American Academy of Pediatrics recommends withholding digital devices till age two and limiting screen time to two hours a day. However, the effect of extended gazing on Meibomian glands in children has not been studied thoroughly. It's feasible that a reduced blink rate at a young age could trigger the early onset of MGD. Since children probably don't

---

Sidebar 6.7
"At Least You Don't Have Cancer"

MGD and Dry Eye sufferers sometimes hear comments like "but your eyes look fine," "they make eye drops for that," or "at least you don't have cancer."

People make these comments because they aren't informed about MGD. They don't realize MGD can present without obvious signs, just like other diseases, for example, high blood pressure or many forms of cancer. They don't know eye drops can't treat the periductal fibrosis commonly found with MGD. Nor do they appreciate the devastating pain MGD can cause.

(and won't) take frequent breaks to blink when they play video games or use handheld devices, the risk exists.

Changes to learning environments during the COVID-19 pandemic might accelerate the onset of symptoms and disease because of the dramatic increase in screen gazing time among children while remote learning from home or otherwise online.

One 2019 study of Meibomian glands in 225 eight- to seventeen-year-olds could not correlate screen time to Meibomian gland dropout specifically, but researchers concluded "it is still unclear what the effects of long-term digital device usage may have as the subjects age." More importantly, in this study researchers unexpectedly found 39 percent of upper and 39 percent of lower lids in the 225 subjects already showed signs of Meibomian gland dropout (seen with meibography). In fact, "most subjects . . . had mild dropout in 1 or both eyelids." These findings highlight the importance of early screening, diagnosis, identification of comorbidities, and the initiation of targeted therapies.

If triggered, will the eight-year-old, or his parents, know how to cope with severe MGD, comorbidities, and the symptoms they can cause?

Suicide and Suicidal Thoughts

Natalia was on the verge of committing suicide because she could no longer bear the pain caused by MGD and comorbidities in her eyes. She had all but lost hope of ever finding relief when she finally found me and began her journey to healing. Dozens of my patients admitted to having made detailed plans to commit suicide for the same reasons. Some of these patients were hospitalized after failed suicide attempts and became my patients only when their families reached out to me. Had these patients not found help, no doubt in time they would have carried out their suicide plans.

One thirty-three-year-old woman living in Southeast Asia could no longer bear the constant stabbing pain in her eyes, but doctors kept saying the pain was all in her head, and her family believed them. She often instant-messaged or spoke with other patients all over the world. She contacted me and my staff, hoping to one day make the trip to the United States for diagnosis and treatment with me. She spoke with Natalia often, including the day before her suicide. We knew her, her pain, her struggles, her frustration with doctors. Her suicide was tragic and we mourn for her. Many others, undoubtedly alone, without support, with eyes too painful to search online or seek help, give up.

In December 2018, we learned of a suicide in Detroit. A mother of two ended her life because of intractable Dry Eye pain and blurred vision after LASIK surgery. She used eye drops every five minutes while awake, without relief. She may have had preexisting occult MGD. We know the cornea can become functionally desensitized from refractive cornea surgery, triggering Dry Eye and causing, or exacerbating, MGD. Could the prompt recognition of the severe impact of her Dry Eye symptoms have prevented her suicide? We will never know.

Frustration, Anger, Hopelessness, and the Nine- to Twelve-Minute Exam

Patients with ineffectively treated MGD, Dry Eye, or comorbidities can become frustrated, hopeless, or angry. After seeing many doctors and trying many treatments that didn't help, they become convinced nothing ever will.

Time may be the issue. In 2011, ophthalmologists spent only nine to twelve minutes on average with each patient, compared to the thirteen to sixteen minutes spent by most other doctors. How can a physician faced with a complex case conduct a detailed exam, formulate a thorough diagnosis, and prescribe treatment in just nine to twelve minutes? Perhaps the answer begins with the formal recognition of Dry Eye as a subspecialty requiring a dedicated training fellowship, such as those that are currently available for glaucoma, refractive surgery, cataract surgery, retina, neuro-ophthalmology, oculoplastics, and pediatric ophthalmology. Solo and multispecialty practices could set up dedicated MGD Dry Eye clinics on their premises staffed with (in the future MGD and Dry Eye fellowship-trained) physicians focused exclusively on MGD and Dry Eye. The physicians would be assisted by patient liaison-educators who would review physician-prescribed therapies, educate on proper at-home care (such as eyedrop administration and personal hygiene), and help patients learn how to triage new symptoms that may arise due to comorbid disease. Under these conditions, doctors with specialized skills could devote more time to the growing population of patients with MGD and Dry Eye and give them hope.

CHAPTER

7

The Last Day of My Life

In addition to working side by side with me on this entire book, here my coauthor Natalia A. Warren recounts the triumphant story of her struggle with Dry Eye and MGD.

I had to gouge my eyes out or this would be the last day of my life. It wasn't a matter of if, but how. A knife would slice into the eyeball and slide out. That wouldn't get it done. A fork would be better. I'd jab the fork into my eye, skewer the eyeball, then twist and yank it out. The thought horrified me, but I had to think it through. I'd need two forks, one in each hand, and a phone by my side to call 911. Surely, an ER doctor would have to remove my eyes if the forks didn't. After a few moments of gruesome torture, I'd be pain-free, but blind. So be it.

My plan had to work. For seven months, I'd lived with my eyes mostly closed because if I opened them for more than two seconds, they felt like raw, gaping wounds. The torturous pain would last until the next morning. Keeping my eyes closed overnight and then all day was the key. I'd wake up, peek out just long enough to point myself in the right direction, and fumble around the house the rest of the day.

As I sat on the sofa scrutinizing each step of the plan, my hope vanished with one lucid thought. I didn't have the courage to stab my eyes with forks. That left me with only one other option. Suicide.

It seemed such a waste, but life with my eyes was unbearable. I blamed my doctors and our health-care system. Why couldn't they find the cause of my pain? Why couldn't they tell me what was wrong with me? Without knowing what was wrong, how could I trust that the pain would end in death? What if the living nightmare persisted in an afterlife? What then?

I pushed past the irrational thoughts that had altered my perception of reality and forced myself to calmly analyze how a suicide would affect my family and friends. It would devastate them. But would they understand, or would they see it as a sin or a sign of weakness? Would they feel I had disgraced them? My husband, a Vietnam army veteran, once told me how soldiers made pacts to shoot each other if they were wounded and couldn't escape the enemy. By now, he'd witnessed the effects of this mysterious disease and my descent into agony for months. He'd driven me to countless doctor appointments, encounters that ultimately offered no relief and no hope. I knew he would understand. But the rest? I worried most about my nieces and nephews. I didn't want to burden their young lives with a suicide in the family.

So I prayed for help and bargained with G-d (the letter "o" is omitted out of respect and in accordance with Jewish tradition), vowing to search online one final time despite the excruciating pain that would strike almost as soon as I opened my eyes.

"YOU'LL LEARN TO LIVE WITH IT"

My eye problems started in June 2009 when I dropped a wire-bristle hairbrush in my right eye while blow-drying my hair. The painful corneal wound would close within a day or two, but then every few weeks reopen, the classic signs of recurrent corneal erosion. My eye doctor, an optometrist who I saw numerous times over the course of a year, prescribed antibiotic and steroid drops, bandage contact lenses, Muro 128® drops, which felt like ocean water in the eye, and other treatments. But the wound refused to heal.

About a year after the hairbrush accident, with the wound reopening more frequently and staying open longer, the optometrist referred me to an ophthalmologist specializing in cornea and external disease. By then, even with the corneal wound, I had been able to complete nearly a year of a master's degree program in health administration while working as a consultant for a technology start-up. (Because of the recession, in April 2009, a few months before the injury, I had lost my position as vice president of global product management at a technology company near Orlando, Florida. So to remain productive during the recession, I chose to consult and pursue a second master's degree.) Between work and school, I had been reading and writing copiously, so my eyes were constantly glued to a screen. (I know now this only made healing more difficult.)

To close the wound in my right eye, the ophthalmologist performed a stromal puncture. With a fine needle, and the eye completely anesthetized, she stabbed my cornea over and over in the area of the wound, pushing the epithelial cells into the basement membrane and deeper. As they healed, the tissues fused, closing the wound permanently. The procedure is successful about 80 percent of the time, but a few weeks later, I needed a second stromal puncture.

Although the wound did finally heal, the foreign-body sensation never stopped completely. It was always in the lower part of my right eye. Then one morning, I woke with excruciating pain in my left eye, feeling like there was a screwdriver in it. It was disorienting. I couldn't understand why the pain had switched eyes. Or had it?

It had. But why?

I returned to my ophthalmologist immediately. She examined me at the slit lamp, diagnosed blepharitis in *both* eyes, and prescribed Restasis® eye drops to control inflammation. I was optimistic, believing the painful eye saga would finally end. But instead of helping, Restasis caused even more pain and burning that lasted all day. I called the doctor and was told it would be several weeks before the drops would take effect. Then one morning as I bent over, a wave of warm liquid engulfed my entire left eyeball. Within seconds, I could feel the outline of the globe in my head as it turned into a sphere of pure and excruciating pain. I reported this adverse reaction to the FDA, stopped using Restasis, and started searching for another doctor.

I saw many. Each tried to help, but they seemed to have few diagnostic options—Schirmer's test for wetness, slit-lamp exams and dyes to reveal ocular surface defects. Treatments were just as limited—lubricating eye drops, topical steroids, oral doxycycline, warm compresses, omega-3 fatty acids, more Restasis (which I declined), or lid wipes. Was there nothing else?

I tried easing my symptoms with lubricating drops. At first, I bought the cheapest ones, not realizing preservatives in these drops could cause damage, especially if used too often and for prolonged periods. Later, I switched to preservative-free drops. Sometimes, especially when waking up with the feeling of a screwdriver in my eye, I would empty the entire contents of a vial into one eye, even though it didn't help much. Soon I was using lubricating eye drops every five minutes. Then the drops stopped helping altogether.

One doctor, throwing his hands in the air, admitted to being stumped. He referred me to a world-renowned university hospital equipped with technology for examining the topography of the ocular surface. It seemed like a reasonable move at the time.

Desperate with the appointment months away, I widened my search for a doctor, asking anyone I knew for recommendations. I saw each one, but none could explain what I was feeling or diagnose the source of my discomfort. All prescribed the usual treatments and some were dismissive. "You'll learn to live with it," one doctor said. After medical school, an internship, a residency program, and how many patients, didn't he know you can't "learn to live with" severe eye pain?

A BIGGER BOX

During that time of endless doctor appointments, my faith in the medical profession eroded deeply despite having several doctors in the family. My grandfather, Wasyl Dmytrijuk, MD, was a general surgeon and otolaryngologist. My sister, Zina D. Hajduczok, MD, is a cardiologist and internist. My brother, Andrew Dmytrijuk, MD, is an oncologist and hematologist. (Now there are even more doctors in my family.)

Once, telling my brother that doctors couldn't explain the cause of my discomfort, I seriously wondered if I was even human.

"Maybe that's why doctors can't figure out what's wrong with my eyes," I said.

"No, you're human." He reassured me. "Your doctors just need to think outside the box."

Hearing that from my brother was a relief.

"Actually," he continued, "it's not so much that your doctors need to think outside the box, because you are in the human box. They just need to get a bigger box."

I wondered if I would ever find a doctor with a really big box.

Years later I was telling my sister how hard it can still be for Dry Eye patients to get help even though now, with Meibomian gland probing, there is a diagnostic and effective treatment device for MGD, plus there are ways to definitively diagnose and treat ocular surface comorbidities.

"Can you imagine if we cardiologists told people with chest pain 'it's all in your head,' or 'at least you don't have cancer' but did nothing further?" she asked in disbelief.

It would be like living in a world where cardiologists eschewed stress tests, diagnostic coronary angiograms, and therapeutic angioplasty and sent patients home with a prescription for a pain killer.

"Our patients wouldn't put up with that, but neither would we," she admonished.

"I DON'T KNOW WHAT TO CALL IT"

By the early spring of 2011, I had been keeping my eyes mostly closed but finally had my first appointment at the university hospital. Technicians there reassured me I was in excellent hands, and because back then I still entertained hope, I was optimistic about feeling better soon and resuming a normal life. I underwent the usual exam and tests, then the doctor ordered a digital topographic map of my ocular surface. With those images, he ruled out the hairbrush injury and the stromal puncture as the causes of the foreign-body sensation in my right eye and instead diagnosed Dry Eye and blepharitis, as did my previous doctors. He prescribed the hospital's preservative-free formula of cyclosporine, the active ingredient in Restasis, and serum tears, eye drops made from my blood, which the hospital formulated into an eye drop. He told me to massage my eyelids and referred me to a colleague.

Several weeks later, I sat crying in the university hospital's waiting room. The pain was too much to bear. Moments after I stopped crying, a resident harvested a teardrop from the corner of my eye, a test for osmolarity, the concentration of solutes in the tear film. I explained to the resident that I'd been crying, but he said it wouldn't affect the test. I couldn't see how that was possible, so I wasn't surprised when the new faculty doctor who examined me and checked the test results declared my eyes weren't dry.

"If they're not dry, what *is* wrong?" I asked.

"I don't know what to call it," he said. "I'd call it ocular neuropathy."

The doctor couldn't explain ocular neuropathy, either, saying only it was a problem with the nerves in my eyes. He prescribed LYRICA® 75 mg twice a day, plus serum tears, a topical preservative-free steroid drop, and oral doxycycline 100 mg twice a day and told me to keep using the cyclosporine drop.

I had no other options, so I followed his advice. Lyrica not only numbed my eyes, it numbed my entire body. I couldn't feel my feet, making the staircase in the house treacherous. Once biting on a baked potato, I realized it was hot only because steam was pouring out of my mouth. From LYRICA commercials, I learned it can cause suicidal thoughts and wondered if the drug contributed to my emotional agony. After a few weeks, I stopped taking it.

The serum tears and steroid drops did nothing.

During the months I was seeing doctors at the university hospital, I was seeing another doctor who diagnosed several other conditions. For nocturnal lagophthalmos, he recommended I sleep with cotton balls taped to my closed eyes. For an overgrowth of demodex mites, he prescribed tea tree oil. Treatment involved swabbing the eyelashes with a strong solution of tea tree oil in the office and then nightly at home for many weeks. Still, my symptoms did not improve. I was getting nowhere.

DETERMINED TO GRADUATE

When I could no longer keep my eyes open, I had to stop working. But friends and family were there to help with schoolwork. (Luckily the classes were held online.) My BFF Dede typed papers while I dictated. My husband read stacks of books out loud to me. But I suffered through the online tests alone.

The master's program required a weeks-long internship. I stayed in bed with my eyes closed an entire weekend before an interview for an administrative position at a hospital, hoping that relief might last longer than a few minutes. It didn't. Before the interview even started my eyes were on fire. Though offered, I declined that position and found one that allowed working remotely, so I could close my eyes periodically. But at the last minute, the hiring manager insisted I work on-site. My father drove me, and I lugged serum tears in a cooler to work, even though the drops didn't help as I sat staring, my eyes in agony, at a computer screen all day.

Graduation day finally came on August 6, 2011. I'd had brilliant professors, learned a lot, and was named co-outstanding student. I was proud of my degree and thrilled that my husband and parents attended the department's private graduation ceremony. But I was in agony, counting the minutes till the next morning when I'd wake without pain.

Less than a week later, I would be sitting on the sofa imagining forks stabbing my eyes, bargaining with G-d and praying for better search-engine results.

THE FINAL SEARCH

I groped my way to the power button on my laptop and listened for the whirring to stop when it had booted, so I could keep my eyes closed as long as possible, then I opened my eyes to navigate online.

I don't remember what I typed into the search engine, but somehow that day I found a blogger in London, England, writing about severe, agonizing eye pain and a feeling like dry tissues stuffed under the eyelids. His words resonated for me because they described another serious symptom I had but hadn't been able to put into words.

"That's me," I thought. "Tissues under my eyelids."

I sat back and closed my eyes, even though it was already too late. The pain had materialized. There was no escaping it now. I wanted to stop reading . . . forever. But to hold up my end of the bargain, I forced myself to open my eyes. The blogger wrote about a doctor who had diagnosed a variety of diseases and treated them successfully. I closed my tortured eyes again, wondering if I should give up now, knowing I couldn't travel all the way to London when

I couldn't even walk across the room. But there was that bargain. I had to keep reading. So I gritted my teeth, opened my eyes, checked the doctor's contact information, and almost fell off my chair. The doctor's office wasn't in England. It was in Tampa, Florida. Desperate, the blogger had crossed the Atlantic to seek help. I would only need to drive one and a half hours to get there.

Within minutes I submitted a question to the doctor's website, and less than two hours later, on August 17, 2011, 11:13 a.m., had a response.

> Suggest evaluation here. May need gland probing to remove obstructions.
>
> *Dr. Maskin*

I made the appointment without hesitating, but in the interim I already had appointments scheduled with other doctors. One cauterized my lower tear ducts deeply to retain any tear film produced by my very dry eyes. Thinking the cautery sites should heal first, I canceled the appointment with Dr. Maskin.

Two days later, he called wondering why I had canceled. When I explained, he said that was reasonable, then asked if I would like to ask him any questions. I most definitely did. Although I don't recall his exact words, I remember Dr. Maskin describing what might be wrong with my eyes, why, and how he diagnoses and treats these diseases. We spoke for forty-five minutes. Afterward I kept wondering about this doctor who spent so much of his valuable time on someone who wasn't even his patient. Why? (We didn't know it then, but that conversation marked my initiation into the study of Dry Eye and MGD and would eventually lead to my work on this book.)

Despite the hope Dr. Maskin offered, I didn't dare take it. By then, hope was my enemy, an unreliable traitor. I'd already seen nearly two dozen doctors, all who initially offered hope. But none had treated the pain effectively or explained its cause. Having hope, I believed, just led to disappointment, so I had stopped my mind from going there, but I did finally reschedule the appointment.

WE WON'T BE DOING THAT TODAY

On September 2, 2011, my father drove me to Tampa for that first appointment with Dr. Maskin.

By the time the technician finished checking my vision, I was in agony and wanted only one thing.

I blurted it out the second Dr. Maskin opened the door and introduced himself.

"Please, Dr. Maskin, take my eyes out. Just take them out," I begged.

"No, no," he answered gently, like a kindergarten teacher soothing a five-year-old who fell and scraped her knee. "We won't be doing that today."

During the five hours of that first visit, Dr. Maskin spent three and half of them with me. First, he asked about my symptoms and medical history, the doctors I'd seen, and the treatments I'd had. He examined my eyes at the slit lamp for a long time and then placed a drop of dye in each. He found the scar of the stromal puncture and evidence of an earlier injury. When I was in my twenties, a tree branch had scratched my eye.

Then he focused on my pain. How did it feel? Where was it located? When did it occur? Did anything trigger it, make it worse, or better? He had me look in every direction while lifting or pressing on my lids. Did it feel worse, better, or the same? When he mobilized my upper lids over the eyeball, the pain emerged and strengthened. When he pressed on my lids, they were sore and tender.

Just like the blogger from London, my chief complaint was the feeling of pain like raw, gaping wounds plus the feeling of having tissues stuffed under the eyelids. But during the exam Dr. Maskin elicited many symptoms that I had discounted because my chief complaint masked the less prominent, though no less important, symptoms:

- Sore and tender lids
- Sticky and dry lids
- Burning
- Stinging
- Sharp pain
- Gritty

- Foreign body
- Photophobia
- Damp and moist outer canthal areas (outer corners)
- Itchy lids
- Pain upon opening the eye in the morning

Then it was time for a fluorescein clearance test (FCT) to evaluate my aqueous tears, first with anesthetic drops, then without. After that, he stimulated my nasal passages just inside the nostrils with a sterile cotton swab to see if my eyes watered. They did.

With the exam and tests completed, Dr. Maskin delivered his diagnoses, providing his rationale for each comorbidity:

- *Obstructive Meibomian gland dysfunction* (MGD), because of lid tenderness and few expressible glands
- *Non-Sjögren's aqueous tear deficiency* (ATD), according to results of the FCT
- *Superior and inferior conjunctivochalasis* in both eyes, visible at the slit lamp and with an elicited change in symptoms when he mobilized my lids over the surface of the eye, and moistness in the outer canthal areas
- *Tea tree oil toxicity,* according to my description of symptoms and signs of eyelid desiccation
- *Demodex mites,* visible in my lashes under a microscope
- *Nocturnal lagophthalmos,* according to my description of symptoms upon awakening
- Possible *recurrent corneal erosion syndrome,* because of the history of trauma to my right eye and, decades earlier, the tree-branch injury to my left eye
- Possible *ocular allergies,* because of symptoms of burning and itching

"Don't I have ocular neuropathy," I asked?

Dr. Maskin said no, because all of my symptoms could be explained by his clinical findings.

Next he described his proposed treatment for each comorbidity and what I could do at home to manage symptoms and support the health of my Meibomian glands and ocular surface.

For MGD, he recommended probing the Meibomian glands right away, a procedure he had developed and had performed on hundreds of patients with excellent results. I could expect improved eye comfort and the lid tenderness to disappear immediately.

For ATD, he recommended cauterizing my upper tear ducts superficially right after Meibomian gland probing and before I left the office that day. I could expect more eye comfort and more moisture.

For conjunctivochalasis, he recommended amniotic membrane transplant (AMT) surgery. He would remove the damaged conjunctiva and replace it with amniotic membrane. Because surgery required medical clearance from my primary care physician and approval by my insurance company, it would be scheduled within a few weeks. (Unfortunately, my circumstances would delay surgery for more than two months.) Although probing and cautery of puncta would treat symptoms of MGD and ATD, symptoms of conjunctivochalasis would persist while I waited for the upcoming AMT surgery.

Dr. Maskin instructed me to stop using tea tree oil because of toxicity. I could expect the menthol sensation to dissipate within a few days. We would tackle demodex mites later because other comorbidities were more pressing.

Wearing Eye Eco silicone moisture chamber goggles (which I could buy in the office) would alleviate the symptoms of lagophthalmos I had when I woke up each morning.

Outdoors I could wear 7eye wraparound sunglasses with silicone shields (I had a pair at home). Protecting my eyes from wind and drafts would help stabilize the tear film and keep my eyes comfortable.

To manage inflammation, Dr. Maskin prescribed low-dose doxycycline, 20 mg daily, and suggested I continue my omega-3 supplement.

For allergies, he prescribed Pataday® topical eye drops, now available without a prescription. (Later I developed sensitivities to these too and had to stop using them and other prescription and over-the-counter topical treatments.) At home, I needed to reduce exposure to allergens, for example, dust, mold, pollen, fumes. He advised that patch tests might reveal common allergies, but cautioned that no allergy test could evaluate every possible allergen.

Dr. Maskin told me to drink plenty of water, get plenty of sleep, and stressed the importance of further testing on my thyroid (I'd already had some preliminary tests showing abnormal thyroid hormone levels) because of the gland's role in ocular surface health.

Finally, he explained that each therapy would yield incremental improvement and, together, a cumulative and synergistic level of relief. I listened, wondering why no other doctor had ever been so thorough.

PROBING THE MEIBOMIAN GLANDS

A short time later, I was prepped for probing. Dr. Maskin put anesthetic drops in my eyes, placed bandage contact lenses over my corneas, and applied jojoba anesthetic ointment to my eyelid margins. I rested my chin on the holder of the slit lamp again and leaned my forehead in, not knowing what to expect.

Dr. Maskin advanced the probe into one gland, then the next. Each time I heard a noise, sometimes a loud *pop,* more often the gritty sound of nails on a washboard. Although numbed, I could feel the probe making a quick pinch each time it entered my glands. He probed the glands of one lid, paused for several seconds to see how I was doing, then probed the other lids.

Next, he inserted a dilator probe into each gland, to expand and prepare them for expression and therapeutic injection. To express the glands, he used a handheld instrument that cradled a lid between two rollers. While applying gentle pressure to the rollers, he expressed the freed-up meibum from inside the glands. Finally, he irrigated the intraductal space of each individual Meibomian gland with a corticosteroid, both to reduce the inflammation and to lavage, or wash out, the glands.

The treatment ended with superficial cautery of the upper tear ducts, and then came my barrage of questions. What do I do at home? Can I expect any reactions? Will my eyes feel better? The fact is, they already did. But still skeptical of doctors and conditioned to disdain hope, I attributed how great my eyes felt to the anesthetic drops.

I kept my eyes closed on the ride home and the rest of that evening. Wary of yet another massive disappointment, I couldn't bring myself to open them. I'd cope for one more night the way I'd coped for the last seven months—eyes closed.

When I woke the next morning, without thinking I opened my eyes. I felt no pain, no screwdriver in the eye. I was tempted to close them and keep them closed all day. Would the pain return? Should I close my eyes before it started? Should I close them now? No. My eyes were open, blinking normally, and comfortable. I didn't need to close them at all.

Around two o'clock that afternoon, Dr. Maskin called to check on me. It was a miracle I'd kept my eyes open that long, but I wondered if the pain-free state would last. Dr. Maskin stressed that I still needed surgery to repair the loose, wrinkled, and inflamed conjunctival tissues. Other conditions, like the allergies and toxicities, needed attention. I would have to keep my lids and lashes clean. I understood but marveled at how much better I felt. Could this be my new normal?

At my follow-up appointment on September 8, 2011, my eyes still felt great. Many more of my glands were expressible, and the lid tenderness had vanished. Today, with ongoing management of comorbidities and annual maintenance probing, I have even more expressible glands and no lid tenderness (see table 7.1).

WAITING FOR SURGERY

Just as Dr. Maskin predicted, the symptoms of untreated comorbidities emerged. Conjunctivochalasis and its effect on my Meibomian glands soon caused me to keep my eyes closed again. Insurance approval for surgery seemed impossibly far off, and other health problems added to my overall frustration: two excruciating kidney stone episodes, weeks waiting to see a rheumatologist and then an endocrinologist before starting treatment for autoimmune thyroid disease. Finally, in the middle of November, over two months since my first appointment with him, Dr. Maskin could go ahead with surgery.

POST-OP MAGIC

The two amniotic membrane transplant surgeries for conjunctivochalasis, one in each eye, were about a month apart. Dr. Maskin

Table 7.1[a]

Overall Status of Meibomian Glands in Lids

Date	Lid	Number of Expressible Glands	Lid Tenderness	Lid Diagnosis
9/2/2011	RU	5	Yes	CPO
(before	RL	9	Yes	CPO
probing)	LU	3	Yes	CDO
	LL	10	Yes	CPO
9/8/2011	RU	>10[b]	No	PDO
(6 days after	RL	>10[b]	No	PDO
first probing)	LU	>10[b]	No	PDO
	LL	>10[b]	No	PDO
8/15/2019	RU	25	No	PDO
(95 months	RL	21	No	PDO
after first	LU	26	No	PDO
probing)	LL	18	No	PDO
8/12/2021	RU	27	No	PDO
(119 months	RL	21	No	PDO
after first	LU	22	No	PDO
probing)	LL	17	No	PDO

[a]This table shows the overall status of the entire population of Meibomian glands in each of my lids upon diagnostic expression, just before my first probing on September 2, 2011, and six days later on September 8, 2011. Note the improvement in expressible glands, lid tenderness, and lid diagnosis just six days after the first probing.

The number of expressible glands in each lid has stayed relatively steady over the years (2019 and 2021 shown), with annual maintenance probing and effective management of comorbidities.

[b]In 2011, Dr. Maskin counted all expressible glands but he did not record how many more than ten were expressible.

(RU: right upper lid; RL: right lower lid; LU: left upper lid; LL: left lower lid; PDO: partial distal obstruction; CDO: complete distal obstruction; CPO: complete proximal obstruction; see chapter 9.)

excised the damaged, loose conjunctival tissue, replacing it with patches cut from amniotic membrane secured in place with glue and sutures. Each eye healed in about two weeks, during which I used an antibiotic ointment, steroid drops, and sterile saline rinses, all preservative-free to aid healing. Although I returned to the office for follow-up appointments, driven by friends and family, Dr. Maskin was always available via phone to recommend methods for easing any transient discomfort.

I called him after the first surgery on Thanksgiving Day, when the topical post-op medications became irritating. It was 10:30 a.m., a time when families crowd in their kitchens or watch the Macy's Thanksgiving Day Parade, but he answered his phone. Dr. Maskin suggested rinsing the eye with sterile saline before using the medications, then keeping both eyes closed for fifteen minutes. It worked. The irritation subsided, and I knew exactly what I'd give thanks for that Thanksgiving.

That wasn't the only time I contacted Dr. Maskin. As my condition improved and symptoms subsided, new unmasked symptoms emerged. It was like peeling back the layers of an onion; as Dr. Maskin diagnosed, treated, and resolved comorbidities, new comorbidities would emerge with their own bothersome symptoms. Early on I phoned, then later sent emails or texts, with questions and concerns about these new symptoms. I discovered quickly that saying "my eye doesn't feel good" was like telling a computer technician "my computer doesn't work." It was too vague. I learned to stop and think how I would describe my symptoms with precision. But even if I used precise terms, my calls often triggered a line of questioning, after which Dr. Maskin would offer his diagnosis and solution. Apparently he could figure out what I needed without always seeing my eyes. Impressively, whether diagnosing my symptoms remotely or in person, Dr. Maskin has always been right.

Burning had constantly plagued my eyes even after the second surgery. They burned incessantly, maddeningly. One day Dr. Maskin instructed me to apply dry, warm compresses to my eyes for two minutes at bedtime. I couldn't imagine how warm compresses would help, but applied them that night. By the next morning, the burning had disappeared.

Over the years, a sharp pain sometimes developed in the upper inner corner of my left eye, but its underlying cause was always different. Constantly irritated by each blink of the upper lid, the pain was unbearable. To offer relief, Dr. Maskin first needed to determine that underlying cause.

Once, a Meibomian gland had swelled up, causing the pain. After a series of questions and a lid exam, Dr. Maskin probed several glands in the left upper lid. Suddenly, soothing meibum filled with gritty bits flooded my eye. The probe had released strictures around a gland duct, allowing its sequestered contents to flow. The instant the gland emptied, the pain subsided. Dr. Maskin then irrigated the eye to flush out the gritty debris.

Another time the cause was folliculitis, inflammation of the eyelash follicle. After he epilated the diseased eyelash, the pain stopped. Once I accidentally poked my eyeball in that spot with my thumbnail, causing a deep abrasion on the ocular surface. Dr. Maskin told me to keep both eyes closed for a few hours. In a few days, the wound healed. A year later, a paper cut in the same spot caused the pain. Again, I kept both eyes closed for a few hours till the wound healed. One time a muscle spasm in the eyelid caused the pain. The eyelid wasn't twitching, I hadn't reinjured anything, and the eyelashes were clean. After a very detailed phone interrogation, Dr. Maskin instructed me to massage the lid gently. Instantaneously, the pain disappeared.

REACHING THE GOAL

After the surgeries for conjunctivochalasis, the feeling of dried tissues stuffed under my eyelids disappeared. My tear film spread normally, so my eyes were much more comfortable again, and were staying that way. But by mid-February 2012, my tear film was overflowing constantly, so Dr. Maskin began increasing the size of the tear duct openings he had superficially cauterized. He opened each a little at a time till he achieved a size that supported stable tear film. (Later, because of comorbidities causing one upper duct to close, and my deeply cauterized lower tear ducts, he referred me to an oculoplastic surgeon to reopen these.)

I was reaching my goal of resuming a productive life, albeit a different one than I had planned. Dr. Maskin compared my convalescence to a journey along a path heading toward the peak of a mountain. Relapses or a flare-up of symptoms might *seem* permanent and arbitrary. But there would be an identifiable reason for each. Treated with targeted therapy, the setbacks would only be temporary, like the mountain path veering downward occasionally as it snakes its way up the mountain. My chronic, comorbid diseases—

anterior blepharitis, demodex mites, distichiasis, trichiasis, ATD, MGD, allergies, sensitivities—would try to ambush me. I would need to counteract proactively with ongoing follow-up diagnosis and treatment. He assured me I would learn to manage my comorbidities and control my symptoms. In time I did, and in doing so learned volumes about them. An aberrant lash or even a speck of residue from cleaning my lashes can still trigger a cascade of symptoms, let alone my autoimmune disease or exposure to fumes. With Dr. Maskin's guidance, for which I am exceptionally grateful, I now have the knowledge and capacity to manage them. My Dry Eye mystery is solved.

NOT A DRY EYE FOUNDATION: KNOWLEDGE, SUPPORT, HOPE

As my eyes improved, I met many Dry Eye and MGD patients who, under Dr. Maskin's care, had overcome intractable eye pain. Others, not yet his patients and suffering with eye pain, called me to consult about their Dry Eye struggles. Some had endured pain for months, others for years, without accurate diagnoses or effective treatments. None knew much about MGD or had heard of comorbidities like conjunctivochalasis. Too many had battled suicidal thoughts and hopelessness. I wanted to restore their hope by closing the massive gap in knowledge of these diseases, but the task seemed Sisyphean.

Then one day, I met Diana Adelman, one of Dr. Maskin's patients with the same dream. We recruited several board members, and in 2014 established Not A Dry Eye Foundation, a 501(c)3 non-profit organization dedicated to raising awareness of Dry Eye. Volunteers built our website (notadryeye.org) and we populated it with comprehensive, credible information about Dry Eye, MGD, and other common comorbidities. Finally, we would be able to help many suffering with these diseases. Since its launch in November 2015, over one hundred thousand people have visited the site.

Today, Diana serves as executive director and treasurer of Not A Dry Eye; Susan Howell, another Dry Eye patient, as secretary; John McAree, MD, an internist and Dry Eye patient, as a board member at large; and I chair the board. Volunteers run the foundation, and we do not accept advertising fees or promote products or services provided by the industry. In 2018, we launched a patient advocacy program, giving structure to a service we had been providing informally for years.

In my volunteer work as a Not A Dry Eye patient advocate, I'm often reminded of my own fragile relationship with hope. Was it G-d answering my prayer? Was it fate or just circumstances that led me to that blogger in London? Regardless, I am now committed to this journey, to staying on top of the mountain, scattered below me the remembered carcasses of horrific pain, beside me the promise of hope.

8

Seven Principles of Meibomian Glands and Meibomian Gland Dysfunction

Myth
*Meibomian glands do little
besides providing oil for the tear film.*
Fact
*Meibomian glands are amazing structures
that play a central role in eye comfort and vision.*

I have observed Meibomian glands up close for over three decades and have distilled these observations into *seven principles* to help you understand my approach to diagnosing and treating MGD.

SEVEN PRINCIPLES OF MEIBOMIAN GLANDS AND MEIBOMIAN GLAND DYSFUNCTION

1. Meibomian glands are barometers of eye and overall health.
2. If Dry Eye were a wheel, MGD would be the hub.
3. MGD often progresses subclinically, in an occult manner.
4. Periductal fibrosis is the proximate cause of MGD and leads to gland atrophy.

5. Eyes perform best when vision is good *and* they are comfortable.
6. Restore Meibomian gland function, then defend the glands from comorbidities and aggravating cofactors.
7. Meibomian glands can be compared to teeth.

PRINCIPLE 1: MEIBOMIAN GLANDS ARE
BAROMETERS OF EYE AND OVERALL HEALTH

Since many systemic comorbidities can affect the health of Meibomian glands, it's not surprising that the glands are a good barometer of not just eye health, but overall health. The common signs of disease in the Meibomian glands—red eyelid margins and tender, sore eyelids or an inflamed conjunctiva—may indicate something is wrong in one of the body's other systems: immune, endocrine, metabolic, nervous, digestive, circulatory, muscular, respiratory, skeletal.

The immune system defends the Meibomian glands and ocular surface against pathogens, but sometimes it can go awry and attack host tissues. The endocrine and metabolic systems exert influence at the cellular and molecular levels, affecting the metamorphosis of meibocytes into meibum. Diabetes can disrupt this process. The metabolic system provides energy for the synthesis of meibum, but it can be slowed by hypothyroidism. The digestive system breaks down the food used by the metabolic system to create usable energy, but it can malfunction and lead to nutritional deficiencies affecting the Meibomian glands. The circulatory system delivers blood and its life-sustaining contents to the Meibomian glands, but it can become sluggish. The eyelid muscles, part of the muscular system, open and close the eyes during blinks, delivering meibum to the ocular surface. But muscle spasms, neurologic problems, and a decreased blink rate can lead to ineffective blinks, exposure, and irritation of the ocular surface. The skeletal system provides structure to the eye socket, but abnormalities of the bony orbit can affect lid anatomy and the quality of blinking.

When these systems are healthy, the Meibomian glands have a much better chance of working properly. If these systems are diseased, they can trigger the onset of MGD or exacerbate it, compromising the quality or quantity of the secreted meibum and initiating the spiral of ever-worsening comorbidities.

For example, a compromised or defective immune system may lead to an infection or autoimmune reaction causing acute or chronic inflammation. Inflammation then leads to periductal fibrosis, constricted glands, increased intraductal pressure, and possible stem cell deficiency, leading to decreased meibum secretion and gland atrophy.

Supporting Overall Health

Adopting a few good habits that support overall health (see chapter 12 for more) increases the likelihood that your Meibomian glands will be healthy too. Namely:

1. Eat healthy.
2. Stay hydrated.
3. Eliminate, or at least limit, caffeine.
4. Limit alcohol to social occasions only.
5. Get plenty of sleep.
6. Exercise.
7. Address any systemic conditions.
8. Adopt healthy eye habits.
9. Avoid tobacco and vaping products.

These may be obvious—every doctor will tell you the same thing about diet, sleep, exercise, drinking water, and taking care of yourself. Well . . . as a medical doctor, I concur. My patients who take care of their health usually complain about far fewer symptoms than those who don't.

PRINCIPLE 2: IF DRY EYE WERE
A WHEEL, MGD WOULD BE THE HUB

If Dry Eye were a wheel, MGD would be its hub, because MGD plays a central role in the disease. The spokes of the wheel would represent ocular comorbidities that can contribute to MGD. The outer

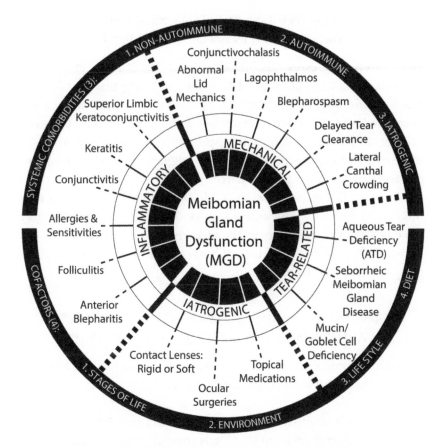

Fig. 8.1. If Dry Eye Were a Wheel, MGD Would Be Its Hub

Although each patient will experience a unique combination of comorbidities and react to cofactors differently, at the core of an interconnected hub and wheel we virtually always find MGD.

Source: Courtesy of Steven L. Maskin, MD.

rim of the wheel would represent various systemic comorbidities and other factors that can also contribute to MGD directly or indirectly. Together, the hub, rim, and spokes of the wheel suggest the interconnected nature of MGD, comorbidities, and contributing factors (see fig. 8.1).

Although each patient will experience a unique combination of comorbidities and react to factors differently, at the core we virtually always find MGD.

PRINCIPLE 3: MGD OFTEN PROGRESSES
SUBCLINICALLY, IN AN OCCULT MANNER

MGD often progresses subclinically, in an occult manner, without obvious signs or symptoms that would indicate diseased Meibomian glands. So, doctors may not look for it. Undetected, thus undiagnosed and untreated, the disease can advance freely. But even in later stages, MGD can be asymptomatic. Then, when it finally reaches a tipping point, MGD either triggers symptoms a patient can feel or signs a doctor can detect.

The subclinical progression of MGD can explain why your eyes might feel fine one day, and the next they hurt. Something may have pushed the disease over the edge, like a lack of sleep, the exhaust of a bus, a cloud of dust. Whatever happened, your MGD finally reached that tipping point.

PRINCIPLE 4: PERIDUCTAL FIBROSIS IS THE PROXIMATE
CAUSE OF MGD AND LEADS TO GLAND ATROPHY

Periductal fibrosis is the proximate cause of MGD leading to gland atrophy through two distinct mechanisms:

1. Fibrosis obstructs the glands with strictures, increasing intraductal pressure that leads to squamous metaplasia in meibocytes, reducing the volume of meibum and leading to gland atrophy. Probing the glands releases the strictures and equilibrates pressure within the glands, dramatically and immediately restoring the glands' ability to synthesize meibum.
2. When periductal inflammation and fibrosis invade the Meibomian gland external duct wall, they may interfere with the functioning of gland stem cells, creating a stem cell deficiency that may cause asymptomatic atrophic MGD. This interference may explain the isolated, discontinuous, or segmental patterns of Meibomian gland atrophy.

Probing glands to release fibrotic tissue appears to activate stem cells. (Meibomian gland stem cells found in the duct walls travel to the acinar epithelium, where they produce progenitor cells that in turn produce daughter cells, called meibocytes, that transform into meibum.) Their reactivation would explain the changes observed in glands after probing: a healthy proliferation of ductal epithelial cells with a thickening of duct walls and growth of tissue in atrophic glands.

PRINCIPLE 5: EYES PERFORM BEST WHEN VISION IS GOOD *AND* THEY ARE COMFORTABLE

The eyes perform their essential service best when vision is good and they are comfortable. If you can't see well, it's difficult to function. If your eyes aren't comfortable, you may not use them, and your entire focus may divert to how they feel. That's why, unless there is an acute vision problem needing immediate attention, I focus on restoring comfort first, because a comfortable, healthy ocular surface is needed for optimal sight.

There are two states of eye comfort. The first is comfort without stressors, such as dust, cold dry air, poor blinking, or allergies. The second is comfort in the presence of stressors. This state depends on the eye's resilience. A resilient eye rebounds, resets itself, and feels little to no nociceptive pain despite exposure to stressors. Both states of comfort are important to patients because they affect the quality of life.

PRINCIPLE 6: RESTORE MEIBOMIAN GLAND FUNCTION, THEN DEFEND THE GLANDS FROM COMORBIDITIES AND AGGRAVATING COFACTORS

For the eyes to be comfortable and have resilience, the Meibomian glands need to be in good working order.

Once the Meibomian glands are functioning normally, with ductal integrity restored after probing, the glands are defended from comorbidities and factors that could cause a rapid return of symptoms, sometimes in as little as two to three months. The aim is maintaining good gland health while preventing the recurrence or onset of diseases. Ongoing diagnosis and treatment remains individualized, specific to a patient's unique set of symptoms and comorbidities. As in earlier phases of treatment, one-size-fits-all does not apply.

PRINCIPLE 7: MEIBOMIAN GLANDS
CAN BE COMPARED TO TEETH

There are several interesting similarities between the anatomy and physiology of teeth and Meibomian glands.

1. We are born with a lot of them, that is, thirty-two teeth and approximately twenty-five to thirty Meibomian glands per lid.
2. Teeth and Meibomian glands are three-dimensional structures.
3. Teeth are near each other, as are Meibomian glands, so it can be hard to figure out exactly where the pain is. If there's a toothache, the problem may be in the tooth, the root, or the gum. If there's eye pain, the problem may be in the gland, lid, tear film, or eyeball. With teeth and eyes, there may even be more than one problem in more than one site, but it might be hard to tell where.
4. Teeth are parallel to each other, as are Meibomian glands.
5. Teeth and Meibomian glands are embedded in tissues that oppose each other: upper and lower jaw, upper and lower eyelids. These tissues move up and down: jaws bite, lids blink.
6. Teeth and Meibomian glands are found near mucosal tissue, where there is liquid flowing nearby: saliva near teeth, tear film near Meibomian glands.
7. Teeth and eyes (corneas in particular, but also the rest of the ocular surface tissue) are highly innervated. When something is wrong, it can hurt a lot.
8. Accumulated debris and inflammatory materials in surrounding spaces can cause disease. Plaque on teeth causes tooth decay, gingivitis, and even heart disease. Bacteria, parasites, and other debris accumulate at the base of the eyelashes near the Meibomian glands, causing MGD, anterior blepharitis, and other diseases. Periductal fibrosis accumulates around the gland duct, causing loss of ductal integrity, stricture, and increased intraductal pressure, as well as possible stem cell deficiency.

9. For maintenance, dentists recommend twice-a-year teeth cleaning to remove plaque and tartar and to prevent disease. Patients with MGD require annual maintenance probing to release strictures, prevent disease, and optimize gland function.

9

The Diagnosis

Myth
*All ophthalmologists perform patient examinations
the same way, and the standardized tests they
administer always provide reliable, actionable results.*
Fact
*The thoroughness of examinations can vary, and results
of standardized tests may be unreliable or of limited use.*

Myth
*Doctors can detect obstructive MGD by pressing on the
eyelids to see if they can express meibum from the glands.*
Fact
*Pressing on eyelids to express meibum
often gives false negative results.*

THE CHALLENGE

Even though diagnosis can be challenging, it's the most important step in treating any disease. Without an accurate diagnosis, treating a patient is like shooting darts at a board while you are blindfolded. You might get lucky and hit the bull's-eye, but chances are you won't. *House,* the TV series about the doctor who faced tough cases every week, and *Diagnosis,* the Netflix series about patients struggling with obscure diseases, illustrate this challenge dramatically.

To improve their chances of hitting the bull's-eye, doctors use various diagnostic tools and administer tests. Often these tests are essential, but sometimes they're unreliable. For example, tests can produce false positive results, indicating disease exists even when it doesn't, or false negative results, failing to detect disease when it exists.

Sometimes diagnoses are challenging because the way patients describe their symptoms may be unintentionally misleading. They may not be able to find words to describe their symptoms accurately, a common problem with friction-induced diseases of the ocular surface like conjunctivochalasis. Or they may hesitate to admit they're feeling pain or discomfort for personal reasons.

Sometimes even when patients describe their symptoms accurately, the symptoms themselves may mask or alter less severe symptoms or masquerade as different diseases. (A stronger symptom in one eye can even mask a less severe, though no less important, symptom in the other eye.)

Furthermore, when patients say they have "pain," the term "pain" alone may not provide enough information to indicate a specific condition for an accurate diagnosis. Nor is it enough to ask patients if they have pain, because they may not associate each sensation they have with the term "pain" (see chapter 6). Both of these approaches might not elicit accurate information from patients, leading to inaccurate diagnoses.

The Consequences of Misdiagnosis and Inadequate Diagnosis

When they are misdiagnosed or inadequately diagnosed, untreated comorbidities can progressively worsen. With symptoms intensifying, the patient's overall status may deteriorate. Sometimes patients switch doctors looking for second opinions. Hopping from doctor to doctor, they waste time and money. They miss out on the benefits of a long-term patient-doctor relationship during which a doctor learns about a patient's comorbidities and how they respond to treatment. As mentioned in chapter 6, with time passing and untreated comorbidities and symptoms worsening, patients sometimes lose hope and develop suicidal thoughts. In the most heartbreaking

Sidebar 9.1
Nonspecific Symptoms, Masquerading
Symptoms, and Other Causes of Eye Pain

MGD can be difficult to diagnose for these reasons:

- The symptoms of MGD, and many comorbidities, are often nonspecific, so they can indicate more than one condition.
- The symptoms of MGD may masquerade as something that's *not* MGD. For example, blinking hard continually (which squeezes meibum out of the glands) to improve comfort can cause facial muscle tightness and pain, symptoms not typically associated with MGD.
- Symptoms may be due to a condition or conditions that aren't MGD but masquerade as Dry Eye or MGD, such as occipital neuralgia, which can cause pain referred to the eye (see chapter 6).

Masquerading symptoms can mislead doctors toward misdiagnoses and confuse patients when treatment isn't going as expected. For example, allergies can cause burning, a symptom usually associated with MGD. But, more specifically, the burning may be due to the allergy, the adverse effect of the allergy exacerbating MGD, or both. If the doctor diagnosis and treats MGD but misses the allergy, the patient will continue to have burning symptoms because the allergy wasn't treated.

cases, patients in severe pain and without hope of finding relief sometimes commit suicide.

Keeping an Open Mind

Doctors avoid misdiagnoses and incomplete diagnoses by keeping
open minds and remembering patients are unique. We make diagnoses specific to patients, not based solely on previous experience
with patterns of symptoms and diseases. Acknowledging your own
uniqueness is important for patients too, so you don't fall into the
trap of comparing your symptoms, treatments, and recoveries with
other patients or become frustrated because your progress seems slow.

Restoring Hope

Patients who suffer a lot sometimes lose trust in doctors. After months
or years of suffering, they become skeptical and can't imagine ever
feeling better. Many who travel long distances to see me, having
exhausted their options with local doctors, think they've tried everything. They doubt I have solutions. If these doctors diagnosed
them with ocular neuropathic pain, they question how anyone
can heal their damaged nerves. (Sometimes even after experiencing complete relief, my patients look at temporary setbacks as permanent reversals, doubting their own experience of healing. Or the
temporary setback might paralyze them with fear because it brings
back memories of horrific pain. Their anguish and terror is real and
justifiable, but over time decreases and resolves as their condition
improves.)

   These patients need their hope restored. So even before discussing their medical histories, I take time to reassure my patients. I explain that I've seen hundreds, or maybe thousands, of patients just
like them with similar chief complaints. After diagnosing and treating numerous less obvious and even occult conditions, symptoms
and pain improve dramatically and even resolve. Although no doctor can predict results with 100 percent certainty, I expect their results will be similar. The key for the best results is compliance with
therapy, good two-way doctor-patient communication, and follow-up
so the doctor can adjust therapy when necessary (see sidebar 9.2).

Sidebar 9.2
Come Back in Two Weeks

Doctors ask patients to return for follow-up appointments to check on them and confirm that prescribed therapies worked. In scientific terms, at the follow-up appointment the doctor evaluates the patient's response to therapy, confirming or disproving the working diagnosis. If the treatment worked and the patient improved, the working diagnosis becomes the definitive diagnosis.

If the patient does not keep follow-up appointments or communicate with the doctor about their progress, the doctor cannot confirm the working diagnosis, adjust existing therapies, or begin therapies for other diagnosed comorbidities. Some doctors may mistakenly believe their patients responded to treatment. If the doctor never learns treatment was ineffective, he may be more inclined than warranted to prescribe it to the next patient.

Requires a Doctor

Patients with MGD need a doctor who can examine their eyes with diagnostic instruments. Social media groups and online forums aren't substitutes for medical exams. Mirrors, even powerful magnifying mirrors, don't reveal everything, and ignoring pain isn't a solution.

I can't stress enough to patients the importance of finding a trusted doctor who can diagnose comorbidities comprehensively, prescribe targeted therapy, and monitor progress to adjust treatment as needed. If you're not getting results, if the explanations you're hearing about your progress make little sense, if you feel your doctor is dismissing your concerns or seems disinterested because you're coming in with yet another symptom, it's probably time to find another doctor.

SIX STEPS TO A COMPREHENSIVE DIAGNOSIS

All doctors have their preferred ways of conducting patient examinations, but their goals are similar: evaluate the patient to formulate a diagnosis and develop a treatment plan. The first encounter between doctor and patient usually lasts longer than follow-up exams. My first encounters can last for forty-five minutes or more, depending on a variety of factors, including the complexity of the following:

- The chief complaint and history of present illness
- Ophthalmic history
- General medical history and current status

Although each patient is unique, I always follow these first five steps during the initial appointment. Thoroughness in each step is crucial so no comorbidity is overlooked. (At subsequent follow-up appointments, I modify the steps: the questions I ask, the exam, the tests I administer, and so forth, based on the patient's response to treatment.)

Step 1: Initial impression
Step 2: The history
Step 3: Initial hypothesis
Step 4: Examination and testing
Step 5: Comprehensive working diagnosis

The final step comes after I see how the patient responds to my recommended treatment.

Step 6: Definitive diagnosis

Step 1: Initial Impression

From my initial impression upon entering the exam room, I get a sense of the patient's health status even without doing a full-body physical exam. I can see if the patient is using cosmetics or may have had cosmetic surgeries or procedures like Botox injections. I can see

---

Sidebar 9.3
The Diagnostic Mosaic

When diagnosing patients, each comorbidity and cofactor I find becomes a single piece in a diagnostic mosaic. Viewing them as interlocking pieces of a mosaic enables me to sort and arrange a complex of comorbidities and cofactors into an organized array that I can easily recall. This approach reinforces that each piece is part of an integrated disease complex that can be considered both individually or as part of the entire mosaic. I keep in mind both the individual pieces and the mosaic while prescribing targeted treatments.

---

red eyes, facial asymmetry and spasms, blepharospasms, lid retraction, the effects of strokes, or other physical disabilities. Inflamed joints of the hands can reveal rheumatoid arthritis. Redness on the face, easily visible when it's not covered by makeup, and rhinophyma, a red and swollen nose, are signs of rosacea, which has been associated with demodex mites, the same parasites linked to MGD. Thin hair, a sign of aging, can also suggest an iron or other micronutrient deficiency or thyroid disease. Bulging eyes may indicate Graves' thyroid disease. These diseases can also affect the eyes and Meibomian glands. Patients with seemingly dry mouths or strained voices may have Sjögren's syndrome or pemphigoid, two autoimmune diseases that can afflict the eyes and contribute to Dry Eye and MGD.

Each comorbidity I find will become a single piece in a diagnostic jigsaw puzzle (see sidebar 9.3).

Step 2: The History

At the initial appointment, I start with the chief complaint, then conduct a thorough review of the patient's ophthalmic and medical

---

Sidebar 9.4
An "Aha" Moment

It happens often. When I ask patients details about their medical histories or what triggered their ocular symptoms, they often say, "No one ever asked me that." When they realize which circumstance triggered the onset or progression of Dry Eye / MGD symptoms, they'll have an "aha" moment, saying they never considered associating that trigger with their disease.

Sometimes patients realize a lifestyle change was the trigger. They may have started binge eating, which can stop meibum production, leaving Meibomian glands dormant. A new job, home, car, pet, or medication might have been a trigger, or exposure to fumes or particulate matter. The possibilities are vast and unique to each individual, sometimes making diagnosis tricky.

---

histories. Patients provide some of this information on medical history forms, and my technicians gather additional information right before I see patients. I ask questions throughout the exam whenever it's necessary.

The Chief Complaint and History of Present Illness

I start with the two questions most important to my patients:

1. What is the chief complaint or the worst symptom?
2. Are there other accompanying ocular symptoms? (Patients should report all symptoms, even mild or just annoying ones, to help their doctor make a thorough diagnosis.)

To better understand the nature of the symptoms, I'll ask follow-up questions like these:

- When did it begin?
- How severe is it on a scale of 0 to 10, with 0 meaning no symptoms, and 10 meaning unbearable pain incompatible with life?
- How does it impact daily life?
- Is it constant or intermittent?
- How often does it occur? Hourly? Daily? Every few days?
- Does it happen at a specific time of day?
- Does it get worse as the day progresses?
- Does something make it better or worse?
- What happens to the symptom when looking up or down, to the left or right, blinking, or with eyes closed?

The questions I ask depend entirely on my initial impression and how the patient answered prior questions (and later on, how the patient is responding to treatment). For example, if a patient presents with facial rosacea, I will ask if the eyes burn or sting. Maybe the person is more comfortable with the eyes closed, or the lid margins get red, itchy, inflamed, and irritated. These are signs and symptoms suggesting MGD.

If patients say their eyes feel gritty, gravelly, or sandy, I ask if they can cry emotional tears. This tells me if the lacrimal glands are producing moisture. I'll also ask if the mouth feels dry and if they have difficulty chewing or swallowing a cracker without water. If yes, the patient may have aqueous tear deficiency (ATD) and Sjögren's syndrome. Once when I entered the examination room, I found a new patient waiting with a finger up her nose. She did this to trigger reflexive tears. This behavior suggested ATD, prompting me to ask ATD-related questions.

I may ask how the patients' eyes feel upon awakening. If they feel dry or scratchy, they may have nocturnal lagophthalmos.

I ask about treatments prescribed by other doctors for the chief complaint and accompanying symptoms, for example, drops, devices, oral medications, surgery. (The number of doctors a patient has seen can indicate how desperate or skeptical they are.) I ask if the patients are still doing any of the treatments. If they are, how often? They might be applying warm compresses, massaging their eyelids, or expressing their glands regularly, without first having their

Meibomian glands probed. Or they might be using drops that can irritate and contribute to symptoms.

I ask if the patient wears or ever wore contact lenses; ever used ACCUTANE® (isotretinoin), finasteride, or other antiandrogens for hair loss or prostate enlargement, or has been exposed to particulate matter.

I ask patients if they use or ever used cosmetics like mascara, eyeliner, eye shadow, or powder foundation that can billow and settle on the lid margins. Liquid and powder foundations can gravitate to the tear film. I ask if they remove their makeup nightly and with what. Do they wear lash extensions—glue-on or magnetic? Have they had any cosmetic procedures, Botox injections, or fillers? Do they use LATISSE® to grow lashes? Do they have eyelid tattoos or permanent eyeliner? All can contribute to symptoms.

Ophthalmic History

While discussing the patient's symptoms, I also note previous diagnoses, such as recurrent corneal erosion, map-dot-fingerprint dystrophy, sty, chalazion, pink eye, or other medical conditions they may have had in and around the eyes and eyelids. The patient may also have a history of trauma and/or surgeries, such as LASIK, cataract, retina, or glaucoma surgeries, or eyelid lifts.

General Medical History and Current Status

After a thorough review of the patient's ocular symptoms, I review the patient's medical history forms, asking for clarification if I have any questions. I look for anything that might be impacting a patient's symptoms or contributing to comorbidities.

1. Allergies: I note any known allergies to medications and environmental allergens. Allergies can play an important role in MGD. (Medications for treating allergies can desiccate the ocular surface.)
2. Nonophthalmic surgeries: I note previous nonophthalmic surgeries, when they were performed, and if there were any complications or lasting effects.

Sidebar 9.5
Answering Questions

Sometimes it's difficult for patients to answer a specific question. They may need time to think about the answer because (1) they aren't sure how to describe precisely what they're feeling, (2) they may never have considered the question before, or (3) the question brings into their conscious awareness something that they've been doing subconsciously, like manipulating their upper eyelids to reduce discomfort (which may be caused by superior bulbar conjunctivochalasis). Sometimes, though rarely, the patient needs a few undisturbed minutes to consider the question and how they will answer. Sometimes the family member, partner, or friend accompanying the patient can answer the question or help the patient find or articulate the answer.

3. Systemic comorbidities and medications: I note any known systemic comorbidities, when they started, how they are being treated, and the patient's response to treatment. I also check medications and supplements, including hormone replacements the patient may be taking.
4. Family history of eye disease and systemic disease: I note the family medical and ophthalmic history. For example, blood relatives with Sjögren's syndrome, connective tissue diseases, cataracts, glaucoma, Dry Eye, and other diseases may indicate the patient's risk for developing conditions that can be a factor in MGD.
5. Social history: Because diet, behavior and lifestyle choices, and the environment can all play a major role in MGD and Dry Eye symptoms, I discuss these with the patient.

Diet

I ask patients to describe their diets and eating habits. Are they on a specific diet or are there any dietary restrictions? Do they binge on sweets or saturated fats? Is their diet healthy? Do they consume caffeine in any form—coffee, tea, chocolate, soda, or other foods containing caffeine? If yes, how often and how much?

Behavior and Lifestyle

Next, we discuss factors in their behavior or lifestyle that can play a role in MGD and Dry Eye. For example, I ask about their line of work. If they use a computer, their blinking can be affected. They may work in areas heavy with dust or particulate matter, in areas where temperatures or humidity are very low or very high, or where their eyes are exposed to sunlight.

We discuss sleep habits. Do they sleep at least six to eight hours each night? (Not sleeping enough can cause elevated blood sugar levels which, like binge eating, can lead to dormant Meibomian glands.) If patients say they awaken with one red, irritated eye, I'll ask if they sleep on that side, and I'll correlate this information with the findings of my examination for floppy lid.

I check if they smoke, vape, or drink alcohol.

Environment

If the environment has not yet come up in our discussion but the patient's symptoms may be affected by it, I ask about the person's home: ambient temperature, humidity, carpeting, ceiling fans, and pets. Where do vents blow? Are vents in the bedroom pointed at the bed, which can irritate the eyes?

Step 3: Initial Hypothesis

There is no substitute for experience when it comes to analyzing patients' symptoms, medical histories, and backgrounds. I draw on over three decades of experience analyzing these to formulate my initial hypothesis. Because comorbidities often cluster, I might the-

---

Sidebar 9.6
Are You Taking Any Medications or Supplements?

Always tell your eye doctor about any medications or supplements you take. Some may contribute to your Dry Eye symptoms. If they do, ask your doctor about taking a different medication that may cause fewer side effects.

---

orize that a patient has several comorbidities. Though at the outset I keep in mind the probability of a patient having a specific condition based on my initial impression and the person's history, ultimately each hypothesis is unique to each patient, based only on our encounter, not on population statistics.

When analyzing symptoms, I first consider the patient's known systemic conditions. Many can play a significant role in MGD. For example, herpes zoster (shingles), a systemic condition, can manifest in any part of the eye and may have caused scarring on one side of the face or scalp, with reduced corneal sensation on that side, which would lead to ATD and MGD.

Next, I establish the nature of the ocular symptoms. Did the patient report one symptom or multiple symptoms? I consider the specific ocular condition(s) or systemic disease(s) that might lead to those symptoms or play a role, always mindful that patients may have a hard time describing their symptoms or may describe them in vastly different ways (see chapter 6).

What Symptoms May Mean

Following general rules that correlate symptoms with diseases can be very helpful for developing the initial hypothesis. I follow these rules, although there are many exceptions. (Note: Although extensive, this is not an exhaustive list of symptoms and the comorbidities they might indicate. There are others.)

Sidebar 9.7
Focal, Global, and Diffuse Symptoms

Focal: A symptom felt in a specific spot
Global: A symptom felt across the entire eyeball
Diffuse: A symptom felt regionally, that is, more than focally, but not necessarily globally

---

FOREIGN-BODY SENSATION

A foreign-body sensation—it feels like something is in the eye—can indicate many conditions. The sensation may be constant or intermittent, and global, focal, or diffuse.

Gravelly, grainy, scratchy, or sandy sensations, whether in a small focal area nasally, diffuse, or global, suggest ATD.

A focal foreign-body sensation can also be trichiasis, a loose eyelash in the eye, a keratinized cap over a Meibomian gland opening and protruding past the lid margin, a muscle spasm in the eyelid, a single internally blocked Meibomian gland, or more. These foreign-body sensations can be sharp or stabbing.

Patients might say they feel dry tissues in the eyes or crushed glass. Possible causes range from trichiasis to conjunctivochalasis.

BURNING OR STINGING

Burning and stinging usually indicate evaporative Dry Eye or meibum deficiency, exposing the underlying ocular surface nerves.

Poor quality blinking and inadequate spreading of tears can also cause burning and stinging. The blinking problem may be iatrogenic. For example, after ptosis repair or blepharoplasty, a patient may not be able to close an eye completely or blink properly, leading to burning or stinging. These symptoms may also be due to an underlying neurologic problem.

ITCHING OR BURNING

Itching and burning are common symptoms of allergies. The eyelids, the eyelid margins, and eyeball can itch or burn. If patients scratch or rub their eyes to relieve the itch, they may exacerbate symptoms by releasing histamine from inflammatory cells (mast cells).

PAIN

Patients often complain of pain. When they use the term, I ask them to clarify and characterize the sensation precisely.

Pain may be focal, diffuse, or global. It can be due to a muscle spasm in the eyelid, conjunctivochalasis and other defects of the ocular surface, ATD, obstructed Meibomian glands, distichiasis, trichiasis, entropion, or abnormalities deeper inside the eye, among other conditions.

Pain may be referred from other parts of the body, for example, occipital neuralgia.

Painful sensitivity to light, photophobia, is a common symptom of Dry Eye or may be due to corneal surface defects. Photophobia may also indicate problems deeper in the eye, such as cataracts, retinal detachment, uveitis, and others.

A condition that often presents as a sharp, stabbing pain at awakening is recurrent corneal erosion (RCE). ATD, nocturnal lagophthalmos (which allows tear evaporation and ocular surface exposure), and MGD (which can cause thickened congested lids) can contribute to RCE. The upper lid adheres to the cornea during sleep. When the eye opens, the thickened lid rips layers off the corneal epithelium. ATD, MGD, conjunctivochalasis, and previous trauma to the cornea can increase the risk and frequency of RCE, as can map-dot-fingerprint dystrophy because of elevated corneal epithelium and thickened basement membrane tissue. RCE is particularly dangerous for post-LASIK patients if the lid adheres to the cornea and tears the flap created during the procedure.

Seemingly benign, misdirected lashes can cause severe pain if they scratch and abrade the cornea and can lead to cornea ulceration, infection, blindness, and permanent loss of the eye.

HEAVINESS AND TIREDNESS

Heaviness and tiredness can indicate conjunctivochalasis or dermatochalasis, as well as delayed tear clearance, MGD, and allergy.

WATERY EYES

Paradoxically, patients with Dry Eye may have reflex tears leading to watery eyes.

Watery eyes may be due to punctal stenosis, a blocked tear duct, or a blocked lacrimal sac, any of which may prevent the continuous drainage of tear film into the punctum, through the lacrimal canaliculus and into the nose.

Watery eyes presenting as dampness or moist sensations at the outer corners (canthus), may be due to conjunctivochalasis if folds in the redundant conjunctival tissue channel tear film to the corners.

Foreign bodies in the eye can cause watering as the eye produces reflex tears to cleanse itself.

Anterior blepharitis due to infections or allergies can cause reflex tears and watery eyes.

TENDERNESS AND SORENESS

Meibomian gland duct walls invaded by periductal fibrosis can lead to loss of integrity and fixed stricture of the central duct lumen, causing elevated intraductal pressure manifesting as lid tenderness (typically upon examination) and soreness.

FREQUENT BLINKING

Blinking more often than every five to seven seconds suggests poor tear film stability, usually due to MGD, possibly ATD, or a mucin deficiency.

BLURRED VISION

Blurred vision suggests a problem from Dry Eye if vision improves after blinking or using artificial tears.

CRUSTING

Crusting near the roots of the lashes and along the lid margins is usually a sign of infectious anterior blepharitis.

LIDS STICK TO EYES

Lids sticking to eyes, especially upon awakening, usually indicates nocturnal lagophthalmos (see sidebar 9.9), but may also suggest MGD and ATD. Lids that stick to eyes can cause painful RCE (see the symptom "Pain").

MUCUS

Mucus discharge in the tear film usually indicates ATD, allergy, or microtrauma.

REDNESS OR INFLAMMATION

Redness is a sign of inflammation. Generally it is a very nonspecific sign indicating that something is happening, but not exactly what. With MGD, redness may be found on the surface of the eye, the lid margin (telangiectasia), or the eyelids.

SAPONIFICATION (FROTHY TEARS)

Patients sometimes report seeing bubbles floating in the tear film and spilling onto the lid margin. Sometimes the tear film looks frothy. Bubbles or frothy tears indicate saponification, the production of soap due to the liberation of free fatty acids from meibum by microbial enzymes. This soap causes burning, irritation, and inflammation.

TWITCHING LIDS

The eyelids might twitch or flutter spontaneously for a few moments or many hours. In my experience, the most common cause is consuming too much caffeine.

PUFFY LIDS / SWELLED LIDS

Puffy or swollen lids are often signs of allergies or MGD, or they may suggest liver or kidney disease. Crying emotional tears can cause puffy lids.

Timing and Severity

Timing is an important consideration. A constant symptom, without variation throughout the day, suggests a constant underlying cause. Symptoms that get worse as the day progresses suggest ATD, although ATD symptoms may remain constant all day. Symptoms triggered when the patient is in the yard with flowers and plants or snuggling with a pet suggest allergies. Nocturnal lagophthalmos, RCE, floppy lid, or MGD may cause symptoms that are worse upon awakening.

Severe symptoms may indicate an advanced state of disease in an eye that is highly sensitized due to chronic low-grade inflammation or an acute disease with severe inflammation. Mild symptoms may be due to reduced sensation from chronic irritation, which may numb the nerve endings. Mild symptoms may also indicate a disease in its early stages or that a stronger symptom is partially masking less severe symptoms.

Adjusting the Initial Hypothesis

Based on what I learn about the patient from my observations and our discussion, I develop an initial working hypothesis. The information I gather next during the examination and from test results will either confirm or refute the hypothesis. If refuted, I may need to adjust it to ensure all the data fit together like evidence in a good murder mystery.

Step 4: Examination and Testing

Thorough examinations lead to accurate diagnoses. Diagnosing and treating only obvious comorbidities won't lead to successfully treated or happy patients if there are significant undiagnosed comorbidities.

Sidebar 9.8
Diagnosing Asymptomatic and Occult Diseases

When a disease occurs with visible signs but without symptoms, it's called asymptomatic. When diseases exist but can't be seen or are unexpectedly found, they're called occult. To confirm its presence, an asymptomatic or occult disease can often be diagnosed with special physical examination techniques. For example, we can elicit lid tenderness from increased intraductal pressure caused by periductal fibrosis by pressing gently on the lid. Similarly, firm, fixed, focal, and unyielding resistance found during intraductal Meibomian gland probing reveals occult periductal fibrosis.

That's why I try to find the cause of every symptom and diagnose every comorbidity.

A Closer Look—External Exam

When I first encountered the patient, I made observations about the patient's general health and external eye appearance. As I continue observing the patient from my desk some four feet away, I note any of the following:

- Skin rashes, flakes, or blisters on the face
- Shiny or dull, dry-looking eyes
- Blink rate
- Conscious or subconscious eye, eyelid, or eyebrow touching, for example, rubbing, scratching, wiping away tears, pushing or pulling on eyelids or eyebrows, or fishing something out of the eyes
- Methods to stimulate tear production, like placing a finger in the nose

Sidebar 9.9
Diagnosing Nocturnal Lagophthalmos

Nocturnal lagophthalmos, eyelids that do not seal completely during sleep, can cause foreign-body sensations, pain, and other symptoms upon awakening in the middle of the night or in the morning. Even a very fine fissure between the eyelids can cause severe discomfort.

Nocturnal lagophthalmos is difficult to diagnose in the exam room because the eyelid fissure may be visible only from below the sleeping patient's chin or chest. One in-office test involves reclining the patient and shining a light on the upper outer part of the closed upper lid near the horizontal lid fold. Light visible between the eyelids suggests the imperfectly sealed lid of lagophthalmos. However, this test does not reproduce the patients' normal sleeping conditions—in their own beds, reclined in their favorite sleeping positions, in the middle of the night, and actually asleep—so it can give misleading results. Plus, the test may be skewed if patients have caffeine or certain types of medications in their systems. Despite the test not being absolute, it may suggest considering this diagnosis.

I ultimately diagnose nocturnal lagophthalmos by history, when patients describe awakening with severe eye pain or dryness, and confirm the diagnosis when patients report that targeted treatment resolved their symptoms.

Conditions in the bedroom can trigger or exacerbate the symptoms of nocturnal lagophthalmos, for example, heating and cooling vents blowing on the face, ceiling fans circulating air and causing drafts, candles or incense releasing particulate matter that sneaks past the fissure and settles in the eyes, low humidity levels that desiccate the ocular surface, or dander from pets that sleep on the bed.

Diagnosing conjunctivochalasis often involves a combination of patient-reported symptoms, questions about those and other symptoms or behaviors, a slit-lamp exam, and a test that elicits symptoms and confirms the diagnosis.

Patients with conjunctivochalasis often report a variety of symptoms. In my experience, heavy and tired eyes suggest conjunctivochalasis tissue is weighing on the lower lid margin. Often conjunctivochalasis channels tears to the outer corner of the eyes and skin, creating dampness and moistness there. (Until I ask about it, patients sometimes think the symptom is insignificant and ignore it, or are not aware of it.) As a result, the entire ocular surface may not be adequately covered with tears, leaving some of it exposed. Conjunctivochalasis can also interrupt the flow of tears from the inferior tear reservoir behind the lower lid into the precorneal tear film. The disruption of the tear film may lead to burning, stinging, and foreign-body sensations.

Sometimes subconsciously, patients manipulate their eyelids to neutralize the effects of chalasis. Patients with superior chalasis, where the upper lid pinches the conjunctival tissue between the globe and the lid, may get temporary symptom relief by lifting the upper lid margin off the eyeball. When I ask, the person accompanying the patient to their appointment will sometimes point out how often the patient touches their eyelids in this manner.

I confirm the conjunctivochalasis diagnosis with the patient seated at the slit lamp and a test that alters the relevant symptoms. (See "Slit-Lamp Exam" under "Step 4: Examination and Testing.") For a diagnosis of inferior conjunctivochalasis, when I evert the lower eyelid, the symptoms should decrease. For a diagnosis of superior conjunctivochalasis, when I gently mobilize the upper eyelid over the eyeball, the symptoms should increase.

- Eyelid symmetry
- Dermatochalasis (redundant eyelid skin tissue around the eyes). If I see dermatochalasis, later during the slit-lamp examination I will look carefully for conjunctivochalasis and lateral canthal crowding (the cluster of comorbidities that includes dermatochalasis, conjunctivochalasis, entropion, trichiasis, and MGD).
- Obvious discharge around the eyes or in their lashes
- Indications of blepharopigmentation or permanent eyeliner

Next, I roll my chair closer to the patient. I check for floppy lids by having the patient look down while trying to evert their upper eyelid. If the lid everts easily, exposing the superior palpebral conjunctiva, the patient has a floppy lid. It may present with redness and irritation upon awakening, although the patient may not be symptomatic.

Next, I feel for preauricular (in front of the ear) or submandibular (under the mandible) lymph nodes. An enlarged, tender lymph node may indicate a viral illness. I inspect ear and nasal cartilage, which if inflamed and tender can be a sign of autoimmune disease.

While sharing their medical history, if the patient described nondescript or atypical pain near the eyes, I will check the back of the head for signs of occipital neuralgia. These types of pain can eclipse the symptoms of Dry Eye, masking them until the occipital neuralgia is reversed.

Visual Field, Motility, and Pupillary Examination

Next I evaluate the patient's peripheral vision using confrontational visual field. I check nine fields of peripheral vision: up and out,

Sidebar 9.11

Diagnosing Allergies and Sensitivities

Allergies can cause a variety of symptoms, often itching and sometimes burning. They can exacerbate other symptoms and cause watery eyes in patients without ATD. Allergens can accumulate on the skin and hair during the day, then transfer to bedding if the patient doesn't shower or wash their hair before bedtime. When allergens are in the eyes overnight, they can make symptoms worse in the morning.

Symptoms that occur or worsen while taking a shower or washing hair may be due to allergies or sensitivities to ingredients in soaps and shampoos. Also, the showerhead may release irritants or fungal spores, and the water may contain irritants like chlorine.

If the symptom happens soon after applying makeup or nail polish or using hair spray, the patient may have sensitivities or allergies to ingredients those products contain.

Sensitivities to fumes, scents, particulate matter (for example, smoke, incense, fine dust) can cause foreign-body sensations, dryness, and burning, and can exacerbate MGD.

Some patients describe extreme sensitivity to changes in humidity levels, prompting questions from me about their environment. Cold winters with dry air or lowered thermostats that pull moisture out of the air can both lead to Dry Eye symptoms. Low temperatures can even alter the fluidity of meibum affecting the spread of tear film with each blink.

straight up, up and in, straight right, straight ahead, straight left, down right, straight down, down left.

Then I check motility, how well the eyes move. Saccades are quick eye movements from one direction to another. Pursuit is following an object, in this case my finger, as I move it into different gaze positions.

Using a penlight, I check the pupils for size, roundness, and symmetry. When I check their reactivity to light and a near target, both pupils should constrict similarly.

Nose, Mouth, and Hands

Keeping the penlight on, if I'm considering a systemic disease, I then look inside the nose and mouth.

Inside the nostrils, I check for lesions such as nodules, blisters, or ulcers.

I look at the tongue, gums, teeth, and palate. Dryness, a lack of saliva, ulcers, blisters, or lots of cavities can be signs of autoimmune disease.

I examine the hands, fingers, and wrist joints and the nail beds. If the patient revealed they have an exposed rash I examine it to identify possible systemic diseases that may impact the patient's eyes or Meibomian glands.

Slit-Lamp Exam

Next, I seat the patient at the slit lamp. The chin rests on a sanitized chin cup and the forehead against a band, so the head is held in a comfortable and relaxed but stable position. The height of the seat and chin cup is adjustable so the patient can look straight ahead while being examined.

The slit-lamp device has a binocular microscope for magnification, with an adjustable angled illumination arm allowing light to cut across the eye at an angle, revealing the depth of lesions.

I begin the slit-lamp examination with an open mind, looking for signs that either support or disprove the initial hypothesis, but I follow a systematic process and these steps consistently to ensure I don't overlook something.

1. TEAR FILM

I evaluate the volume and clarity of the tear film. It should be at least 0.3 millimeters in height and clear, without signs of debris, mucus, white blood cells, makeup, or foam.

2. LID MARGIN

I check for abnormalities of the lid margin and Meibomian gland orifices. Notches, grooves, or a thickened or rounded posterior lid margin indicate MGD. The orifices should be anterior to the muco-cutaneous junction but may have been pulled by scar tissue anteriorly (forward) or posteriorly (back). A waxy cap sometimes covers the orifices and the underlying still-liquid meibum. Telangiectasia indicates MGD.

If the lids turn inward (entropion) or outward (ectropion), the lid margin may rub the eye or be overexposed.

Permanent eyeliner (blepharopigmentation) is also associated with MGD.

Parallel folds of bulbar conjunctival chalasis tissue resting on the lower lid margin can obliterate the tear film and exacerbate symptoms. When I see this, I ask the patient if their eyes feel heavy or tired. If yes, I evert the lower lid, allowing the chalasis tissue to drop. Then I ask the patient if the heaviness or tiredness changed. If yes, the chalasis is symptomatic, and ocular surface reconstruction will likely reduce or eliminate those symptoms. Even if the change was slight, symptoms can improve significantly after reconstruction surgery.

3. LASHES

Next I examine the lashes, looking for discharge, aberrant growth, trichiasis (eyelashes growing toward the eyeball), lash ptosis (straightening of lashes), or distichiasis (an extra row of lashes). Crusting indicates bacterial infections. Cylindrical deposits suggest demodex mites. I may find the residue of artificial tears or cosmetics adhering to the lashes.

4. PALPEBRAL AND BULBAR CONJUNCTIVA

With the patient's eyes in an upward gaze, I evert the lower lid to examine the inferior palpebral and bulbar conjunctiva tissues. (The bulbar conjunctiva is the transparent tissue that covers the white part of the eye; the palpebral conjunctiva covers the inner lining of the eyelid that touches the eye.) They should be smooth and free of inflammation and scarring. The bulbar tissue should be colorless and the palpebral tissue should be slightly pink.

5. FORNIX

With the lower lid still everted, I ask the patient to look higher so I can check the lower fornix for foreign bodies, mucus strands, and other abnormalities. Sometimes patients have loose eyelashes in the fornix that can cause foreign-body sensations. I may find symblepharon (fibrotic adhesion of the palpebral conjunctiva to the bulbar conjunctiva), a foreshortened fornix (a fornix with reduced depth) as can be seen in ocular cicatricial pemphigoid, or a tissue reaction indicating infections or allergies.

6. PUNCTUM

I check if the lower punctum is apposed to the eyeball and tear lake or everted. The punctum may be open, closed, stenotic (narrowed), or have a plug inserted. I push in the nasolacrimal sac on the side of the nose, checking for discharge from the puncta, which could be a sign of dacryocystitis or canaliculitis. Inserted deep in the canal, patients sometimes have "smart plugs," a type of punctal plug that may be visible under transillumination (lighting tissue from behind to reveal the plug).

7. PLICA SEMILUNARIS AND CARUNCLE

If the plica semilunaris, the semilunar fold of conjunctival tissue at the inner corner of the eye, or the caruncle, the ball of tissue, are scarred, they may appear flattened as seen in ocular cicatricial pem-

phigoid or other cicatrizing diseases, such as previous viral infection, chemical or thermal injury, and Stevens-Johnson syndrome.

8. SUPERIOR EYEBALL AND LID EXAM

The patient looks down. I raise the upper lid and proceed with
the same examination superiorly, examining the upper lid margin,
lashes, superior punctum, bulbar conjunctiva, cornea, and the superior limbus for evidence of superior limbic keratoconjunctivitis
(SLK, redness, filaments, and erosions). I may find conjunctivochalasis or subconjunctival orbital fat prolapse in the superior temporal quadrants. Subject to friction from the movement of the upper
lid, the superior conjunctival tissue can be loose, redundant, and
inflamed.

I release the lid. While the patient looks down, I lightly mobilize the upper lids, without applying significant pressure, over the
superior part of the eyeball to test if symptoms can be re-created or
increased, suggesting the abnormal tissue is a likely causative factor
of this symptom.

Next, I evert the upper lid and inspect for redness, foreign bodies, and fibrotic tissue reactions suggestive of current or previous
infections and allergies, as well as microtrauma and growths.

9. CORNEA

Next I examine the cornea. A healthy cornea is clear, transparent,
and compact, without edema, inflammation, or growths.

10. INTERNAL STRUCTURES OF THE EYE

Then I examine the internal structures of the eye, including the
anterior chamber, iris, pupil, lens, and posterior segment, including
the retina and optic nerve, for abnormalities.

Vital Dye Staining

Next, I check the ocular surface for defects and assess tear film stability. I place a drop of sterile saline on a strip of paper saturated

with fluorescein dye, evert the lower lid, and let the drop of saline, now suffused with dye, land in the inferior fornix.

The fluorescein stain reveals any epithelial cell defects on the surface of the eye and on the lid wiper of the everted lid. Each staining pattern indicates a specific problem. (Decoding these patterns is beyond the scope of this book.) Occasionally I use rose bengal stain to reveal dead and devitalized cells lacking mucin, or lissamine green stain to reveal dead and degenerated cells.

After checking for surface defects, I ask the patient to blink five times, then keep the eyes open to test the tear breakup time (TBUT). I monitor the tear film and count the seconds before it breaks up. Tear film that breaks up in less than five seconds is unstable, usually indicating a lipid deficiency in the tear film and, less often, aqueous or mucin deficiency. The peaks and valleys of an irregular corneal surface will also lead to an unstable tear film because the tear film is thinner over elevated tissue, as with Salzmann's nodular degeneration.

Meibomian Glands

As part of a comprehensive evaluation of the Meibomian glands, I apply mild to moderate pressure with a sterile cotton swab to the eyelids just beyond the eyelashes, count the number of glands secreting meibum, and grade its quality. I also ask the patient to note any sore or tender spots. (Tenderness indicates elevated intraductal pressure from glands obstructed with periductal fibrosis.) An assisting technician records these findings on a Meibomian Gland Classification Form (MCF) provided by MGDi® (see fig. 9.1).

I anesthetize the ocular surface with a drop of tetracaine before administering this test, to ensure any tenderness is not emanating from the cornea or ocular surface but from obstructed glands in the lid.

The five attributes of meibum I record are as follows:

1. Clarity: Is the meibum clear or cloudy?
2. Fluidity: Is the meibum fluid? Is it thick or thin?
3. Color: Is the meibum colorless, amber, yellow, white, or pearl?
4. Particulate matter: Is there particulate matter suspended in the meibum?

5. Volume: In qualitative terms, is the overall volume of meibum expressed from the entire population of glands in the lid reduced or within normal ranges?

Healthy meibum is clear, thin, colorless to pale amber, and contains minimal particulate matter. With gently applied pressure, the secreted droplet should be at least approximately the diameter of an orifice, about 100 microns. Other variations may indicate some degree of MGD.

Next, I examine *the lids* for these *three indicators of gland obstruction.*

1. Lid tenderness in at least one-third of a lid
2. Four or less expressible glands in the lid
3. Visible obstruction at the orifice (pertinent when there is no lid tenderness and five or more glands are expressible)

Based on the indicators found, I assign a functional classification to each lid as a meibum-secreting unit. (The key indicators, for example, tenderness, may only impact a minority of glands, but clinically and for the purposes of classification, represent the status of the entire lid as a meibum-secreting unit.)

The functional classifications that I typically assign for each lid as a meibum-secreting unit are as follows (see also fig. 9.2):

1. Normal (not shown)
   - Five or more expressible glands
   - No tenderness (normal intraductal pressure)
2. PDO: Partial distal obstruction (not shown)
   - Visible threadlike keratin may be noted within the orifice (orifice metaplasia)
   - Five or more expressible glands
   - No tenderness because obstruction is partial and does not cause elevated intraductal pressure
3. PDO-NF: Partial distal obstruction–nonfunctional (not shown)
   - Visible threadlike keratin may be noted within the orifice (orifice metaplasia)

- Four or fewer expressible glands
- No tenderness because obstruction is partial and meibum is not being produced, as though the glands were dormant (observed in nearly a dozen cases of binge eating; see table 5.10 and sidebar 5.2)

4. CPO: Complete proximal obstruction
   - Five or more expressible glands
   - Tenderness due to increased intraductal pressure from blockage deeper within the gland

5. CPO-PA: Complete proximal obstruction–partial atrophy
   - Five or more expressible glands
   - Decreasing tenderness as meibum synthesis decreases behind the blockage
   - Truncated, short glands later visualized with infrared meibography and or transillumination

6. CDO: Complete distal obstruction
   - Four or fewer expressible glands
   - Tenderness due to increased intraductal pressure

7. CDO-NF: Complete distal obstruction–nonfunctional
   - Four or fewer expressible glands
   - Decreasing tenderness as meibum synthesis decreases behind the blockage

Whole gland atrophy (WGA) can be diagnosed later with transillumination or infrared meibography.

MCF information is qualitative and helps to explain and summarize exam findings. For example, expressible meibum with a tender lid suggests occult obstruction with elevated intraductal pressure deeper within the gland, beyond at least the first acinus. A lack of expressible glands with a tender lid suggests complete obstruction between the orifice and the first acinus with elevated intraductal pressure (see sidebar 9.12).

As an example, the patient's MCF (fig. 9.1) shows the left upper lid had eight glands that were expressible with the application of moderate pressure. The expressed meibum was generally cloudy, amber-colored, had a thick consistency, and contained particulate matter. The volume of meibum expressed was normal. The patient reported lid tenderness as I pressed on the lids to express the glands.

A *healthy* Meibomian gland synthesizes and secretes meibum freely and adequately. If five or more glands in a lid are expressible and there is no lid tenderness (suggesting a lack of complete obstruction), the lid has adequate meibum secreting functionality (the lid produces sufficient oil necessary for tear film) and the diagnostic classification for the lid is within *normal* limits.

For classifying the Meibomian gland disease states, lid tenderness is an important finding. In our classification, lid tenderness was considered positive when at least one-third of a lid was tender to mild or moderate pressure. *Complete proximal obstruction* (CPO) and the buildup of meibum behind the obstruction leads to an increase of intraductal pressure, which causes lid tenderness and *cystic changes to acini* deeper within the glands. If not released with probing, elevated pressure can lead to *atrophy* of the affected acinar-ductular units, known as *complete proximal obstruction with partial atrophy* (CPO-PA). CPO is the lid's diagnosis when there are five or more expressible glands and at least one-third of the lid is tender. Truncated glands due to partial atrophy may be confirmed later with meibography.

Complete distal obstruction (CDO), characterized by obstruction somewhere between the orifice and the first acinus, increases intraductal pressure behind the obstruction, causing lid tenderness. A lid with four or fewer expressible glands and tenderness in at least one-third of the lid is diagnosed as CDO.

If not released with probing, elevated pressure can lead to *cystic changes to acini* within the entire gland and a *di-*

lated duct. The gland then stops synthesizing meibum, becomes a nonfunctional gland (CDO-NF), and lid tenderness gradually diminishes. A lid with four or fewer expressible glands and no lid tenderness is diagnosed as CDO-NF.

Over time the entire complex of acini along the length of a duct with CDO may atrophy, known as *whole gland atrophy* (WGA). If the orifice is visible, the duct generally remains intact. Because the acini no longer synthesize meibum, there is no expressible meibum and no lid tenderness. WGA can be confirmed later with meibography. (See fig. 9.2 for the diagnostic classification of lids just mentioned.)

Not shown in fig. 9.2, *partial distal obstruction* (PDO), is characterized by partial obstruction possibly due to orifice squamous metaplasia and/or mildly constricting occult periductal fibrosis. A lid with five or more expressible glands and no elevated intraductal pressure, therefore no lid tenderness, is diagnosed as PDO.

Also not shown, *partial distal obstruction–nonfunctional* (PDO-NF) differs from CDO-NF in that patients with PDO-NF have a history of binge eating episodes with possible insulin resistance and elevated blood sugar. The glands appear to be in a dormant state. When normal eating resumes, the glands resume their normal function and return to PDO.

Because there were more than five expressible glands and lid tenderness, my diagnosis for the lid was complete proximal obstruction (CPO). On the other hand, the diagnosis I gave for the patient's right upper lid was complete distal obstruction (CDO), because there were fewer than five expressible glands (four in this case), and the patient reported tenderness while I pressed on the lids. Not enough meibum was expressible to evaluate its quality.

MGD₁ *(MGD1)*

MEIBOMIAN GLAND CLASSIFICATION FORM

Name: ▮▮▮▮▮▮▮▮▮▮

Previously Probed   Yes   (No)   Date: 02/21/2020

RIGHT UPPER LID

# Expressible Glands	4		
Expressibility	Mild		Moderate
Clarity	Clear		Cloudy
Color	Clear	Pearl	White
	Amber		Yellow
Consistency	Thin	Thick	Ribbon
Particulate Matter	Yes		No
Volume	↓	Normal	↑
Tenderness	(Yes)	No	See VAS

Diagnosis: CDO

LEFT UPPER LID

# Expressible Glands	8		
Expressibility	Mild		(Moderate)
Clarity	Clear		(Cloudy)
Color	Clear	Pearl	White
	(Amber)		Yellow
Consistency	Thin	(Thick)	Ribbon
Particulate Matter	(Yes)		No
Volume	↓	(Normal)	↑
Tenderness	(Yes)	No	See VAS

Diagnosis: CPO

RIGHT LOWER LID

# Expressible Glands	3		
Expressibility	Mild		Moderate
Clarity	Clear		Cloudy
Color	Clear	Pearl	White
	Amber		Yellow
Consistency	Thin	Thick	Ribbon
Particulate Matter	Yes		No
Volume	↓	Normal	↑
Tenderness	Yes	(No)	See VAS

Diagnosis: CDO – NF

Other Details: _____

LEFT LOWER LID

# Expressible Glands	15		
Expressibility	Mild		(Moderate)
Clarity	(Clear)		Cloudy
Color	Clear	Pearl	White
	(Amber)		Yellow
Consistency	Thin	(Thick)	Ribbon
Particulate Matter	Yes		(No)
Volume	↓	(Normal)	↑
Tenderness	Yes	(No)	See VAS

Diagnosis: PDO

Other Details: _____

Fig. 9.1. A Patient's Meibomian Gland Classification Form (MCF)

The MCF is used to record the number of Meibomian glands per lid that are expressible, meibum quality (clarity, color, consistency, and particulate matter), volume, and lid tenderness. The number of expressible glands and lid-tenderness findings provide a basis for each lid's diagnosis: CDO, CPO, etc.

Source: Courtesy of Steven L. Maskin, MD.

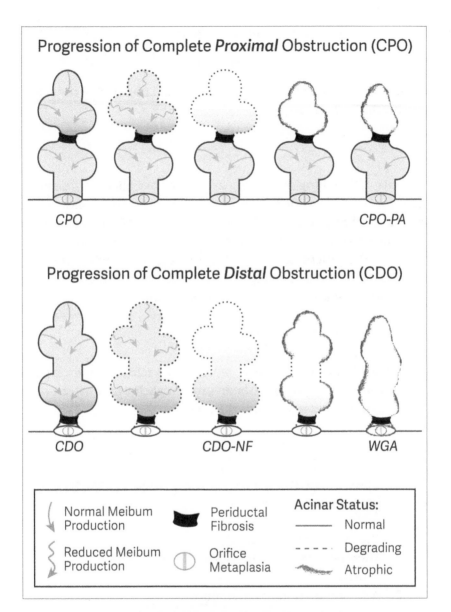

**Fig. 9.2. The Diagnostic Classification of Lids
with Meibomian Gland Dysfunction**

The diagnostic classification of lids with MGD, showing two routes of disease progression in a gland. Complete proximal obstruction (CPO) develops deeper than the first acinus of a Meibomian gland and leads to partial atrophy (CPO-PA). Complete distal obstruction (CDO) develops at the orifice or before the first acinus of a gland, leading to a nonfunctional gland (CDO-NF) and eventually to whole gland atrophy (WGA).

Source: Adapted by permission from BMJ Publishing Group Limited. From Steven L. Maskin and Whitney R. Testa, "Growth of Meibomian Gland Tissue After Intraductal Meibomian Gland Probing in Patients with Obstructive Meibomian Gland Dysfunction," *British Journal of Ophthalmology* 102, no. 1 (2018), 59–68.

Other Tests

Depending on a patient's symptoms or what I find during the exam, I may administer more tests.

ALLERGIES

Patients with itching or burning eyes may have allergies. To aid diagnosis, I perform a quick allergy test by placing a drop of fast-acting topical antihistamine in each eye. If within two minutes, and often just thirty seconds, these symptoms markedly diminish or disappear, it's likely the patient has an allergic component to their symptoms. (I evaluate for allergies before administering the anesthetic drops in preparation for Meibomian gland classification.)

INTRAOCULAR PRESSURE

I check the intraocular pressure, which if elevated can indicate glaucoma. After placing an anesthetic drop in each eye, I use an ophthalmic tonometer to measure the pressure.

FLUORESCEIN CLEARANCE TEST

The fluorescein clearance test (FCT) measures aqueous tear secretions under three different conditions:

1. The eye is anesthetized
2. After the anesthetic has worn off and sensation has returned
3. With stimulation of nasal mucosa

FCT also tests the eye's ability to clear irritants from the tear film.

First, I anesthetize each eye with one drop of tetracaine. Once anesthetized, I blot the fornices with a cotton-tipped applicator to prevent false negative results. Then, using a micropipette, I place 5 microliters of Altafluor Benox, 0.25% fluorescein sodium with 0.4% benoxinate hydrochloride (another anesthetizing agent), into the inferior fornices. After ten minutes, a Schirmer filter paper wetting strip is bent and hung over the lower lid margin of each eye at the junction of the outer and central third of the lower lid. The strips are left there for precisely one minute, then removed. The distance moisture traveled along the strips is recorded. Wetting less than 3 millimeters indicates ATD.

Ten minutes later (when the anesthetic has worn off) another strip is placed over the lid margin of each eye. After one minute, the strips are removed and the level of wetness is recorded again. As before, wetting less than 3 millimeters indicates ATD. Cobalt-blue light shined from a flashlight reveals any residual fluorescein dye on the strips, indicating delayed tear clearance, the eye's inability to remove irritants effectively.

Finally, if testing suggests ATD, then ten minutes later, a cotton thread extending from the end of a cotton-tipped applicator is placed just inside the patient's nostril, on the side with the lower Schirmer's test result, against the mucosal tissue to stimulate tears, while a final wetting strip hangs over the lid margin of each eye. After one minute, the strips are removed and the level of wetness is compared to the previous strips. If the patient produces no tears with nasal stimulation beyond what was produced previously, the result suggests severe ATD as seen with Sjögren's syndrome.

I test both eyes and may find one eye is dryer than the other.

SERIAL SCHIRMER'S TEST WITH ANESTHESIA

At the first visit, I administer the FCT to evaluate aqueous tear production and delayed tear clearance. At follow-up visits, if I need to evaluate tear volume, I usually administer the Schirmer's test with an anesthetic eye drop. For my patients, the serial Schirmer's test has been an important and sensitive indicator of aqueous deficiency that I have used for over two decades in my practice. (Some physicians forgo the Schirmer's test, using instead newer tests, such as osmolarity and MMP-9. Because these other tests are nonspecific, they are of limited value for my patients; see "Other Diagnostics.")

I may repeat the test several times (hence *serial* Schirmer's test) in immediate succession to avoid false negative readings, meaning even though the disease exists, the test does not register it. (Many patients have come to me for a second or even tenth opinion, after being told they had normal watery tear production according to Schirmer's test results. Then, when I tested them using the *serial* Schirmer's test, I found ATD.)

Sidebar 9.13
Serial Schirmer's Test Reveals Aqueous Deficiency

This story adapted from my previous book, *Reversing Dry Eye Syndrome,* illustrates the high sensitivity (ability to correctly identify the presence of a disease) of the serial Schirmer's test.

Matthew was a forty-five-year-old electrician suffering with many symptoms of ATD, especially scratchiness and a grainy sensation experienced throughout the day. Convinced he had Dry Eye, he saw several doctors who examined his eyes and ran a standard Schirmer's test. Each of these doctors found that his eyes were normal. Still, Matthew experienced severe eye pain. Over-the-counter drops gave him no relief, and he remained convinced he had Dry Eye.

Finally, a friend recommended that he see me. Matthew's description of his symptoms and my examination led me to believe he had ATD. To confirm my hypothesis I administered a Schirmer's test with anesthesia, already thinking I might have to administer serial tests because of Matthew's history of normal Schirmer's test results. As I anticipated, the first test did not indicate ATD. So while the eyes were still anesthetized, I immediately administered a second test, taking extra precautions to minimize reflex tearing by testing only one eye at a time. This second round of tests revealed inadequate aqueous tear production in each eye, confirming my original hypothesis.

To retain his tears and improve comfort, I cauterized his tear drainage ducts with superficial punctal occlusion. Today he is pain-free.

Table 9.1
Serial Schirmer's Test

Test Strip Number	Test Result	Action	Diagnosis
1	>10mm	Repeat test.	Inconclusive
2 through X[a]	>10mm, but less than the previous test	Repeat test. Stop when the result plateaus or increases.	There is no ATD if test result never drops below 10mm.
Any	<10mm	Stop testing.	ATD

[a]X is the number of the subsequent test.

For the test, one anesthetizing drop of tetracaine is placed in each inferior fornix. The patient closes the eyes for thirty seconds or until irritation from the anesthetic drop stops, indicating the anesthetic has taken effect. The fornices are blotted with a cotton-tipped applicator, and a Schirmer's strip is hung over the lower lid margin of each eye. After five minutes, the strips are removed and the distance moisture traveled is recorded. Any result less than 10 millimeters suggests ATD.

To minimize altering test results due to reflex tearing, I may test only one eye at a time. In fact, if the FCT results are contrary to what I expect, I will administer the serial Schirmer's test on one eye at a time.

If I suspect the patient has ATD but the first Schirmer's test result was greater than 10mm, I retest.

As long as subsequent Schirmer's tests have a value lower than the previous test, but greater than 10mm, I retest until the value increases, plateaus, or drops below 10 millimeters, revealing ATD. As with the FCT, I may find that one eye is dryer than the other and may need to retest only one eye.

If the first or any repeat test result falls below 10mm, I conclude the patient has ATD and there is no need for further testing.

Microbiology Workup

Depending on what I see during any part of the exam, I may test for microbes on the lashes, lid margins, or conjunctiva.

If I suspect demodex mites, I check for telltale cylindrical deposits at the base of the eyelashes, epilate a few of those lashes, and examine them under a desktop pathology microscope. If I don't find deposits (the mites don't always leave them), I may remove several random lashes for examination under the microscope. With magnification, live mites can sometimes be seen wiggling their limbs. I let patients who show interest look at the mites through the microscope themselves.

If I suspect a bacterial infection, I may culture the lashes, lid margin, and conjunctiva. I take samples with a sterile cotton swab dipped in trypticase soy broth (TSB), a growth-enhancing medium, and incubate the culture at 37 degrees Celsius in the office. If something grows, the sample is shipped to an outside lab to identify the strain of bacteria and determine which antibiotic will be most effective, that is, the antibiotic sensitivity. (While waiting for the lab's definitive results, I may start the patient on a broad-spectrum antibiotic ophthalmic ointment and/or topical drops.)

Infrared Meibography

Infrared meibography reveals the anatomy of the entire Meibomian gland population of an everted lid. The patient sits at a Mediworks S390L WDR FireFly Digital Slit Lamp from Eyefficient (Aurora, Ohio), a device that has a color video camera with an infrared filter. After anesthetic drops are placed in the eyes, I evert the lid to do the meibography.

Viewing the captured meibography video, I look for any signs of Meibomian gland abnormalities. The glands may be distorted. The ducts may be dilated, suggestive of elevated intraductal pressure. I may see cystic changes (that is, ballooning out) in the acini or evidence of acinar-ductular atrophy. Atrophy may be distal, close to the orifice at the lid margin, or proximal, at the far end of the gland, creating a truncated or shortened gland. Atrophy may be discontinuous with a segment of the gland absent, suggesting focal atrophic

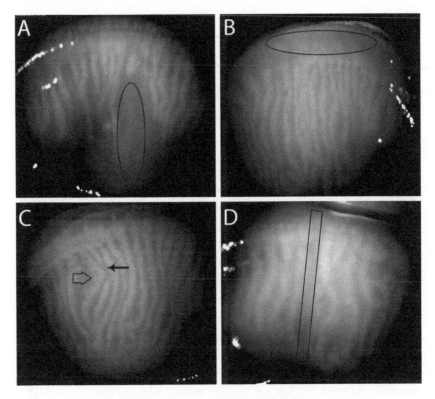

Fig 9.3. Types of Gland Atrophy

Four upper lids (A, B, C, D) with different types of gland atrophy visible with infrared meibography.

A. Truncated glands with acinar-ductular units closest to the fornix missing (vertical oval), called proximal gland atrophy.

B. Acinar-ductular units missing near the lid margin, called distal gland atrophy.

C. A focal segment of acinar-ductular unit dropout in the middle of a gland (black arrow), which creates a discontinuous gland. A tortuous gland (open arrow) showing ballooning cystic changes of acinar-ductular units.

D. A completely atrophied gland without acinar-ductular units along its entire length, called whole gland atrophy (WGA). The duct channel may still be present but not visible without the surrounding clusters of acini along its length.

Source: Courtesy of Steven L. Maskin, MD.

acinar-ductular units. Or the entire gland may be atrophic, called whole gland atrophy.

Meibography can reveal tortuosity of the glands, meaning that rather than aligning parallel to each other, they bend and twist randomly. Bent and twisted Meibomian glands are common with chronic inflammatory diseases such as allergic blepharoconjuncti-vitis. I have hypothesized that chronic inflammation weakens peri-glandular support tissue, allowing gravitational forces to affect gland anatomy. Because the gland is anchored to the lid margin at its ori-fice, gravity may tug on the rest of the gland, leading to microscopic rotations, twists, and tortuosity.

Confocal Microscopy

The confocal microscope enables evaluation of Meibomian gland ducts at the cellular level, up to about 150 microns deep. It can reveal periductal fibrosis, inflammation, and atrophic changes of the distal excretory duct, which is likely to indicate similar changes deeper within. (Suspected fibrosis deeper within can be confirmed later with Maskin® Probing; see chapter 11.)

I use a Heidelberg Engineering HRT3 Rostock Cornea Module (RCM) confocal microscope to examine the distal duct area. The pa-tient sits in an office chair looking down, and the microscope is di-rected to a gland orifice on the upper lid margin. The orifice lumen (the main channel through which meibum flows) is checked for internal stricture formation. It may be wide open, closed, partially collapsed, or clogged. Loss of ductal integrity with periductal fibro-sis and sometimes fibrovascular growth onto the external duct wall and invasion through it can be noted. Then the microscope is di-rected toward the palpebral conjunctival surface to evaluate acinar epithelium.

Periductal fibrosis, appearing like a sheet, an organized circum-ferential scar, or a flattening or scalloping of the normally oval-to-round external duct wall, is nearly ubiquitous at this microscopic level, visible in most of my patients with MGD (see fig. 4.1).

Other Diagnostics

The FDA has approved other devices for diagnosing Dry Eye that give insight into tear film. However, except for lipid interferome-try, these tests are relatively nonspecific and of limited use in my practice.

TEAR OSMOLARITY

The TearLab® Osmolarity System is a device used to aid the diagnosis of Dry Eye. A small amount of tear film is collected from the outer corner of the eyes for analysis. The higher the osmolarity, or concentration of "salts" in the sample, the lower the aqueous tear volume. Some doctors use osmolarity to monitor the ongoing status of Dry Eye, for example, if osmolarity goes up, Dry Eye may be getting worse.

Unfortunately, the test does not differentiate between causes of increased osmolarity, such as ATD and evaporative Dry Eye. There is also a question about the reproducibility of test results, and at least one study showed normal eyes with elevated osmolarity.

MMP-9 ENZYME TEST

InflammaDry® tests for the MMP-9 enzyme, an inflammatory marker found in tear film. A sample is collected from the inferior palpebral conjunctiva and placed in a test cassette for ten minutes. A positive test result, indicated by a red line no matter how faint, suggests an inflammatory cause of Dry Eye. However, the test does not specify the source of the inflammation (for example, within the Meibomian glands, on the ocular surface), or its cause (for example, an allergy or ATD).

LIPID INTERFEROMETRY

Interferometers take measurements of targets by shining beams of light that interfere with each other, enabling the measurement of the average thickness of the tear film lipid layer and its spreadability. This information can be used when diagnosing and managing MGD. (The TearScience® LipiView® Ocular Surface Interferometer also evaluates the completeness of blinks during the 20-second interval when it measures the lipid layer.)

Step 5: Comprehensive Working Diagnosis

Once I have a complete picture—I've talked to the patient, reviewed the medical history, examined the patient's eyes, administered tests, and interpreted the results—I arrive at a comprehensive working diagnosis. At this point, the comorbidities and cofactors underlying and explaining the patient's symptoms fit together like a mosaic.

I review and explain to the patient the pertinent exam findings and test results and show how these led me to the list of working hypotheses. I then tie everything back to the patient's symptoms.

With the diagnosis established, or usually diagnoses, we move on to discussing treatment options and their priorities. Sometimes in acute cases, if patients have traveled long distances to see me, or if they're in so much pain that they're having suicidal thoughts or begging me to remove their eyes, treatment starts immediately. For these patients, relief from painful, debilitating symptoms is paramount.

For treatment, I focus first on abnormalities in the three major systems—aqueous tears, meibum and Meibomian glands, and the ocular surface tissue—while immediately treating infections or allergies. Administering effective treatments for diseases in these three systems can provide immediate and dramatic improvements in symptoms, vision, and ocular surface health. This diagnostic and treatment approach has proven to be uniformly successful for my patients for decades.

Step 6: Definitive Diagnosis

When patients return for follow-up appointments, I review their symptoms, examine their eyes, and assess the effects of treatment. Treatment that succeeds indicates that the working diagnosis was accurate. If not, I reevaluate. I may need to return to step 2, delving further into the patient's medical history, which may reveal a missed comorbidity or cofactor. Sometimes treatment isn't effective because patients aren't compliant with at-home therapies. Sometimes they adopt habits that can be detrimental, like the patient who decided to irrigate her eyes with tap water from the showerhead instead of using preservative-free vials of sterile saline solution (see sidebar 10.11, "Don't Use the Tap Water!"), or the patient who administered drops by letting them slide down his nonsterile eyelid into the eye rather than dropping them directly into the fornix behind his lower lid.

Sidebar 9.14
Ocular Neuropathic Pain, Part 2:
Diagnosis or Misdiagnosis?

A mismatch in signs and symptoms can prompt a diagnosis of ocular or corneal neuropathic pain, emanating from the peripheral or central nervous system. The patient typically feels burning pain or other severe discomfort, but the doctor sees little to no signs and finds no cause for the pain. Ocular neuropathic pain is sometimes called "pain without stain" because even vital staining reveals no abnormalities accounting for the patient's pain.

The diagnosis of neuropathic pain is considered a diagnosis of exclusion, reached by the process of elimination, ruling out every other possibility. This requires a rigorous evaluation, ensuring there are no occult diseases at the core of these patients' symptoms.

I believe neuropathic pain is overdiagnosed. In thirty-plus years, I have seen many Dry Eye patients who had received neuropathic pain diagnoses from eye doctors all over the world, those in private practice and those working in departments of ophthalmology at major universities. In fact these patients that came to me for help were suffering with nociceptive pain. My rigorous examinations, including tests that elicited symptoms to re-create the patient's chief complaint, indicated nonobvious and occult diseases. These patients had highly sensitized ocular surface nerves from inadequately treated ocular surface diseases. With targeted treatment, their pain diminished significantly and often vanished.

Some doctors use confocal microscopes to examine corneal nerves in patients suspected of having neuropathic pain, suggesting abnormal nerves observed under the microscope indicate the condition. However, there are many discrepancies and inconsistencies reported with this test.

Some doctors test for ocular neuropathic pain by placing anesthetic drops in the eyes, believing pain that persists in the anesthetized eyes definitively indicates neuropathic pain. I disagree with this approach for several reasons.

First, anesthetizing drops do not penetrate the eyelid tissue or reach the Meibomian glands and eliminate symptoms emanating from them. Next, because the external parts of the eye are near one another, a patient may misidentify the location of pain resistant to anesthetizing drops. What seems like corneal or surface pain, for example, may instead emanate from the lids or Meibomian glands where sensory nerve endings are found around their ducts and acini. Furthermore, I have found that hypersensitized nerves, irritated for weeks, months, or years by MGD, ATD, and other comorbidities, may not respond to an anesthetizing agent but can respond to targeted treatment. Thus, anesthetic drops may not eliminate deep-seated nociceptive pain on the ocular surface. Finally, the test may be flawed because anesthetic drops can lose potency in as little as three weeks if left at room temperature, rendering inconclusive test results.

There may be patients who do suffer with true neuropathic pain, but in my opinion, they would be exceedingly rare. Even so, I believe the existing diagnostic or established tests are inconclusive. For an indisputable definitive diagnosis of ocular neuropathic pain, we need better, more specific tests. For now, simple awareness that various diseases of the ocular surface can cause painful, debilitating, and severe nociceptive symptoms that respond poorly to anesthetic drops should trigger doctors to perform rigorous diagnostic evaluation.

Haunted by an "Ocular Neuropathy" Diagnosis

A patient who found me after being misdiagnosed with ocular neuropathic pain retells her story.

By 2019 the relentless searing, burning pain in my eyes forced me to put my life on hold. Having seen two other ophthalmologists whose treatments offered no relief, I found a third one. This one prescribed five different oral and topical medications and instructed me to apply warm compresses to my eyes twice a day. Instead of improving, my symptoms grew worse (I couldn't even keep my eyes open unless they were directly over a humidifier), leading the doctor to conclude my problem was ocular neuropathy. He explained that my ocular nerves were damaged and stuck in a feedback loop, signaling pain without an actual underlying cause. He recommended scleral contact lenses to heal the nerves and stop the pain.

I was skeptical. I had entrusted my eyes to this doctor wholeheartedly at first. But now, five months later, he refused to consider any other possibilities. I researched scleral contact lenses and learned they would be expensive and might be difficult to fit, plus there were no guarantees they would help. While researching the lenses, I found information about Dr. Steven Maskin and Meibomian glands. Could these glands be the problem, and would they benefit from probing?

No, the doctor insisted, Meibomian gland dysfunction was not the cause of my pain. My Meibomian glands were expressible and therefore, he reasoned, mostly open. Instead, my ocular surface nerves, autonomously signaling pain, were the problem.

Because of the pain, I started keeping my eyes closed

for long stretches. It was a difficult time for me and my family. Because my grandmother was blind for the second half of her life, my family had experience adjusting life for someone with vision loss. So they began preparing for me to live life with my eyes mostly closed, using dictation software to read and write. But I wasn't prepared to accept this fate, and neither was my family.

My mother and I decided to travel to Tampa, Florida, to seek out Dr. Maskin for yet another opinion. After a thorough examination, he diagnosed combined tear deficiency—both ATD and MGD—and conjunctivochalasis. When he probed my Meibomian glands, he found about 90 percent constricted with scar tissue. Within a day of probing, the searing, burning pain disappeared. He later cauterized my tear ducts and performed AMT surgery [see chapter 10].

I came to realize that warm compresses had not helped, because my Meibomian glands had been obstructed. My previous doctor had only been expressing oil produced near the openings of my glands. Deeper within, invisible to the doctor, the glands were obstructed.

Although today I lead a pain-free, normal, and very busy life, I am haunted by the ocular neuropathy diagnosis. Not only did it disrupt my income and career as an art historian, my efforts to come to terms with a life filled with constant, searing pain and limited eye use also triggered profound anxiety and depression, which I am still processing. Given the extreme pain I had been in, and on the verge of losing hope of ever finding help, I was facing a bleak future. Dr. Maskin's treatment saved my life in its broadest sense, my physical and mental well-being, my relationships with friends and family, and my rewarding career.

Ruthie Dibble, PhD

10

Treating Meibomian Gland Dysfunction and Comorbidities

Myth
*All patients respond well to commonly
prescribed treatments for MGD.*
Facts
*Unless comorbidities are addressed effectively, MGD patients
may continue to suffer with symptoms despite treatment.
Commonly prescribed treatments are often ineffective, or only
partially effective, because they don't target the periductal
fibrosis found in the vast majority of glands with MGD.*

TREATMENT STRATEGY

Honed over thirty-plus years of clinical practice, my approach to the treatment of Dry Eye, MGD, and ocular surface disease is

- individualized for each patient
- targeted at specific identified diseases
- prioritized for maximum effectiveness and efficiency

I aim to administer therapies that produce the greatest results and give the most relief in the shortest time frame. When I find diseases, I generally treat them in the order listed as follows. However,

I adjust this general treatment approach according to each individual patient's comorbidities and symptoms. In fact, I often start most patients on multiple therapies simultaneously and always treat allergies and infections at once. Of course, an acute or vision-threatening disease, such as corneal ulcer or perforation, acute glaucoma, or retinal detachment, will take priority.

PRIORITIZING TREATMENTS

1. Aqueous tear deficiency (ATD)
2. Ocular surface abnormalities
3. Meibomian gland dysfunction (MGD)
4. Allergies and sensitivities
5. Anterior blepharitis and conjunctivitis
6. Floppy lid and other abnormal eyelid mechanics
7. Lagophthalmos
8. Eyelash irritants
9. Delayed tear clearance (DTC)
10. Blepharospasm
11. Rosacea
12. Side effects from systemic medications
13. Systemic diseases

Treating common comorbidities associated with the three major systems—aqueous tears, ocular surface, Meibomian glands and meibum—as well as allergies, infections, and altered lid mechanics, including lagophthalmos, often resolves up to 90 percent or more of a patient's symptoms.

Although new treatments may be available one day, in this chapter I discuss the treatments I routinely use in my practice today. These treatments can quickly and consistently make an enormous difference for someone suffering with Dry Eye and MGD.

See chapter 12 for personal hygiene, behavioral, nutritional, and environmental tips that can provide additional help with symptoms.

1. AQUEOUS TEAR DEFICIENCY (ATD)

Because tear film volume plays such an important role in eye comfort, ocular surface health, and quality of vision, I address it first when aqueous tear deficiency (ATD) is present. Treatments range from over-the-counter artificial tears and prescription drops to in-office procedures and outpatient surgery.

Often by the time they first see me, my patients have already tried many treatments, for example, lubricating, anti-inflammatory, immunosuppressant, and blood-product drops, or punctal plugs, but have had inadequate or insufficient improvement in symptoms. So once I've established that they have persistent ATD, I move on to other treatments for increasing aqueous tear volume, such as punctal occlusion using thermal cautery, amniotic membrane transplant surgery, and secretagogues (medications that stimulate moisture-producing glands).

Over-the-Counter Artificial Tears

Artificial tears are over-the-counter supplements or replacements for natural tears. They work palliatively to reduce symptoms and improve comfort, rather than treat and reverse a condition like ATD. New drops occasionally find their way to the market, adding to the dizzying array of drops already available today.

Artificial tears are not perfect replacements for natural tear film, because they contain only some minerals and elements found in natural tears and, unlike tear film, they do not replenish continuously.

Some artificial tears contain oils that substitute for the secreted meibum of patients with lipid deficiency. Some contain a viscosity-enhancing cellulose compound that helps with moisture retention and adherence to the eye's mucous membrane. The higher the concentration of this cellulose compound, usually hydroxypropyl methylcellulose or carboxymethylcellulose, the longer the drop tends to remain in the eyes. Eye drops containing these compounds can leave a gooey, sticky residue in the eyes and eyelashes. If the drops cause irritation, try drops with a lower concentration of these ingredients, clean lashes thirty minutes after use with water, or avoid cellulose compounds altogether.

Preservatives in artificial tears can irritate and can cause inflammation. Over time, patients may become sensitized to them or experience toxic reactions. Benzalkonium chloride, a preservative commonly found in lubricating and other eye drops, can cause toxicity and eventual corneal melting. Therefore, it's always best to avoid eye drops with preservatives, especially for long-term use.

Generally, preservative-free artificial tears are safe to use up to four times per day. But using them more often, and not just temporarily, can cause irritation, dilute and wash out important components of the natural tear film, and suggests a need for more advanced therapies.

If ATD is due to a side effect from a medication taken for a short term, such as BENADRYL® or another antihistamine for an acute allergy, I prescribe preservative-free artificial tears for the duration of the treatment, instruct the patient to use them frequently, and monitor the outcome closely. In these short-term cases, frequent use of artificial tears can prevent friction-induced inflammation of the ocular surface due to transient ATD.

Some patients may not tolerate one, or sometimes any, type of artificial tear.

Immunosuppressant and Anti-Inflammatory Topical Medications

Patients with aqueous tear deficiency may respond to treatment with topical medications that suppress the immune system. These medications are thought to increase tear production through improving lacrimal gland function by reducing inflammation. Patients who experience pain or other side effects from these medications should stop using the drops to avoid further aggravating already irritated nerves. Some doctors suggest storing drops in the refrigerator or using a concomitant topical steroid to limit irritation from the drops.

Cyclosporine

Prescription eye drops containing cyclosporine, an immunosuppressant used for years to prevent organ transplant rejection, is commonly prescribed for ATD. Patients are instructed to allow a six-month trial to evaluate efficacy, a long time, particularly for a patient with debilitating eye pain.

Restasis®, approved by the FDA in 2003, contains 0.05% cyclosporine in a solution containing glycerin and castor oil. The castor oil can be irritating to some patients. According to the product information sheet, Restasis was shown to increase Schirmer's scores 10 millimeters at six months in 15 percent of patients, compared to 5 percent in vehicle-treated patients. ("Vehicle" is the term for a liquid to which a medication is added. In this case, the vehicle is everything in the solution minus the cyclosporine.) Tear production did not improve in patients on Restasis using topical anti-inflammatory medications or punctal plugs.

Klarity-C Drops®, available since 2018 from the compounding pharmacy Imprimis, contains 0.1% cyclosporine, twice as much as Restasis, plus lubricants (dextran, glycerol, and hydroxypropyl methylcellulose) in a chondroitin sulfate emulsion. The compounding pharmacy can customize ingredients for each patient.

CEQUA™, another available cyclosporine treatment, contains 0.09% cyclosporine in a nanomicellar solution that delivers the active ingredient to the ocular surface without an emulsion.

Lifitegrast

Lifitegrast, the active ingredient in Xiidra®, though not a steroid, reduces inflammation through interrupting the inflammation cascade by decreasing inflammatory cell binding. The FDA has approved it for the treatment of Dry Eye. Patients use the drops twice a day, twelve hours between each dose.

Topical Steroid Drops

FLAREX®, PRED FORTE® (prednisolone acetate), and FML FORTE® suspensions are among the topical corticosteroid drops that doctors sometimes prescribe to treat the inflammation associated with ATD. However, I have not found topical steroid drops to be a good long-term solution for ATD, because use for longer than ten days can increase intraocular pressure and reduce the host's defense against microbes, while longer than a few months can cause or advance cataracts. If my aim is simply to reduce inflammation in the short term, I may prescribe a compounded preservative-free steroid for a short course of treatment while focusing on increasing tear volume with other treatments.

Punctal Occlusion

Punctal occlusion is a method for blocking tear outflow ducts. It prevents the outflow of tear film into the nose, keeping the tear film on the surface of the eye to increase tear volume. One technique involves placing a foreign body, usually a plug acting like a dam, directly into the tear punctum and duct. Another technique uses thermal cautery, laser, or other means to create a nonvisible scar that closes the punctum.

Punctal Plugs

Punctal plugs come in different shapes and sizes. They are usually made of silicone, but sometimes of slow-dissolving collagen. Although they can be easily inserted into the puncta by a doctor, the plugs have drawbacks.

For example, not all patients tolerate plugs. Even very small plugs can cause foreign-body sensations. Patients can have allergies or sensitivities to the plug material. The plugs can rub against the conjunctival tissue, causing trauma to the delicate surface tissue and reflex tearing that wells up and overflows to the lid and cheek. The plugs can harbor bacteria, increasing the risk of infection in the tear duct, known as canaliculitis, or in the nasolacrimal sac, known as dacryocystitis.

As with shoes, it might be hard to find a perfect fit. If the plugs are too small, tears can drain around them. If not secure, they can slip deep into the canal, where they can cause scarring and then be difficult to remove, sometimes requiring a surgical procedure. Often the plugs simply fall out. About 40 percent of the time, punctal plugs are lost.

Punctal Cautery

Punctal cautery, an effective alternative to punctal plugs, is an in-office procedure done with local anesthesia. After anesthetizing the area with either 4% topical lidocaine solution or an injection of 2% lidocaine with epinephrine, an electrical current running through a wire is applied to close the tear punctum. Cautery takes a split second and feels like a pinch, though the subsequent small scar is not felt. The patient applies antibiotic drops for about a week while the cautery site heals.

TOTAL, DEEP CAUTERY

Total, deep cautery blocks the punctum and canaliculus duct completely. It stops all tear outflow and is unlikely to reopen spontaneously. Afterward, if there are too many aqueous tears and epiphora, or tear overflow, the cautery may need to be reversed. But reversing deep cautery can be difficult, requiring the skills of an oculoplastic surgeon with experience in tear duct reconstruction.

SUPERFICIAL AND PARTIAL CAUTERY

Superficial cautery, meaning cautery that is shallow and near the surface, is the technique I prefer. It has worked very well for my patients, including those who tried punctal plugs without success. As with deep cautery, I can still close the duct completely, but later if tear volume becomes excessive, 90 percent of the time I can easily enlarge the opening in the office. (Before reversing the occlusion, I first rule out other causes of increased tear volume.)

Although superficial cautery can spontaneously open (recanalize), the opening is typically smaller than the original and can be reclosed easily if necessary. Unlike deep cautery, superficial cautery allows some control over the size of the opening to accommodate the volume of tears produced by each eye. For example, if a cauterized patient with excess tears blots their eyes every hour, I enlarge the opening. If a patient with a history of severe ATD blots three times a day or less, the opening is approximately the right size. I may increase it slightly to improve the patient's comfort, but not so much that the eyes become dry again. It's a question of finding a balance between a patient's comfort and tear production.

If the patient isn't blotting their eyes but still has symptoms, a repeat FCT or serial Schirmer's test can reveal persistent insufficient tear volume, the likely cause of those symptoms. If, however, the test shows adequate tear production, I look for different causes of the symptoms.

Sidebar 10.1
Pioneering Superficial Cautery:
An Innovative Breakthrough

About fifteen years ago, Sarah, a forty-year-old woman who had undergone LASIK more than a year earlier, arrived in my office complaining of reduced contrast sensitivity, with halos, and pain. Although her lower puncta had been totally closed, on examination her tear meniscus appeared inadequate. My preliminary finding was soon confirmed by a serial Schirmer's test that showed mild to moderate persistent ATD. Sarah was producing some aqueous tears, but not enough. She needed to retain more tear film in her eyes, but closing her upper puncta 100 percent with deep cautery would have caused irritating epiphora. Instead, I tried superficial cautery, achieving about 90 percent closure. Sarah's tear volume improved and her symptoms disappeared. I realized that controlling the size of the opening with superficial cautery—a breakthrough, innovative approach to treating ATD—could help many patients, and I have used it ever since.

Amniotic Membrane Transplant (AMT) Surgery

In 2007, I published a paper in the medical journal *Cornea* showing a trend toward increased tear volumes in patients with temporal conjunctivochalasis who had ocular surface reconstruction with amniotic membrane. I theorized that the improvement in measured tear volume could be related to improved tear flow across the surface of the eye toward the nose instead of being misdirected by chalasis toward the outer corner of the eye.

Because of its positive effect on tear volume, flow, and reduction of symptoms, I recommend AMT surgery to my patients for symptomatic conjunctivochalasis and persistent ATD (see "Frictional Disease" later in this chapter).

Secretagogues

Secretagogues are prescription oral medications that stimulate acetylcholine receptors in lacrimal glands and sweat glands, as well as vital tissues and organs in the cardiac, pulmonary, and gastrointestinal systems. The two most widely prescribed secretagogues are cevimeline, sold as Evoxac®, and pilocarpine, sold as Salagen®. These are commonly used by patients with Sjögren's syndrome to combat dry mouth because they also stimulate salivary glands.

Although both work well in a significant number of ATD patients, exactly who might benefit is difficult to predict. For example, patients with low tear volume who can produce emotional tears, indicating their lacrimal glands can synthesize tears, should benefit. But not all do.

On the downside, secretagogues can overstimulate glands causing excessive sweating and salivation, which may lead to drooling. They can also cause headaches, cardiac symptoms, intestinal cramps, and exacerbate asthma.

Because of the risk of side effects, before prescribing secretagogues, I obtain clearance from my patients' other medical doctors to ensure no contraindications.

Blood-Derived Eye Drops

Eye drops derived from blood are sometimes prescribed to patients with ATD. These eye drops are usually made from autologous (meaning the patient's own) serum or platelet rich plasma (PRP). Sometimes the drops are made from donated blood or donated umbilical-cord blood.

The blood is spun in a centrifuge to isolate various blood components, including growth and anti-inflammatory factors present in tear film but not found in commercial eye drops. The beneficial components are combined with a vehicle, such as a 0.9% sterile saline solution, to a desired concentration. Usually these drops are preservative-free and can be soothing without causing irritation. Because they do not contain preservatives, they are easily contaminated by microorganisms. They are expensive to produce and should be processed only under sterile conditions to ensure safety.

Although I sometimes prescribe blood-derived eye drops to my patients, I believe they are overprescribed. I consider them only for patients who have ATD despite 90 percent or greater closure of both upper and lower puncta, who had surgery to correct ocular surface defects such as symptomatic conjunctivochalasis, and have not benefited from topical treatment with cyclosporine or anti-inflammatories such as Xiidra, and treatment with secretagogues if they were candidates. In fact, patients who start using blood-derived eye drops before seeing me often stop or reduce their use after I initiate other targeted therapies.

Because some patients do benefit from autologous serum drops, I am licensed to prepare and dispense them in my office. I have a small lab with a sterile, certified hood where I spin blood and formulate the drops to a concentration usually between 20 and 50 percent. Batches of a patient's eye drops are separated into vials that they then store in their freezers. Thawed vials are refrigerated and, if necessary, carried in a portable cooler on ice packs. Once thawed, a vial lasts ten to fourteen days. Then it's discarded and replaced with a new vial. Drops that develop an odor or change color may have become contaminated while a patient was using them and should be discarded.

Stimulation of the Trigeminal Nerve

Stimulating the trigeminal sensory nerve triggers aqueous tear secretions. In fact, during the fluorescein clearance test for severe ATD (like that seen with Sjögren's syndrome), this nerve is stimulated by the cotton thread twirled inside the nose.

The iTear® 100 system is a neurostimulator device held against the side of the nose for about thirty seconds to stimulate the trigeminal nerve, which activates the parasympathetic nerve to trigger aqueous tear secretions. The most common side effects are headaches and dizziness in about 2–3 percent of patients. According to

Sidebar 10.2
Treatments in Development

This chapter and chapter 11 cover therapies available now that I use regularly to treat specific comorbidities with great results. Although I and my patients welcome advances in treatment, I see no reason to brush aside tried-and-true methods simply because a new treatment has hit the market, particularly if the treatment doesn't target comorbidities or its mechanism of action is not fully understood. (Note: This book does not include treatments available only outside the United States, since I have no access to them.)

Nevertheless, here are several products for Dry Eye, MGD, or related comorbidities recently released, in development, or undergoing clinical trials. How well they perform or whether they receive FDA approval, as of this writing, remains to be seen.

- CyclASol® water-free and preservative-free vehicle for cyclosporine from Novaliq. Currently in development.
- Eye Lipid Mobilizer™ resonant frequency to liquefy meibum, from Eyedetec. Currently in development.
- Anti-hyperkeratinization topical therapy, from Azura. Currently in phase-2 clinical trial.
- Lubricin drop for reducing surface friction, from Lubris BioPharma. Currently in phase-2 clinical trial.
- Tyrvaya™ acetylcholine nasal spray for neural stimulation of tears, from Oyster Point Pharma. Currently available.
- TP-03, topical treatment for demodex mites, from Tarsus. Currently in phase-3 clinical trial.

Sidebar 10.3
A Finger in Her Nose?

Years ago, a patient named Paula from California came to me for help with painful Dry Eye. When I walked into the exam room, she was holding her index finger inside her left nostril. Her chief complaint was a scratchy, sandy sensation in each eye despite using preservative-free lubricating eye drops with such frequency it was preventing participation in normal social activities.

I examined Paula and found a decreased tear meniscus and fluorescein vital dye staining of the nasal bulbar conjunctiva suggesting ATD. The first two conditions of a fluorescein clearance test showed an ATD pattern. During the third condition of the test, while Paula twirled a cotton swab just inside her nostril to produce aqueous tears, she had a revelation. That was why her eyes felt better when she put her finger in her nose. It made her eyes water.

Paula's treatment was straightforward. I performed superficial punctal cautery on the inferior puncta of both her eyes to increase tear volume. Finally, she could stop using artificial tears, keep her index finger out of her nose, and resume a normal life.

the iTear website, the device has been optimized to provide a safe amount of mechanical stimulation over a period of thirty days.

Scleral Lenses

Unlike a contact lens that covers primarily the cornea, a scleral lens covers both the cornea and a significant part of the sclera where it rests on the conjunctival tissue. Scleral lenses are made by several

---

Sidebar 10.4
Improving Symptoms, Building Trust

It is *extremely* important that patients experiencing significant psychosocial upheaval due to Dry Eye and MGD, experience a *significant reduction in symptoms soon* after their first visit. It is also important that these patients understand the causes of any residual symptoms and that a step-by-step, systematic approach to ongoing treatment typically provides additional relief incrementally and cumulatively. Going through this process restores hope even in those patients planning drastic measures to end their unbearable pain and unimaginable discomfort.

---

manufacturers. They can be expensive, must be fitted by a trained optometrist, and finding a comfortable pair can be difficult. As a rigid lens, a scleral lens can restore vision if the cornea surface is irregular.

Some scleral lenses have reservoirs for lubricating drops to bathe the cornea. These are used to treat severe ATD and cicatrizing conjunctivitis caused by ocular cicatricial pemphigoid and Stevens-Johnson syndrome.

Sometimes doctors prescribe scleral lenses to Dry Eye patients with chronic pain, often when the doctor can't find a treatment that provides relief or has diagnosed neuropathic pain (using what I believe is the inconclusive test described in chapter 9). In my experience, scleral lenses can be helpful but are widely overprescribed for Dry Eye pain management. Instead, I successfully manage many of these cases typically by looking for occult MGD and other insufficiently treated tear and ocular surface diseases.

2. OCULAR SURFACE ABNORMALITIES

A comfortable eye with optimal vision typically has a smooth, healthy surface without physical abnormalities. The fornix, the pouch behind the lower eyelid, should be the right depth—neither too shallow nor too deep. An abnormal ocular surface may prevent the even distribution of tear film, leading to discomfort, surface erosions, and reduced vision. Conditions characterized by irregular, raised, or elevated tissue of the cornea (for example, map-dot-fingerprint dystrophy, Salzmann's nodular degeneration, pterygium), or conjunctival growths (for example, pinguecula, ocular surface squamous neoplasia, which can also involve the cornea) and those involving broad areas of friction between the eyelids and the ocular surface (for example, conjunctivochalasis, SLK) may prevent the even distribution of tear film leading to discomfort, inflammation, and reduced vision. These diseases can be extremely painful and cause burning or foreign-body sensations.

Therapy depends on the nature and extent of disease and its underlying cause. To restore comfort and improve vision, the patient may need surgery that involves removing the abnormal tissue and resurfacing the eye to correct physical abnormalities. Sometimes lifestyle changes are necessary. To fully achieve the goal of treatment—minimizing the incidence of corneal erosions, managing pain, and improving vision—it is also essential to evaluate for comorbid MGD and ATD.

Cornea Surface Irregularities

Treatment for map-dot-fingerprint dystrophy may range from lubricating or hypertonic saline drops to surgical removal, plus wearing a bandage contact lens to aid healing, or a PROKERA® bandage lens containing a disc of amniotic membrane attached to a polycarbonate ring.

Treatment for Salzmann's nodular degeneration may involve excision or peeling off of the nodule, followed by wearing a bandage contact lens for several days to aid healing. Alternatively, a PROKERA lens may be placed over the nodule.

Pterygium treatment ranges from lifestyle changes—wearing UV blocking sunglasses and wide-brimmed hats—to surgical removal of the fleshy pink tissue and placement of a tissue graft if inflammation cannot be controlled, if it progresses toward the pupil, or shows signs of malignant transformation.

Conjunctival Growths

Treatment for inflamed pinguecula aims to stop or prevent the sources of chronic irritation and may include surgery to remove the abnormal tissue.

In 1994, I discovered what may be the first medical cure for ocular surface squamous neoplasia (a type of cancer of the eye surface), comprised of topical interferon alpha-2b 1 million IU/ml applied four times per day for two months. Without surgery or side effects from therapy, the cancerous lesion regressed. My findings were published in the *Archives of Ophthalmology* that year and selected for republication in the Spanish and Chinese editions of the journal. Subsequent studies by others confirmed its efficacy. Prior to attempting surgical excision, this therapy is now a mainstay of treatment for the disease and can eliminate the need to remove large amounts of tissue.

Frictional Disease

Repairing sections of abnormal bulbar conjunctiva and reducing the friction between it and the lining of the lid is a highly successful treatment for conjunctivochalasis and superior limbic keratoconjunctivitis (SLK). Because this friction also appears to be the underlying cause of a condition associated with eye irritation known as lid wiper epitheliopathy, adequate treatment of frictional disease, including optimizing the tear film and treating MGD and ATD, in my experience, also treats lid wiper disease.

My preferred method—resurfacing with amniotic membrane transplant (AMT) surgery—replaces diseased tissue with a smooth, healthy amniotic membrane. The smooth surface reduces friction during blinking and eye movement and restores proper tear flow across the surface of the eye toward the nose. After surgery, my patients often note improved ocular moisture and better vision. I've done thousands of these surgeries with great success.

Surgery to excise and replace damaged superior, inferior, and temporal conjunctival tissue with cryo-preserved amniotic membrane is done in an outpatient setting under IV (intravenous) sedation with topical anesthesia. I prefer this method of ocular surface reconstruction for several reasons:

- All the diseased, loose, or excessively redundant tissue is removed and replaced with healthy amniotic membrane.
- The amniotic membrane contains no viable (living) cells, so it is unlikely that the tissue will be rejected.
- The membrane contains growth factors that help to reduce inflammation and suppresses redness, blood vessel growth, and scar tissue formation.
- Healing is relatively fast, usually within just two weeks, so the possibility of achieving relief isn't delayed by many weeks or months.
- Relief is often dramatic when a smooth ocular surface is restored.

AMT surgery takes about an hour per eye. The loose and wrinkled diseased tissue is removed and replaced with a graft, tailored to fit into place, and fixed with both adhesive and sutures. (Fixing the graft with adhesive alone and without sutures risks displacement of the graft and would require a return to the operating room.) To avoid inflammation that self-absorbing sutures can create, I use nylon sutures, which I later remove in the office.

For repair of damaged nasal conjunctiva, I prefer to use limbal-conjunctival autograft, harvesting the graft from the patient's own eyes. The graft includes conjunctiva and the attached section of limbus, which contains stem cells. If autografting tissue is not an option, I may apply topical chemotherapy with mitomycin-C (MMC) and then perform AMT surgery.

After surgery on the superior bulbar region, patients wear a bandage contact lens to aid healing and reduce awareness of the sutures. Patients with significant comorbidities often use preservative-free steroid drops (made under a sterile hood in my office laboratory) to control inflammation, and antibiotic drops to prevent infection. If needed, patients will sometimes irrigate their eyes daily with sterile preservative-free saline or use allergy drops. Sometimes I prescribe antibiotic ophthalmic ointment to prevent lash crusting during healing. Patients sleep with a shield to protect the postoperative eye unless they have lagophthalmos, in which case they sleep with their moisture chamber goggles. I tell patients not to touch or rub their eyes, except when they wash their face and eyelids with a mild cleanser and rinse with water.

Once conjunctival epithelium has crossed the junction of the patient's old tissue and the new amniotic graft, usually in seven to ten days, I take out the stitches after numbing the eye with a drop of topical anesthetic. Complete healing usually takes ten to fourteen days. The most common potential adverse reaction is a sensitivity to preservatives in steroid and antibiotic drops, which is why I often prescribe preservative-free therapeutic drops.

Other treatment methods for conjunctivochalasis involve excision alone of redundant tissue, as well as thermal cautery or ablation with radiofrequency to shrink tissue. These methods are likely to leave behind abnormal tissue on the ocular surface without providing the therapeutic anti-inflammatory benefits of the grafted amniotic membrane. Some doctors treat SLK with a bandage soft contact lens that acts as an interface between the two rubbing surfaces to reduce friction. The bandage lens can be effective palliatively but does not eliminate the underlying problem.

3. MEIBOMIAN GLAND DYSFUNCTION

Conventional treatments for MGD have not been consistently effective, leading to frustrated patients and doctors. I attribute this inconsistent effectiveness to inadequate diagnoses that overlook the major cause of gland obstruction—occult, fixed, periductal fibrosis—and miss other ocular surface diseases that contribute to symptoms (see sidebar 10.5).

The Maskin® Probing Protocol (see the following section and chapter 11) releases this fibrotic tissue, which prepares the Meibomian glands for conventional MGD treatments—warm compresses, lid hygiene, topical or oral antibiotics, and anti-inflammatory medications—thus optimizing their effectiveness.

Sidebar 10.5
Why Conventional Treatments for MGD Often Fail

Conventional treatments for obstructive MGD were based on historically accepted models, attributing disease progression to thickened meibum secretions and excessive deposits of protein, namely keratin. These models gave rise to treatments that thinned the meibum with heat and used pressure to squeeze oil and keratin sequestered within the ducts out through the orifice.

Today there are more treatments for MGD, but too often they are based on the thick meibum and excessive keratin models while missing the critical role of periductal fibrosis in the development and progression of MGD.

Conducted over the last fifteen years and published in peer-reviewed journals, our research has shown that occult periductal fibrosis, seen using confocal microscopy, invades the Meibomian gland's external duct wall. This invasion leads to reduced duct wall thickness and loss of ductal integrity as the duct lumen becomes constricted, creating *fixed resistance* that blocks meibum flow through the central duct and out through the orifice while increasing intraductal pressure. The location of the fibrotic invasion is important because the external duct wall is thought to be the site of Meibomian gland stem cells and therefore a likely factor in the development of asymptomatic, as well as symptomatic, atrophic MGD.

Consequently, to be truly effective, any treatments for MGD must target periductal fibrosis directly.

With intraductal Meibomian gland probing, fixed obstructions can be diagnosed definitively and simultaneously treated in the way angiogram and angioplasty are used to find and reverse blockages in the arteries of the heart. For many patients, the news gets better. In some cases after probing, even atrophied Meibomian glands can be revived and show tissue growth.

Intraductal Meibomian gland probing, the breakthrough diagnostic and therapeutic procedure that releases periductal fibrosis and restores gland functionality, is discussed in more detail in chapter 11.

Maskin® Probing

Maskin Probing is a breakthrough diagnostic and therapeutic device that safely and effectively releases periductal fibrotic strictures, reversing the course of disease (see chapter 11). After probing it is important to quickly and effectively treat comorbidities to support newly restored gland function.

Nonpharmaceutical Conventional Therapies

Achieving and maintaining a healthy microenvironment helps to suppress comorbid disease and is essential to establishing a full, functioning, healthy, and resilient Meibomian gland population. This healthy microenvironment depends on the fundamentals: good quality blinking, lid hygiene, and nutrition, in conjunction with Meibomian gland probing to release periductal fibrosis and restore, confirm, and maintain ductal integrity. Other therapies, such as lid massage or gentle expression, may also be beneficial in some cases after Maskin Probing.

Effective Blinks

Effective blinks are complete and frequent. The eyelid margins meet, touching without leaving gaps, every five to seven seconds.

Taking breaks periodically during gazing activities is just as important as complete blinking. Look off into the distance, away from what you're doing, and blink hard a few times. While you're taking a break from gazing, stretch and loosen your neck muscles and drink some water to stay hydrated.

Any eyelid anatomic or physiologic comorbidity that impedes effective blinks—Graves' disease, Parkinson's disease, blink lagophthalmos, and others—may need treatment ranging from medications to lid oculoplastic surgery, or from radiation to orbital surgery for Graves' disease.

Lid Hygiene: Warm Compresses and Cleansing

Warm compresses thin out meibum, enabling it to flow through an open or partially occluded central duct and into the tear film. They can provide palliative relief depending on the extent of periductal fibrosis and loss of lumen integrity.

However, patients sometimes report warm compresses exacerbate symptoms. This can happen in glands constricted by periductal fibrosis, because the increased blood flow to glands caused by heat can increase intraductal pressure behind the stricture. If warm compresses cause symptoms to worsen, patients should discontinue therapy. After probing the Meibomian glands, releasing constrictions, and restoring ductal integrity, therapy with warm compresses can usually resume if needed to provide additional comfort.

The frequency of warm compress treatment for MGD that I prescribe to patients is dependent wholly on severity of symptoms, comorbidities, and willingness to adhere to treatment, and can vary from five minutes two times a day, to as little as two minutes once a day. To treat chalazion or hordeolum, compresses may be applied more frequently and directly to the inflamed nodule, then less frequently as inflammation resolves.

There are many eye masks and techniques for applying warm compresses at home. One simple technique is described in chapter 12.

Cleansing is one of the most important therapies for improving the microenvironment of the Meibomian glands and preventing comorbid anterior blepharitis. Washing lids and lashes removes organic material such as oils, dirt, pollen, allergens, dead skin, microbes, and other irritants. These irritants can cause inflammation, leading to lid margin congestion, periductal fibrosis, and subsequent MGD. The entire face, including the area around the eyes, should be cleansed twice a day as well. (For more information about cleansing, see "Lid and Facial Hygiene" in the "Anterior Blepharitis and Conjunctivitis" section to come.)

Nutrition

Nutrition plays a significant role in ocular health. Consuming a healthy diet rich in a variety of minerals, vitamins, and other nutrients, while avoiding simple sugars and saturated fats, helps to maintain the health and proper functioning of Meibomian glands and surrounding tissues. (For more information, see chapter 12.)

Lid Expression and Massage

Therapeutic expression and manual massaging of lids are ways to squeeze meibum out of the Meibomian glands with external force usually after warm compresses are applied.

With massage, mild to moderate pressure is applied to the entire eyelid, usually in a circular motion. With therapeutic expression, pressure is applied vertically from the proximal end of the gland— below the brow for the upper lid or above the cheek for the lower lid—toward the orifices. (Expression is sometimes called "milking" the glands.) Doctors may perform lid massage or expression in the office. Patients may be instructed to massage or express their eyelids at home.

In my opinion, massage is not generally necessary, because under healthy conditions, blinking naturally squeezes the glands correctly. When blinks are frequent, complete, and effective, my patients usually don't need eyelid massage after gland probing and treatment that targeted their comorbidities. Still, a handful of my patients find mild lid massage useful on occasion.

I am also not an advocate of office-based therapeutic expression, that requires an excessive sustained force to evacuate ductal contents. Excessive force applied to the lids causes severe pain, elevates intraductal pressure, and may damage glands (see the section "Risks of Therapeutic Expression"). On the other hand, gentle ex-

---

Sidebar 10.6
Expressing When Glands Have
Complete Proximal Obstruction (CPO)

In my experience, patients with MGD who say they benefit from therapeutic expression have fixed obstruction deeper in the gland, what I have called complete proximal obstruction (CPO). After expression, these patients may describe feeling *simultaneously more lubrication and more inflammation.* Because the obstruction is proximal (deeper) in the gland, there is at least one distal (near the surface) acinus in communication with the orifice, so meibum can reach the tear film, causing the soothing sensation of lubrication. However, simultaneously, behind the periductal fibrotic obstruction, the external pressure applied during expression increases intraductal pressure, exacerbating inflammation and symptoms. The increased pressure can lead to loss of gland tissue behind the obstruction and short, truncated glands.

---

pression of the glands after Maskin Probing to restore ductal integrity is safe. It can help to remove any sequestered ductal contents liberated by probing without significant risk, provided mild pressure is applied in the right direction.

DEVICES THAT HEAT, MASSAGE, OR EXPRESS LIDS

Devices that heat and massage or express the eyelids may be of limited therapeutic value because they do not target periductal fibrosis. Nevertheless, if these devices are used after probing establishes and confirms the patency of Meibomian glands, they may be viable complementary therapies. Otherwise, therapeutic expression can drive meibum farther back into the gland, further increasing pressure on the acinar-ductular units, increasing inflammation, and possibly leading to gland atrophy.

The following devices use heat and expression as part of the treatment protocol.

LipiFlow®

LipiFlow aims to remove nonfixed obstructions from within the duct. Paddles cradle the lids, heating them from the conjunctival side while pulsating pressure is externally applied to the lids from the outside. Treatment lasts for twelve minutes per eye. Sometimes therapeutic expression is done after the treatment. Contraindications include the more common corneal disorders that present with Dry Eye symptoms, such as recurrent corneal erosion and map-dot-fingerprint dystrophy, as well as systemic diseases that cause dryness, such as Sjögren's syndrome.

IPL (Intense Pulsed Light) with Therapeutic Expression

Used for years in dermatology to treat a variety of skin conditions, like age spots, sun damage, rosacea, birthmarks, and freckles, IPL followed by therapeutic gland expression is now used to treat MGD.

IPL's original role in treating Dry Eye was heating lids in preparation for therapeutic gland expression, though some now theorize IPL itself may have a role in treating MGD by reducing lid margin telangiectasia and inflammation.

The IPL beam emitted through a handheld device is usually applied for four ten-minute sessions to the lower lid, with the upper lid receiving only indirect light and heat. (Some doctors are experimenting with treating upper lids directly.) Patients may need corticosteroid and other eye drops to control posttreatment inflammation. After the initial set of treatments several weeks apart, patients return once or twice a year for maintenance.

IPL is not suitable for everyone, for example, patients with dark skin. Patients have reported that the therapeutic gland expression after IPL can be painful (see sidebar: 10.7, "Maskin® Probing and IPL").

Systane® iLUX®

iLUX is an in-office handheld thermal pulsation device. The eyelids are assessed and treatment zones are identified. The zones are

Sidebar 10.7
Maskin® Probing and IPL

Although IPL and other therapies using heat and pressure do not target the periductal fibrosis that causes elevated intraductal pressure and stem cell deficiency (the apparent underlying causes of atrophic MGD), these therapies can play a supportive and complementary role in the treatment of MGD after Meibomian gland probing.

Researchers in China illustrated this effect in a 2019 randomized controlled trial comparing Maskin Probing (for physically releasing fixed obstructions and restoring ductal integrity) to IPL (for reducing telangiectasia). They compared both stand-alone treatments to a combination therapy; Meibomian glands were probed first, then three weeks later patients received IPL.

Each of the two treatments alone showed statistically significant improvement for the seven parameters studied: SPEED scores (symptoms), TBUT, cornea erosions, meibum quality, lid telangiectasia, orifice abnormality, and lid tenderness. When comparing probing to IPL results for each parameter, probing showed statistically significant ($p < 0.001$) improvement over IPL in reducing lid tenderness. (P-value, short for "probability value," indicates if data is statistically significant or not. A p-value less than or equal to 0.05 indicates data is statistically significant.) Combination therapy produced the greatest statistically significant improvements in SPEED scores, TBUT, meibum quality, and telangiectasia.

When discussing their results, the authors expressed reservations about administering IPL without first probing, because

". . . instead of showing reduction in symptoms, two patients (14.8 percent) in the present study reported even more serious symptoms at the end of the IPL treatment course. It can be speculated that this deterioration may be related to obstruction sites within the glands . . . heat released by IPL and the pressure caused by the forceps might paradoxically increase the intraductal pressure and exacerbate the inflammatory response; thus, treatment with IPL alone may not alleviate disease symptoms but instead irritate the condition. This effect can be indirectly observed in the present data in terms of the post-treatment lid tenderness of the IPL group, despite showing symptom alleviation compared with baseline, still being significantly higher than the MGP and MGP-IPL groups."

It's important to note that a single IPL treatment requires three separate IPL sessions, typically followed by manual expression, which, if applied with excessive force, could potentially damage glands. For years, I have been seeing new patients who had undergone six or more IPL sessions but who continued to experience persistent and severe symptoms. Remarkably, in recent months I have seen a few new patients with persistent symptoms despite undergoing eighteen or more IPL sessions over the course of two years.

heated with the device and the gland contents expressed. Treatment takes about eight to twelve minutes per eye. A recent study showed iLUX and LipiFlow (mentioned earlier) produced similar improvements in clinical parameters.

eyeXpress™

eyeXpress, a temperature-controlled goggle that heats the eyelids to 110 degrees for about fifteen minutes, prepares the Meibomian glands for expression. The hands-free device requires no assistance by office staff or the patient.

MiBo Thermoflo

MiBo Thermoflo, a handheld device with two small pads that are placed on the patient's closed eyelids, heats the eyelids to 108 degrees. Pressure is then applied via a thermoelectric heat pump to soften and evacuate the Meibomian glands.

TearCare®

TearCare paddles heat the eyelids while the patient blinks, theoretically increasing the delivery of meibum to the tear film. After several minutes of heating and blinking, the eyelids may be expressed.

NuLids

NuLids is a handheld device with an oscillating tip; it is used at home to massage the Meibomian glands and clean the lid margin.

RISKS OF THERAPEUTIC LID EXPRESSION

In my opinion, office-based therapeutic lid expression poses risks. External pressure won't always direct meibum to flow toward the gland's orifice. For example, when Meibomian glands have fixed fibrotic blockages deeper within (which happens over 90 percent of the time in my patients with MGD), or an unopened orifice, external pressure can force healthy or stagnant and unhealthy meibum deeper into the gland or acini, exacerbating any already built-up pressure. How meibum might flow in tortuous glands that are U-shaped is another concern.

Furthermore, therapeutic expression can require the application of significant force, typically at least 5–40 psi of sustained pressure (see sidebar 10.8). That much pressure applied to the eyelids can be extremely painful. In one study (Korb and Blackie, 2011), "only 7 percent of the patients could tolerate the pressure necessary to administer complete therapeutic expression along the entire lower eyelid."

That much pressure may also cause an ischemia-reperfusion event. This occurs when blood supply returns to tissue (reperfusion)

Sidebar 10.8
How Much Pressure is 5–40 PSI?

If you've ever had your blood pressure taken, you know how uncomfortable a fully inflated blood pressure cuff can be. To find your systolic blood pressure (the pressure when the heart contracts) the cuff is inflated to the level required to stop blood flow through the artery. At that point it's immediately released to restore blood flow.

Systolic pressure is measured in millimeters of mercury (mmHg), and normal pressure is approximately 120 mmHg.

In a study measuring how much pressure needs to be applied to eyelids during therapeutic expression of Meibomian glands, researchers had to apply anywhere from 5 to 40 psi (pounds per square inch), with a mean of 25.6 psi applied to the glands, to evacuate the glands.

How would that much pressure feel in an inflated blood pressure cuff if 1 psi is roughly equivalent to 51.71 mmHg?

Using 51.71 as a multiplier, the pressure in the cuff at 5–40 psi, with a mean of 25.6 psi, would range from 258 mmHg to 2,068 mmHg, with a mean of 1,324 mmHg.

258 mmHg in a blood pressure cuff would be intolerable, 2,068 mmHg unimaginable.

---

after a period of reduced oxygenation (ischemia). In this setting it is conceivable that therapeutic expression may further increase lid inflammation and exacerbate periductal fibrosis.

Finally, neither expression nor massage can remove or release the fibrotic tissue constricting the Meibomian gland outflow tract. These mechanical occlusions require an appropriate mechanical resolution rather than potentially harmful therapeutic expression.

Conventional Therapy: Anti-Inflammatory Medications

Topical and oral anti-inflammatory medications reduce both acute and chronic inflammation. To a significant extent, these medications help palliatively, relieving symptoms without treating the root cause of inflammation.

Topical Corticosteroid Drops or Ointments

Topical steroids reduce inflammation but should only be used for short periods because of potential side effects. They can cause cataracts and increase risk of infection. Patients can have allergies and sensitivities to other ingredients in the medications. Topical steroids can raise intraocular pressure, leading to glaucoma and vision loss. Whenever they are prescribed, doctors must check intraocular pressure regularly.

Other Topical Anti-Inflammatory Drops

Restasis, other forms of cyclosporine, and Xiidra (lifitegrast) are discussed earlier in this chapter. Besides reducing ocular surface inflammation, they may reduce inflammation associated with the Meibomian glands.

Oral Omega Fatty Acid Supplements

Essential fatty acids are some of the essential nutrients that the body requires but does not synthesize by itself and therefore must be included in the diet. These include the omega-6 linoleic and omega-3 linolenic families of polyunsaturated fatty acids (PUFAs) and highly unsaturated fatty acids (HUFAs).

The antioxidant and anti-inflammatory properties of two of the main omega-3 fatty acids (eicosapentaenoic acid, EPA, and docosahexaenoic acid, DHA) may improve TBUT and symptoms for patients with MGD. However, one study showed omega-3 supplements were no more effective than olive oil in improving signs and symptoms of Dry Eye.

Within the omega-6 family of fatty acids, gamma-linolenic acid

(GLA) is also recognized as having anti-inflammatory properties. One study found omega-3 (EPA and DHA) plus GLA taken for six months improved ocular symptoms to a statistically significant degree.

Because both omega-3 and omega-6 are essential fatty acids, it's important to make sure you are consuming appropriate amounts of each. One supplement that contains both omega-3 and -6 is Hydro-Eye® by ScienceBased Health.

Before seeing me, most of my patients tried omega fatty acid supplements. Some found no improvement and others felt their symptoms improved. If their eyes felt better after taking omega supplements, I tell patients to keep doing so, or they can try omega supplements if they haven't already, as long as there are no contraindications, such as easy bruising.

Oral Antibiotics

Doxycycline and minocycline are antibiotics. At higher doses they have antibacterial properties. At lower doses, experts believe they have a neutralizing effect on free radicals and show anti-inflammatory properties.

Azithromycin can be an effective treatment for posterior blepharitis. A 2011 study in Brazil of patients with posterior blepharitis taking a pulsed course of 500 mg oral azythromycin showed improvement in signs and symptoms, except in those patients with lid swelling, eyelid hyperemia (excessive redness), photophobia, and foreign-body sensation. The antibiotic can only be taken for a short period because of the risk of increasing bacterial resistance.

To protect their gut microbiomes while taking any antibiotics, patients should eat foods such as yogurt rich in probiotics or take probiotic supplements (with a span of at least six hours between the medication and the probiotic), and continue for at least a week or two after stopping the antibiotic.

Topical AzaSite® (azithromycin)

Topical AzaSite® gel drops, a prescription containing azithromycin, is an antibiotic with anti-inflammatory properties. The antibiotic is thought to improve the quality of meibum in a vehicle delivery system, which stabilizes and sustains its release to the ocular surface.

4. ALLERGIES AND SENSITIVITIES

Topical antihistamine drops like Pataday® (OTC), ZADITOR® (OTC), LASTACAFT®, or ZERVIATE™ can help with allergy symptoms, as long as patients aren't sensitive or allergic to ingredients in the drops. In 2020, the FDA approved the first over-the-counter preservative-free antihistamine drop, Alaway® Preservative Free, containing ketotifen 0.035%.

I instruct patients to irrigate with preservative-free 0.9% sterile saline solution at least once a day to flush eyes and remove allergens, toxins, and sensitizing agents. Irrigating eyes is especially important if DTC (delayed tear clearance) is a comorbidity.

Sometimes I refer patients to allergists for allergy testing to identify the triggering allergens. However, patients sometimes do not test positive with skin patch or blood tests for allergies but do have ocular allergies. The fact is, there are infinite potential allergens and no way to test them all. In these cases I treat patients with refrigerated topical antihistamines if tolerated, instruct them to irrigate and possibly apply cold compresses, and suggest lifestyle changes (see chapter 12) that can also help reduce symptoms.

If allergy symptoms persist, I ask when symptoms are at their worst. Sometimes itching and burning peak upon awakening or in the middle of the night, suggesting an allergic reaction during sleep. Allergens may have collected in the patient's hair, face, and body during the day. When the patient went to bed, allergens transferred to the pillowcase and from there to the eyes. Shampooing the hair and washing the face and eyelids with mild soapy water at bedtime helps eliminate allergens and accumulated toxins and irritants.

Some patients may need to increase tolerance to certain allergens so they can avoid allergic reactions and related symptoms altogether. Treatment may include sublingual allergy therapy and immunotolerance injections.

Sidebar 10.9
Allergy Testing and Desensitization Therapy

Allergy testing may be an option for some patients, although treatment for allergies can be tricky. There are literally countless potential allergens in everyone's environment. So it's impossible to test for each one.

Because oral anti-allergy medications like BENADRYL®, ZYRTEC®, and Claritin® can be drying, exacerbating Dry Eye symptoms, if a patient tests positive for allergies, desensitization therapy may be an option for them. But even if a patient undergoes allergy desensitization therapy for one allergen, they may still have allergic reactions to something they weren't tested for.

---

5. ANTERIOR BLEPHARITIS AND CONJUNCTIVITIS

Anterior blepharitis is characterized by inflammation at the anterior half of the lid margin and the base of the lashes. Along with allergies and ATD, it is among the most common comorbidities to adversely affect Meibomian glands, leading to increased obstruction and reduced gland expression. Infectious anterior blepharitis is usually bacterial or parasitic, but can also be viral or fungal and may be accompanied by infectious conjunctivitis. Alternatively, inflammation may be noninfectious due to allergies and/or sensitivities. Treatment depends on the cause of inflammation.

No matter the cause, it's important to quickly and effectively treat any comorbidities that may arise which otherwise could exacerbate MGD. Early treatment of these comorbidities can allow glands to function well. If treatment of comorbidities is not administered promptly, glands treated with Maskin probing will reobstruct and may require early repeat probing.

General Lid and Facial Hygiene

Lid and facial hygiene—cleansing the lids, lashes, brows, and area around the eyes—is important for preventing and managing anterior infectious and noninfectious blepharitis. Skin disorders on the face, especially the eyelids and area around the eyes, and the forehead, can contribute to MGD. Eczematous flakes of skin from these areas can fall into and irritate the eyes. Demodex mites infesting the fine hairs of the lid skin can also irritate the eyes.

Cleansing the eyelids is not enough. The entire face, including the entire area around the eyes, should be cleaned twice a day with mild soapy water. Products like Dove Sensitive Skin Beauty Bar or Éminence Stone Crop Gel Wash remove organic debris, microbes, chemicals, toxins, and airborne irritants.

Alternatively, you can try a commercially prepared cleanser, or cleansing pads, formulated specifically for the area around the eyes, like OCuSOFT® cleansers and lid wipes or products containing hypochlorous acid, such as Avenova® or Zocular® cleansers that contain an okra-infused surfactant. Find a cleanser that your eyes can tolerate and works for your skin, and purchase the product from a reputable dealer to help ensure its safety.

Lather the lids gently but firmly. Hard scrubbing is not only unnecessary, it can be detrimental. Avoid hot water. It can burn, irritate, or cause skin to flake. Washing excessively can desiccate the lid margins, leading to unhealthy duct orifices and MGD. A few of my patients went a little overboard, using several lid cleansers, each at least once per day.

Patients sometimes make these other mistakes:

- Not washing the face regularly
- Not washing, or avoiding, the area around the eyes or the lids
- Washing the face or the lids without soap or cleanser, that is, using water only
- Washing the lids only and avoiding the lashes
- Using too much soap or cleanser or washing too long, which can desiccate the lid margins

Some patients are sensitive to soaps and even mild cleansers. For them, lid hygiene can be very challenging but still necessary.

Besides explaining proper facial hygiene and its importance to my patients, I might prescribe a short course of over-the-counter hydrocortisone cream or LOTEMAX® ophthalmic ointment to treat noninfectious flaking eyelid skin. If they wear makeup, I discuss eye cosmetics, as these can pose significant problems for the ocular surface. Patients should avoid makeup with irritating ingredients, such as alcohols, benzalkonium chloride, EDTA, formaldehyde, and parabens. Makeup should not be waterproof, shared, or applied to the posterior lid margin. (For more information, see "Practice Good Eyelid Hygiene" in chapter 12.)

Treatment for Bacterial Infections

I treat bacterial infections of the lid margin with a topical antibiotic ophthalmic ointment. If there is comorbid conjunctivitis, I add a topical antibiotic drop. All my patients with anterior blepharitis start on broad spectrum topical antibiotics but may change to a more selective antibiotic if they're not improving. The different antibiotic is based on a lab culture that analyzes the susceptibility of isolated bacteria against a panel of antibiotics. Knowing the organism's sensitivities to antibiotics is also helpful if a patient has, or develops, concomitant dacryocystitis, which usually requires a systemic oral antibiotic.

Folliculitis, inflammation in the eyelash follicle, is treated with warm compresses and broad spectrum antibiotic ointment if there's evidence of infection. Epilation, removing the infected follicle, can help by reversing the microabscess and improving access to the lids and lashes for hygiene.

Treatment for Parasitic Infections: Demodex Mites

Demodex mites are found on the shafts and roots of lashes and in the Meibomian glands. They have approximately a three-week life cycle and reproduce prolifically. When they die, their bodies release bacteria to the lid margins. Treating demodex mites may be difficult but not impossible. Topical treatments can be very effective.

I advise my patients to cleanse eyelid margins, brows, the scalp, neck, and hairs at the openings of the nostrils, as well as external parts of the ear with shampoo or other products containing tea tree oil, for two months. Patients should wash bedding and pillowcases in hot water immediately after their first tea tree oil treatment and use the hot dryer setting to kill the mites. Bedding should be washed at least once a week thereafter. Significant others, or anyone who lives with the patient, should be examined for demodex mites and treated.

Cliradex® foam and towelettes contain a component found in tea tree oil shown to kill the demodex parasite and can be very effective therapy. Initially, patients use the product twice a day, then adjust frequency depending on their response.

If patients cannot tolerate tea tree oil compounds, I have prescribed with great success topical antiparasitic compounded ivermectin ointment, applied to the lashes nightly.

Some patients may not tolerate any topical treatment, so I prescribe oral ivermectin. These patients need to be under the care of their primary care physician, infectious disease specialist, or other doctor to monitor their progress and any adverse reaction to the medication. Metronidazole, also taken orally, may increase the effectiveness of oral ivermectin against demodex mites.

6. FLOPPY LID AND OTHER ABNORMAL EYELID MECHANICS

Patients with floppy lid disease can awaken with a red, irritated eye after an upper lid everts against the pillowcase during sleep.

Such a patient can try sleeping on the back and wearing an aluminum eye shield or moisture chamber goggles (see the next section, "Lagophthalmos") to prevent the upper lid from everting. The definitive treatment, a lid-tightening procedure performed by an oculoplastic surgeon, prevents the lid from everting.

Other eyelid mechanics that require repair by an oculoplastic surgeon include spastic entropion with trichiasis; symptomatic ectropion; lid override or imbrication; lower lid laxity with drooping and visible white sclera (above the inferior lid margin), which stretches and thins the tear film; and lid retraction, sometimes seen with Graves' disease, which causes exposure with lagophthalmos and ineffective blinking. Patients who have had cosmetic lid surgery may have altered eyelid mechanics affecting the blink and tear film.

Sidebar 10.10
Biofilm

Some doctors believe biofilm, a thin film of bacteria adhering to a surface, can build up on the lid margin and at the base of the eyelashes, causing anterior blepharitis. Their recommendations typically focus on removing this biofilm by scraping or exfoliating the lid margin.

I have concerns about the potential side effects of excessive or aggressive exfoliating and lid margin scraping, because of the following:

- There is evidence that the lid margin contains stem cells which may be important for the proliferation and differentiation of eyelid skin, the conjunctiva, and possibly Meibomian gland cells.
- Excessive exfoliation with inadvertent removal of lid margin epithelial cells may increase permeability, allowing microscopic toxins, irritants, allergens, and microbes access to epithelial and dermal-epithelial junction tissues (rete ridges), leading to periglandular inflammation and periductal fibroses of the Meibomian gland outflow tract.
- Exfoliation may subsequently expose the base of eyelashes to bacteria, leading to folliculitis—infection at the base of the lashes and within the follicle's sebaceous gland and shaft areas.

Instead of scraping or exfoliating the lid margin, I advise my patients to establish a regular program of good lid and facial hygiene habits at home, which includes a safe, tolerable, and effective cleanser, with additional topical treatment in cases of infectious anterior blepharitis, such as antibiotic ointment for bacterial infections, and antiparasitics for demodex mites. For excessively keratinized lid margin surfaces, I prescribe a small amount of vitamin A ointment. These are safe and proven topical treatments, which I have been prescribing for over thirty years and which have been very effective for my patients.

If the patient uses Botox or fillers, I discuss risks and precautions. Excessive or poorly placed Botox can cause poor, incomplete blinks and even lead to reduced aqueous tear and Meibomian gland secretions. Fillers can alter the lower lid contour and affect the quality of blinks. Patients who experience these side effects may need to adjust their use of these agents.

7. LAGOPHTHALMOS

The two types of lagophthalmos (incomplete closure of the eyelid) I see most often in patients are nocturnal lagophthalmos (eyes open while sleeping) and blink lagophthalmos (incomplete blinks).

Protecting Eyes While Sleeping

Air flowing across the eyes during sleep can desiccate the cornea, conjunctiva, and lid margin when there is a slight gap between closed lids. If a patient wakes with Dry Eye symptoms and suffers from nocturnal lagophthalmos or floppy lids, I recommend protecting the eyes and eyelids from exposure to airflow while sleeping.

What I prescribe depends on the degree of exposure during sleep and if the patient has comorbidities like allergies to the materials in the devices.

Moisture Chamber Goggles and Sleep Masks

Eye Eco makes reusable moisture chamber goggles and masks in a variety of styles and sizes, so most patients can find a suitable pair.

The goggles are made of soft silicone and slip on easily. The Onyix™ Hydrating Sleep Mask model works well for patients with floppy lid or sleep apnea who wear CPAP masks. The Tranquileyes® model includes foam inserts that can be soaked in water to create a moist environment for the eyes.

To increase moisture during the night, a preservative-free lubricating eye drop or a quarter-inch bead of ophthalmic lubricating ointment can be used right before slipping on the goggles. These ointments typically contain varying concentrations of mineral oil and petroleum, and may contain lanolin. Some patients cannot tolerate these ingredients or high concentrations of them. Some patients may be allergic to lanolin. Find one you can tolerate by trial and error.

Moisture chamber goggles and masks should be washed and dried after each use, according to the manufacturer's instructions.

Disposable Eye Shields

EyeLocc™, a sterile lid dressing slightly larger than the eye socket, is designed to protect the eye during general anesthesia. It has a clear oval film surrounded by an opaque border with adhesive on the inside. The dressing prevents air access and locks the upper lid into a closed position. Before using, wash your face to remove natural oils and makeup, and dry thoroughly so the shield can adhere properly.

EyeLocc shields may not adhere properly for patients who use lubricating ointment, though patients sometimes can stop using lubricating ointment when wearing these shields.

Some patients may be sensitive to the adhesive and unable to tolerate it.

Other Methods

Patients who cannot tolerate the materials in commercial eye shields may be able to tolerate materials like Saran wrap. The clear, plastic film is stretched over the closed eye and adhered with a thin film of lubricating ointment applied to the brow and cheekbone. A blindfold or sleep mask may be worn over the plastic wrap.

Other single- or multiuse nighttime eye protection can be found online.

Redirect Airflow

Whether sleeping, watching TV, working, or sitting in a restaurant, it's important to keep airflow directed away from the eyes. Avoid ceiling fans. Pick your seat in restaurants carefully.

If you have nocturnal lagophthalmos, direct ceiling fans and HVAC vents away from the bed, toward a wall or across the ceiling.

Blinking

Remember to blink every five to seven seconds. The eyes need to close completely each time. Try blinking exercises while looking in a mirror, or ask someone to pay close attention to your eyes when you blink. Is it less or more than every five to seven seconds? Do your eyes close completely? Ask a friend to video your face when you aren't paying attention so you can monitor your progress. (See chapter 12 for a simple blinking exercise.)

8. EYELASH IRRITANTS

Many conditions can afflict the eyelashes. Treatment may be as simple as improving eyelid hygiene or epilating a few lashes, or it may require the skills of an oculoplastic surgeon, for example, to repair lid entropion.

Eyelash cosmetics like mascara, cosmetic treatments like LATISSE®, and procedures such as permanent eyeliner, can cause irritation, which can increase lid-margin inflammation. I advise patients with ocular surface disease and MGD to minimize or avoid their use.

I often find lashes colliding at the outer corner of the eyes as part of a cluster of comorbidities I call lateral canthal crowding. Simply epilating lashes on the upper and lower lids at the outer corners of the eyes keeps the lashes from colliding and preventing complete blinks. In recurrent cases, the lash follicle(s) may have to be removed or may require surgery for a malpositioned lid. Besides contributing to symptoms and affecting blinks, these lashes can cause irritation leading to blepharospasm and increased surface inflammation. Lashes in this area may also strike the temporal conjunctival tissue, inflaming and exacerbating preexisting chalasis.

Good lid hygiene is extremely important for controlling inflammation that can lead to scarring of the lash follicle and an alteration of the trajectory of the growing lashes, such as trichiasis. See chapter 12 for tips to improve lid hygiene.

9. DELAYED TEAR CLEARANCE (DTC)

A healthy ocular surface clears and replenishes older tear film continuously. When tear clearance is delayed, irritants, allergens, toxins, and sensitizing particles that can cause inflammation and discomfort remain in the stagnant tear film, leaving debris like a dirty bathtub ring on the ocular surface.

If I find a patient has delayed tear clearance (DTC), usually diagnosed using the fluorescein clearance test (FCT), I immediately start the patient on a daily regimen of irrigation with preservative-free 0.9% sterile saline solution, available with a prescription. The saline solution comes in single-use vials, one hundred to a box, and is usually covered by insurance.

To irrigate effectively, I recommend directing five to ten good squirts into the inner pouch of each lower eyelid. Each squirt should produce a stream of saline, more like a miniature garden hose rather than an individual drop.

When DTC is due to edema and inflammation within the tear drainage system, often seen with ocular rosacea, I prescribe a one-week course of 1% preservative-free methylprednisolone, a steroid-containing eye drop to reverse the condition at least temporarily.

If DTC is due to allergies, in addition to irrigation I may prescribe steroid and antihistamine nasal sprays as well as topical antihistamine drops.

10. BLEPHAROSPASM

Blepharospasm is the uncontrolled, involuntary spasm or twitching of the eyelid muscles with closing of the eye.

Benign essential blepharospasm (BEB) is not life threatening, has

Sidebar 10.11
Don't Use the Tap Water!

Susanne, a fifty-year-old woman with delayed tear clearance and a history of ATD, had initially responded well to punctal occlusion and AMT surgery for conjunctivochalasis, but she returned to my office with red and irritated eyes. She'd been having the symptoms for about two months. A slit-lamp examination suggested exposure to toxins or other irritants.

I then reviewed the therapies I had prescribed, including daily irrigation, which she had continued religiously since her last exam. Nothing seemed out of the ordinary. So I sat back, deciding we needed a detailed chat about her eye-care routine.

When it came to irrigation, Susanne said she had stopped using the vials of sterile saline solution I had prescribed. Instead, she irrigated her eyes daily with shower water. For several seconds, she forced herself to open her eyes and gaze at the showerhead. No wonder her eyes were irritated!

I explained that shower water, containing chlorine and other chemicals, was too harsh for her eyes. Susanne would have to switch back to sterile saline. Once she did, her eyes felt and looked much better.

---

no known cause, and is not associated with other diseases. Secondary blepharospasm is associated with one or more underlying diseases that trigger the spasm. Often blepharospasm is mixed: BEB and secondary occur simultaneously. The usual treatment for BEB is BOTOX®, injections of botulinum toxin produced by the bacterium *Clostridium botulinum* to paralyze the eyelid muscles.

I approach blepharospasm the same way I approach signs and

symptoms of other ocular surface diseases. First, I identify the underlying diseases that may be triggering the lid spasm, then I prioritize their treatment and incrementally target each disease to reverse symptoms. Consequently, I do not support routinely injecting BOTOX for blepharospasm, the usual treatment, without first searching for and treating underlying causes. These causes can range from cornea inflammation to the usual suspects, for example, ATD, MGD, allergy, anterior blepharitis, conjunctivochalasis, and lagophthalmos. Diet and especially caffeine consumption can play a significant role.

I have had success eliminating or reducing the frequency and severity of blepharospasms with this approach, greatly improving my patients' clinical status, and reducing the BOTOX needed.

11. ROSACEA

Rosacea leads to inflammation on the ocular surface and can also lead to blood vessel invasion of the peripheral cornea, often in the setting of DTC. Rosacea may be difficult to diagnose in darkly pigmented individuals. When present, rosacea is often accompanied by MGD.

Traditional treatments for rosacea include an oral tetracycline derivative and treatment for MGD and DTC. Dietary and environmental factors can also be addressed to reduce the severity and frequency of symptoms, for example, avoiding inflammatory foods, limiting sun exposure.

Childhood rosacea can be treated with oral erythromycin if the patient is younger than eight to ten years old. Tetracycline and related antibiotics can irreversibly stain teeth in children under age ten.

12. SIDE EFFECTS FROM SYSTEMIC MEDICATIONS

On the rare occasions when I think it is necessary or beneficial to adjust the dosage of a systemic medication or try a replacement medication, I discuss the medication(s) with a patient's other physician(s).

Often when MGD and Dry Eye symptoms subside, we can re-evaluate the use of medications that can cause or exacerbate symptoms, such as antidepressants, anxiolytics (antianxiety), or pain medications. Patients may be able to reduce the dosage or stop taking them altogether.

13. SYSTEMIC DISEASES

A wide range of systemic diseases can play a role in a patient's Dry Eye symptoms. Diagnosing and treating each of the systemic conditions is as important as treating the eyes.

Sometimes patients don't even know they have a systemic condition until they see me, in which case I work with their primary care or other doctors to initiate treatment. For example, Alan, a forty-five-year-old male patient, presented with episodic severe ocular surface inflammation and redness. He had undergone treatment for Dry Eye with other doctors, but his symptoms persisted. I diagnosed episcleritis, inflammation of the tissue between the conjunctiva and the sclera, and ordered screening blood tests. The test results showed elevated serum uric acid levels, indicating the patient had a high risk for gout, even though the patient had no nonocular symptoms of gout. I discussed Alan's case with his primary care doctor, who treated him with allopurinol. Treatment lowered Alan's uric acid level and also eliminated his red-eye episodes.

PRIORITIZING AND ONGOING TREATMENTS

As I've explained, a patient's symptoms determine the course of treatment. I prioritize the treatments together with my patient based on a variety of factors, including

- which symptoms are the worst
- how quickly a treatment will take effect (often my patients have already been suffering for months or even years when I first see them)
- when, where, and how treatment is administered, for example, in the office, at home, in hospital outpatient surgery
- how far the patient traveled and any logistics related to travel arrangements

Sidebar 10.12
Ocular Neuropathic Pain, Part 3: Treatment

As I explained in "Ocular Neuropathic Pain, Part 1" and "Part 2" (see chapters 6 and 9), some of my colleagues have used the term "ocular neuropathic pain" to explain the cause of pain that can't be attributed to an obvious nociceptive eye disease. I have seen dozens of patients wrongly diagnosed with this condition who were prescribed a variety of treatments and whose cases I then successfully managed by identifying and treating occult ocular surface diseases that were the true sources of pain.

Treatments typically prescribed for neuropathic pain are autologous serum drops and topical steroid drops. But these treatments may not be effective, because they treat ocular surface disease in a nonspecific way—with a tear replacement and an anti-inflammatory pharmaceutical—without targeting the underlying cause of pain.

Sometimes doctors prescribe scleral lenses. These can be very effective for severe ocular surface diseases, such as advanced mucin-deficient Stevens-Johnson syndrome. However, scleral lenses can also interrupt the normal tear film, irritate the conjunctiva, change the ocular microbiome, and add frictional stresses to the Meibomian glands of the upper lid.

If pain persists, these patients may be referred to a pain management doctor or put on systemic nerve-altering drugs that may have debilitating and profound side effects, including

- Lyrica® (pregabalin), which may increase "the risk of suicidal thoughts and behavior"
- Gabapentin, which may increase "the risk of sui-

cidal thoughts and behavior" and increase the risk
of acute narrow-angle glaucoma

- antidepressants, which can cause or exacerbate
ATD and MGD and can cause erratic behavior.
They can also lead to suicidal thoughts in children
and young adults

These pharmaceuticals can mask pain. But they also
increase the risk of suicidal thoughts in patients who may
be without hope because they can't find relief, while an
underlying nociceptive pain condition worsens.

Rather than expose my patients to these risks and the
potential adverse side effects of these treatments for neuropathic pain, I conduct rigorous examinations, identify
occult and previously unrecognized diseases, and appropriately treat my patients for those. When there is evidence of fixed, obstructed Meibomian glands, ATD, conjunctivochalasis, a pinched nerve in the neck, or other
untreated problems, I treat these comorbidities. In fact,
I've found that the nerves of patients with heightened
sensitivities from prolonged inadequately treated nociceptive pain calm down significantly when comorbidities
are targeted and treated effectively. Then, if I instill an
anesthetic eye drop (the test many use to detect neuropathic pain), the patients' eyes as expected, and for the
first time since being told they had neuropathic pain, become numb. With proper care, over time the patient can
become symptom-free.

If I find ATD, and the typical conventional therapies have not
helped, I usually recommend doing punctal occlusion using thermal cautery. If the patient has MGD, I explain why probing the
Meibomian glands is essential and important. If I find ocular surface

All too often patients come to me desperate and in pain, with diagnoses of ocular neuropathic or neurologic pain. After I diagnose the causes of their ocular pain and treat them with targeted therapies, their symptoms consistently resolve. With her permission, I have included one such story posted as a review of my practice on Google, from my patient Shellace James.

> In September of 2018 I developed severe burning eye pain. It seemed to start as allergies but became a burning that did not numb with anesthetics. My eye doctor of over twenty years tried allergy drops and steroids, but nothing changed. He referred me to a specialist locally and he said I had blepharitis. After getting no relief from warm compresses, I was given steroid and antibiotic eye drops and doxycycline. At this point I was getting desperate and started researching on my own. I started to express my Meibomian glands, which offered a small bit of relief. I was told it looked like I had a neurological problem, which didn't make sense, because the surface of my eyes was looking more and more unhealthy. I kept finding papers written by Dr. Maskin about Meibomian gland dysfunction and gland probing. I went to another local clinic and tried LipiFlow, which did nothing. I then went several hours away to an eye hospital, which is one of the top eye hospitals in the world. I left with a tube of antibiotic eye ointment and was referred back to my family doctor to try nerve pain meds. At this point I decided to take a huge leap of faith and make an

appointment with Dr. Maskin. The first day he ran tests and closed off my lower tear ducts, and the second day he did the probing, which stopped the burning pain. The surface of my eyes is looking less dry and I am finally hopeful that I will recover completely. I can get a good night's sleep and not spend every waking moment thinking about how much I hurt. I am very thankful to Dr. Maskin and everyone in his office for their help and compassion.

Sidebar 10.14
Patients Who Try to Diagnose and Treat Themselves

Dry Eye patients who try to diagnose and treat themselves may not succeed. Since they can't examine their eyes under magnification or administer tests, they can't diagnose all of their comorbidities. Without knowing which comorbidities they have, they don't know which treatments to use. Or they may need treatments like prescriptions or surgeries that they can't prescribe or administer themselves. So it's always best to find a good doctor to both diagnose and treat your comorbidities.

Recognize that what you read on the Internet in all likelihood does not pertain to you precisely. Maybe part of someone's experience sounds familiar, but it's impossible to know where the similarities and differences begin and end. Forgoing the care of a doctor or relying on the Internet only can lead to confusion, poor choices, and disease progression.

defects, I consider a procedure to correct the defects. If the ocular surface defect is minor and not contributing significantly to symptoms, I defer the procedure and monitor the patient's response to other treatments first.

I prescribe topical and oral medications as necessary and go over tips for managing symptoms and comorbidities at home. I discuss ways the patient might improve his or her personal environment by adjusting humidity, temperature, lighting, exposure to particulate matter, and other factors (see chapter 12). If necessary, I order blood tests to evaluate possible systemic diseases and may recommend the patient see their primary care doctor or a specialist.

Once treatment starts, I monitor patients closely, adjust treatment when necessary, and keep an open line of communication so

---

Sidebar 10.15
Suicidal Thoughts

Sometimes my new patients confess that I'm their last hope, admitting to suicidal thoughts. Sometimes they describe the detailed plans they have made to end their lives. They divulge this right away or toward the end of their initial visit when they've become comfortable sharing their deepest personal fears. Sometimes I hear it third-hand, from a friend or a loved one.

If you're desperate and losing hope because treatment hasn't improved your symptoms, you may need a more rigorous examination, a more comprehensive set of diagnoses, or a different treatment strategy.

Within this chapter and chapter 11, I focus on the most effective and efficient treatments that I commonly use to consistently restore comfort to patient's eyes. However, other treatments are available. This is why I can't stress enough that you, the patient, should never lose hope.

Sidebar 10.16
A Note to Families and Friends

If your loved one continues to experience pain after treatment for Dry Eye and MGD, trust them even if their eyes don't look bad to you. They may be suffering with comorbidities invisible to the naked eye. You can help in several ways:

- Read this book to them and reassure them.
- It may be a matter of finding a doctor who knows how to diagnose and treat their condition(s). Find that doctor (see chapter 12) and take your loved one to their appointments, especially if driving has become difficult for them.

Whatever you do, don't give up hope, and don't let your loved one give up hope. In my experience, something almost always can be done to improve symptoms.

---

patients can keep me informed. In time, once they are stable and have comfortable eyes, my patients learn how to avoid triggers and manage symptoms. I ask them to return at least once a year for a thorough exam and maintenance probing to support the health of their Meibomian glands.

11

Intraductal Meibomian Gland Probing

The Maskin® Probe and Protocol

Myth
*New and commonly prescribed therapies for MGD
consistently resolve the signs and symptoms of disease.*
Fact
*Many new and commonly prescribed treatments may be ineffective
because they don't target and release the periductal fibrosis found
at different depths in 90 percent of glands in lids with MGD.*

Myth
*Once Meibomian glands are atrophied,
they are gone for good.*
Fact
Meibomian gland probing can restore glands.

Hidden within the eyelid beneath the surface of the lid margin, periductal fibrosis constricting and invading Meibomian glands has been difficult to detect and very difficult to treat. Maskin® Probing provides physical proof of fixed blockages and restores the integrity of the intraductal space.

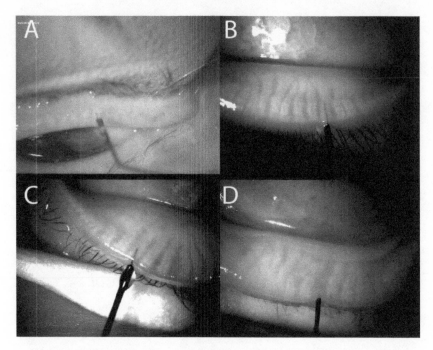

Fig. 11.1. Maskin® Probes and MicroTubes Inside Meibomian Glands

A. 1 millimeter Maskin Probe entering an orifice in an upper lid.

B. 2 millimeter Maskin Probe safely inside the intraductal space (infrared meibography).

C. 1 millimeter Maskin MicroTube dispensing therapeutic medication into the intraductal space.

D. 1 millimeter Maskin Probe advanced through an orifice into a gland that shows a complete loss of acinar-ductular units (whole gland atrophy, WGA), confirming the central duct channel remains intact in this setting.

Sources: A and D: Courtesy of Steven L. Maskin, MD; B and C: Reproduced from Steven L. Maskin and Sreevardhan Alluri, "Meibography Guided Intraductal Meibomian Gland Probing Using Real-Time Infrared Video Feed," *British Journal of Ophthalmology* 104, no. 12 (2020), 1676–1682, with permission from BMJ Publishing Group Ltd.

PART I: THE HISTORY

Patient Zero

The first time I inserted a sterile probe into a patient's Meibomian gland, I heard the characteristic *pop*. My patient heard it, too, the same way you can hear your teeth grinding inside your head. It was the mid-2000s, and at the time I wondered what caused that sound.

Right before the *pop*, the probe had encountered fixed resistance. There was something firm and unyielding inside the gland, blocking it and preventing it from secreting meibum. Clearly, this was not thickened meibum, keratin, or cellular debris.

Immediately after the *pop*, meibum oozed out of the probed gland, along the wire probe through the opening at the lid margin, like a miniature uncapped oil well.

I inserted the probe into a second gland. Again, it encountered something firm and unyielding. When the probe pushed through, I heard another *pop*.

My patient sat back and I asked him how he felt. Already, he felt meibum soothing his eye and localized relief from the pressure that had built up inside his eyelid.

I asked if he wanted me to keep probing.

Without hesitating, he said yes, and we wondered if the next gland would make a popping sound, too.

Early Experience with Meibomian Glands

Since 1988 during my fellowship at the Bascom Palmer Eye Institute of the University of Miami medical school, I hoped to one day find new treatments for MGD, the ubiquitous disease characterized by obstructed Meibomian glands. After entering private practice in Tampa in 1991 and focusing exclusively on nonrefractive cornea and external disease, I began seeing countless patients with MGD and Dry Eye. These diseases, although very common, had been notoriously difficult to treat, so many doctors referred their patients to me. Demand for my services was so high that I even wrote a book about Dry Eye in 2007.

Most of these patients suffered not only with Dry Eye and MGD, but with a variety of ocular surface comorbidities, each requiring timely and accurate diagnosis. Early on in my practice, I had discovered that eliciting a change in the severity or quality of Dry Eye symptoms through physical manipulation of tissue during an examination would help localize the disease (as is the case in other areas of diagnostic medicine). Based on this discovery, I developed relatively simple, though highly accurate, diagnostic techniques. For

Sidebar 11.1
Eliciting a Change in Symptoms

Eliciting a change in symptoms is something doctors often do when diagnosing. For example, if a patient complains of abdominal pain, the doctor will push on the abdomen to locate the source of pain. Increased pain in the right lower quadrant of the abdomen may suggest appendicitis.

However, to my knowledge, diagnostic techniques at the slit lamp using physician manipulation of ocular tissue to elicit a change in symptoms have not been widely used by eye doctors to diagnose Dry Eye, MGD, and other ocular surface comorbidities, such as conjunctivochalasis. These techniques help both with diagnosing the presence of a disease and its impact on a patient's symptom complex.

example, by simply mobilizing the upper eyelid over the eyeball with the patient looking down during a slit-lamp exam, I could determine if the patient's symptoms were in part due to friction-related superior conjunctivochalasis. Other simple tests helped with the diagnosis of comorbidities. A fast-acting antihistamine drop could confirm in seconds if allergies were a factor. The serial Schirmer's test proved to be more sensitive and ultimately more accurate than a single Schirmer's test. The fluorescein clearance test, which I had used since my fellowship, indicated delayed tear clearance.

With definitive diagnoses, I could take a proven, straightforward approach with treatment: AMT surgery for conjunctivochalasis; antihistamine eye drops, hygiene and lifestyle changes, and so forth, for allergies; punctal occlusion for ATD; irrigation for delayed tear clearance. I still use these highly effective diagnostic techniques and treatments today.

Questions Without Answers

MGD proved more elusive. Patients complained of pain and tenderness in their eyelids and burning in their eyes sometimes with photophobia. But those of us treating this disease back then could only guess at what was happening inside the Meibomian glands to cause these symptoms. Plus the usual treatments, such as oral and topical antibiotics, eyelid cleansing, warm compresses, eyelid massage and/or expression, and topical steroids, offered patients little, largely inconsistent, relief.

At the time, and even to this day, some doctors believed excess keratinization and meibum thickening within the ducts were the major proximate causes of obstructive MGD. They theorized these nonfixed ductal contents caused elevated intraductal pressure leading to cystic changes, squamous metaplasia, fibrosis, and gland atrophy (see chapter 4). Although seemingly logical and widely accepted, to me this explanation was insufficient. Why did transillumination show that parts of some glands atrophy while other parts don't? Why did some neighboring glands atrophy while others remained intact? Why did the lid become tender, whether or not meibum was expressible? As the years passed, I wanted answers to these nagging questions even more. (Eventually these questions led me to develop and propose a new classification system for obstructive MGD, based on probe findings plus transillumination or meibography results; see fig. 9.2.)

Early on I hypothesized that the answers and the source of my patients' persistent pain would be found inside the Meibomian glands themselves. And so, in the early to mid-1990s, I began thinking about exploring the internal duct space. No one had done this before, perhaps fearful that the glands would be permanently damaged. But I had handled rabbit Meibomian glands during my fellowship training in the late 1980s. To prepare the rabbit glands for culture, under a microscope I surgically isolated sections of lids containing three glands, then placed these sections into a digestive enzyme to loosen the glands from their connective tissue. Once loosened, I surgically separated the acinar-ductular units from the whole ducts. Whereas the delicate acinar-ductular epithelium often disintegrated, the duct tissue proved more durable and remained largely intact. Thus, having witnessed firsthand the durability of the rabbit Meibomian gland ducts, I expected no less from human ducts (see fig. 1.1).

Many of my patients had mild to moderate MGD. With their other comorbidities resolved, they were improving 20–70 percent, but because MGD persisted, they weren't improving 100 percent. I had to fix this problem. By the early 2000s, as I and my MGD patients grew increasingly frustrated, my plan began to crystallize. Somehow I would have to enter a patient's glands to explore them from the inside.

The Ideal Patient

One day in the mid-2000s, the ideal patient arrived at my office. He was a middle-aged man with severe, obstructive MGD and extremely painful lids. Despite seeing many ophthalmologists and trying many treatments, nothing had worked. Because of the pain, he couldn't do the simplest task. As it happens, Patient Zero had turned up in my office and he desperately needed help.

It was time to act, to enter the human Meibomian gland duct, explore the intraductal space, and search for the root cause of a difficult medical diagnostic problem. I began by fashioning the first sterile prototype Meibomian gland probe. I showed the tiny probe to the patient and described the procedure. This would be an investigative, fact-finding exploration of the glands, based on my years of experience handling rabbit Meibomian gland tissues back in the late 1980s. I would push the tip of the probe into a few outer glands of the left lower lid for starters. We would observe from our distinct vantage points as doctor and patient, and report our findings. I didn't know what we might learn but I was hoping for information that might help explain this disease. Without hesitating, the patient signed an informed consent document.

After I applied a topical anesthetic to his eyes, the patient rested his chin and forehead on the supports at the slit lamp. While a technician held his head steady from behind, I inserted the probe into one obviously blocked gland in the lower lid until I felt firm resistance. Then I pushed on the probe a little harder.

Pop!

The probe relieved the resistance and meibum flowed. I inserted the probe into another gland. We heard another *pop,* and I watched meibum flow again. At the third gland, the probe encountered something gritty, making a sound like nails on a washboard. With each subsequent gland, the probe encountered resistance, making either a popping sound or the gritty nails-on-a-washboard sound when it released.

When I finished probing all the glands, plenty of meibum flowed, relieving pressure inside the entire lid. Patient Zero was ecstatic.

I asked if we should continue. He told me to keep probing.

So I probed the rest of the glands in the other three lids. When I finished, Patient Zero jumped out of his chair and hugged me. His suffering had ended, but my work was just beginning. This probe might help other patients with MGD, but first I needed to know how it worked and why.

Periductal Fibrosis

At the time, I only knew the probe had encountered fibrosis, or scar tissue, inside Patient Zero's Meibomian glands, rather than the thick meibum, excess keratin, or cell debris that was typically associated with MGD. If the obstruction consisted of these, the probe would have slid through easily. Instead, the obstruction was fixed, firm, and didn't yield immediately. It resisted and released when probed, just like scar tissue sometimes found in the lacrimal punctum (tear drainage duct) or canaliculus (tear drainage canal).

But I didn't know the nature of the fibrosis, because I couldn't see it hidden within Patient Zero's lids. I could only feel it with the probe, hear and feel its release, and then watch freed meibum flow out through the orifice. The fibrosis was growing in an occult manner, hidden within the tissue of the lids, close enough to the glands to obstruct them, but I couldn't say if it grew within the lumen (hollow channel through which meibum flows), inside the duct wall, around the duct wall, or some combination of these.

While reviewing the relevant literature, I came across the 1997 book with a chapter by Ivan Cher, MD, an ophthalmologist at the University of New South Wales in Australia, in which he described dimpling and other changes of the gland orifices associated with

MGD and observed at the slit lamp. In the article, without the insights provided by intraductal probing, he speculated "strangulation by fibrosis may contribute to 'drop-out.'" I found this intriguing. Further research uncovered published images using confocal microscopy of periglandular and periductal fibrosis.

Taken together—the published confocal images, slit-lamp findings, and my probe findings—it became clear that the scar tissue causing glandular obstruction was periductal in location. We now know unequivocally, periductal fibrosis wraps around the duct wall like a python coiling around its prey, and we have evidence that it also invades the external duct wall and stem cell zone. It causes stricture and loss of ductal integrity, and plays a significant role in the vast majority of MGD cases.

It also explains the sounds we hear when probing. A *pop* indicates the release of a single band of fibrosis, like the snapping apart of a tight rubber band. The gritty, nail-on-a-washboard sound indicates the snapping apart of several bands at different depths.

Meibomian Gland Probing—Early Research and Outcomes

The sound of probing a blocked Meibomian gland is hard to forget, the hug of a grateful patient even harder. Patient Zero finally had relief from obstructive MGD, the most common factor in debilitating Dry Eye. I realized probing Meibomian glands might be a viable treatment for MGD. If it worked for him, it might work for others.

I had expected probing the glands would be straightforward and safe because central ducts are flexible and have intrinsic structure. Like the sleeve of a cotton shirt when an arm slips in, the Meibomian gland naturally yields and straightens when a blunt probe enters. But I had three questions:

1. Would probing work for anyone else?
2. Would the benefits last?
3. Was it safe?

With their approval, I began probing the glands of patients with obstructive MGD regularly, meticulously recording the results. I worked with the probes for many months, probing patients' glands and collating data to study the long-term safety and efficacy of the treatment. I presented my findings at ophthalmology and optometry meetings and published them in peer-reviewed journals.

The first presentation was a poster delivered at the 2009 ARVO (Association for Research in Vision and Ophthalmology) meeting, with a subsequent 2010 manuscript published in the journal *Cornea*, entitled "Intraductal Meibomian Gland Probing Relieves Symptoms of Obstructive Meibomian Gland Dysfunction." These reports showed that immediately after probing, patients with obstructive MGD displayed marked improvement in symptoms. Of the twenty-five patients who had complained of lid tenderness or soreness as well as lid margin congestion (lid heaviness, stickiness, gumminess, and awareness of lids), twenty-four experienced immediate relief, with all twenty-five patients having sustained relief within one month after probing.

Importantly, patients reported that many previously unrecognized and subclinical symptoms (which had not been reported during their preprobing visits or may have been simply tolerated) had also improved (see fig. 11.2). In addition to the relief of the chief complaint with probing, I wrote in 2010 that "patients offered unsolicited comments during follow-up visits [about other symptoms that also improved]. But interestingly, these other symptoms were not reported during preprobing visits. These symptoms were subclinical. Only after these symptoms had resolved did patients recognize having tolerated the symptom. This supports the notion that chronic MGD may create gradual onset of subtle subclinical disease. After probing, subclinical symptoms became apparent by their improvement."

None of the twenty-five patients reported adverse effects or sequelae (the medical term for downstream adverse effects). In the manuscript, I described how the probe often encountered variable resistance within the gland, and the nature of that hidden resistance— sometimes fixed and firm, producing an audible *pop* or a gritty sensation, while other times a mild resistance. I speculated that obstructive MGD can progress subclinically and occultly, that is, undetectably. I concluded that *"Intraductal fibrotic and neovascular changes may explain the persistence of obstructive MGD despite exhaustive therapies directed at the lid margin and orifice and the inconsistent*

Cornea • Volume 29, Number 10, October 2010

TABLE 3. Postprobing, Newly Recognized, and Previously Subclinical Symptoms Improved With Meibomian Gland Probing

Subclinical Symptom	No. Patients
Smoother lid surface	8
↑ Lubrication	6
↑ Vision	4
↓ Pain	4
↓ Burning	3
↑ Comfort	3
↓ Artificial tears	3
↓ Dry	3
↓ Foreign body sensation	3
↓ Photophobia	2
↓ Redness	2
↓ Soreness	2
↓ Tearing	2
↑ Moist	2
No friction between lid and eye	2
↓ Mucus	2
↓ Itching	1
↓ Tired eye	1
CTL not dry	1
↑ Lid excursion	1
Eye feels cooler	1
↓ Aching	1

Fig. 11.2. Surprising Improvements in Newly Recognized and Previously Subclinical Symptoms After Meibomian Gland Probing

Patients reported improvements in previously unrecognized symptoms after treatment with Maskin® Probing. CTL = contact lens, ↑ = increase, ↓ = decrease.

Source: Steven L. Maskin, "Intraductal Meibomian Gland Probing Relieves Symptoms of Obstructive Meibomian Gland Dysfunction," *Cornea* 29, no. 10 (2010), 1145–1152, https://journals.lww.com/corneajrnl/Abstract/2010/10000/Intraductal_Meibomian_Gland_Probing_Relieves.13.aspx.

effect of warm compresses and lid massage. Intraductal Meibomian gland probing appears highly effective in quickly relieving inflammatory symptoms of obstructive MGD."

(Quote from Steven L. Maskin, "Intraductal Meibomian Gland Probing Relieves Symptoms of Obstructive MGD," poster presented at the annual meeting of the Association for Research in Vision and Ophthalmology, May 2009, Fort Lauderdale, FL. Abstract published in *Investigative Ophthalmology & Visual Science,* April 2009, 4636.)

Although the early data suggested probing would be a game changer for thousands upon thousands of patients suffering with obstructive MGD, I needed more proof before the procedure could be broadly adopted.

Vulnerable Patients

Through word of mouth, news about my research and the remarkable relief my patients experienced began to spread. More and more patients with severe comorbidities and MGD gravitated to my practice, sometimes referred by colleagues who had seen the journal article or heard me speak about probing at a conference. Other patients found me via online chats, blogs, and forums. Some had read my previous book, *Reversing Dry Eye Syndrome.* Many traveled long distances to see me—from Singapore and Australia, all over Europe, the United States, and every continent except Antarctica. Sometimes during their first visits, these patients would describe intractable, horrific pain. Incapacitated by the pain and without hope of finding relief, many had considered suicide. Others had become depressed and suicidal. Some had been hospitalized after attempting suicide.

I was ready even for these patients. Over the years, I had honed my techniques for diagnosing and treating other ocular surface comorbidities. I also discovered that persistent lid tenderness after an anesthetic drop indicated elevated intraductal pressure, a sign of obstructive MGD. I realized this finding could be used as a simple, reliable, and repeatable diagnostic test.

Now I would hone probing as a reliable treatment and diagnostic tool for MGD. For me and my patients, anything less was unacceptable. With the desperate pleas of my most vulnerable patients resonating in my thoughts, I challenged myself to rise to this task. Although the work would be demanding for me, a physician in a solo private practice, my patients' dramatic turnarounds after this simple office procedure were compelling and energizing.

Two Response Curves

Early on, as I studied patients' responses to probing, I began using the visual analog scale (VAS), a standardized measurement tool for recording patients' subjective evaluations of the severity of their symptoms. (VAS is a reliable tool for subjectively measuring severity of symptoms. With VAS, patients make a handwritten vertical mark on a horizontal line 10 centimeters long, with 0 representing no pain and 10 representing the worst pain they have ever experienced.)

Some patients experienced dramatic relief immediately after probing, and others would come back a few months later with greatly improved symptoms. However, I couldn't explain the reason for the different timing of symptom relief. Then one day in my clinic as I was walking between examination rooms and puzzling over this mystery, I stopped in my tracks. It suddenly hit me: all the patients who had immediate relief had suffered with lid tenderness, whereas the ones with delayed relief had different symptoms of MGD, like burning or stinging. These two distinct responses meant somehow probing was addressing more than one type of problem in the glands. But what were they?

By 2010, the VAS data I had been collecting from patients confirmed these two distinct response curves to (see fig. 11.3). One response curve, an immediate, dramatic, approximately 80 percent improvement in lid tenderness, occurred within the first twenty-four hours of probing and lasted about twelve months. I interpreted this improvement in lid tenderness to the equilibration of the intra-ductal pressure imbalance caused by fixed fibrotic obstruction. With the fixed obstruction released and ductal integrity restored, meibum flow resumed, relieving eyelid tenderness and inflammation. The process is analogous to clearing an intestinal obstruction. With the obstruction cleared, normal flow resumes, quickly reducing abdominal tenderness and inflammation.

The second response curve was associated with symptoms such

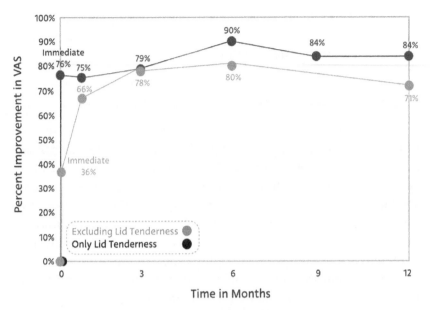

**Fig. 11.3. Results of Meibomian Gland Probing on
Visual Analog Scale for Symptoms of MGD**

Patients rated their symptoms immediately after probing and then again every
few months for a year on a visual analog scale (VAS).

The X axis shows time in months, with zero as the moment immediately after
probing. The Y axis shows the percent of improvement in symptoms.

Source: Steven L. Maskin and Kelly Kantor, "Intraductal Meibomian Gland Probing to Restore
Functionality for Obstructive Meibomian Gland Dysfunction." Poster presented at the annual
meeting of the American Academy of Ophthalmology, October 2011, Orlando, FL.

as burning and photophobia, but not lid tenderness. Improvement
in these symptoms was more gradual, with an immediate improvement of 35 percent on average, increasing to approximately 80 percent two to three months after probing. I concluded these symptoms
improved due to overall improved gland health and functionality,
rather than relief of intraductal pressure, although I did not, at the
time, have any specific insight into what was happening at the cellular level to cause it.

More recent studies have suggested the second curve may have
been related to the glands' postprobing biologic response to releasing periductal fibrosis. Several weeks to months after its release, together with a decrease in symptoms, we have seen a proliferation of
ductal epithelial cells with a thickening of duct walls, suggesting

stem cell activation. These cellular and symptom improvements were consistent with the growth of Meibomian gland tissue seen in as little as five months after probing.

First, Do No Harm, and Lasting Results

Primum non nocere, "First, do no harm," the driving principle behind all biomedical research and product development, has guided my work from day one. Probing Meibomian glands could help many patients, but the procedure had to be safe, causing neither immediate harm nor long-term adverse effects. By the 2011 ARVO meeting, I had compiled enough data from probing and follow-up appointments of the original cohort of twenty-five patients (forty-nine lids) to present an updated poster describing the two response curves (fig. 11.3) and promising findings about longer-term efficacy and safety. I was able to follow up and obtain data on twenty-one (84 percent; forty-two lids) of the initial twenty-five patients. Sixteen patients had follow-up exams in the office, three by phone, and two by email. Two patients were unavailable, and two others had died.

I presented the following information:

- The entire cohort of twenty-one patients (forty-two lids) reported ongoing improvement in symptoms at their last follow-up appointment more than two years after probing (overall average follow-up was 28.3 months).
- Seven patients (fourteen lids) had retreatment (33.3 percent) and fourteen patients (twenty-eight lids) did not require retreatment (66.7 percent).
- No patients reported worsening symptoms or adverse consequences.
- VAS scores remained markedly improved for at least nine months.

I drew the following conclusion:

Intraductal Meibomian gland probing appears highly effective in safely and rapidly reducing standardized VAS patient scores of a variety of symptoms associated with MGD.

Clearly, Meibomian gland probing was a safe and effective treatment for my patients with MGD, but still more research was needed with a much larger pool of patients.

Other Studies from Around the World

Motivated to ensure that every patient with obstructive MGD could access the treatment, I contracted with a Tampa-based manufacturer of ophthalmic devices to produce the probes. Some ophthalmologists and optometrists quickly recognized the benefits and started using the probes following my protocols. Some even conducted their own studies and clinical trials.

I had no influence over the independent research conducted globally. Probing has been studied in Massachusetts (2020, 2017), China (2019, 2016, 2014), Turkey (2019, 2016), India (2019), Cuba (2017), Japan (2015), Mexico (2015), Russia (2013), and New York State (2012).

The studies, published in peer-reviewed journals and listed here chronologically (most recent first), uniformly report the safety and efficacy of intraductal Meibomian gland probing used as a treatment to restore ductal integrity in obstructive MGD. Although studies deviated from my recommended protocols in a variety of ways, all reported improvement in patients refractory (not responding) to conventional treatments. If my protocols had been followed, we could expect even better results.

INDEPENDENT RESEARCH STUDIES, CONDUCTED GLOBALLY AND PUBLISHED IN PEER-REVIEWED JOURNALS

"Meibomian Gland Probing in Patients with Meibomian Gland Dysfunction"
Nirupama, D., et al., *Indian Journal of Clinical and Experimental Ophthalmology* 5, no. 1 (2019), 78–81.

"Dynamic Intraductal Meibomian Probing: A Modified Approach to the Treatment of Obstructive Meibomian Gland Dysfunction"

Syed, Zeba A., and Francis C. Sutula, *Ophthalmic Plastic and Reconstructive Surgery*, July/August 2017, 307–309.

"Efficacy of Intraductal Probing in the Dysfunction of the Meibomian Glands"
Cárdenas Díaz, Taimi, et al., *Revista Cubana de Oftalmologia*, [S.1.], v. 30, n. 2, 2017.

"Effectiveness of Intraductal Meibomian Gland Probing for Obstructive Meibomian Gland Dysfunction"
Sarman, Zuleyha Sik, et al., *Cornea*, June 2016, 721–724.

"Analysis of Meibum Before and After Intraductal Meibomian Gland Probing in Eyes with Obstructive Meibomian Gland Dysfunction"
Nakayama, Naohiko, et al., *Cornea*, October 2015, 1206–1208.

"Sondaje intraductal de las glándulas de Meibomio para el tratamiento de blefaritis posterior severa" [Intraductal Meibomian gland probing for the treatment of blepharitis]
Fermon, S., Hindi I. Zaga, and Alvarez D. Melloni, *Archivos de la Sociedad Española de Oftalmologí*, February 2015, 76–80.

"Efficacy of Physiotherapy and Hygienic Procedures in Treatment of Adults and Children with Chronic Blepharitis and Dry Eye Syndrome"
Prozornaia, L. P., and V. V. Brzhevskiĭ, *Vestnik oftalmologii*, May–June 2013, 68–70, 72–73.

"Intraductal Meibomian Gland Probing in the Management of Ocular Rosacea"
Wladis, Edward J., *Ophthalmic Plastic and Reconstructive Surgery*, November–December 2012, 416–418.

Clinical Trials

To date, three randomized clinical trials in China, one in the United States, and one in Turkey have evaluated the safety and efficacy of Meibomian gland probing.

Clinical trials are typically rigorous studies that compare a treatment to a control or no treatment. Patients enrolled in the clinical trial receive either the treatment, a placebo, or, in the case of a procedure, a sham treatment—one in which it appears as if the patients undergo the procedure when in fact they don't. The outcomes of patients who received treatment are then compared to the control group of patients who did not receive treatment.

Clinical trials are usually double-blind, meaning that to control for biases, the patient and evaluating doctor don't know if the treatment or placebo is being administered.

Randomized clinical trials put patients randomly in treatment or placebo/sham groups.

Here is a chronological listing (most recent first) of clinical trials that have evaluated the safety and efficacy of Meibomian gland probing. Although these studies also deviated from my recommended protocols in a variety of ways, all reported improvement in patients refractory to conventional treatment. Here too, if my protocols had been followed, we could expect even better results.

INTRADUCTAL MEIBOMIAN
GLAND PROBING CLINICAL TRIALS

"A Randomized, Sham-Controlled Trial of Intraductal Meibomian Gland Probing with or Without Topical Antibiotic/ Steroid for Obstructive Meibomian Gland Dysfunction"
Kheirkhah, Ahmad, et al., *The Ocular Surface,* October 2020, 852–856 (see sidebar 11.2).

"Effectiveness of Intraductal Meibomian Gland Probing in Addition to the Conventional Treatment in Patients with Obstructive Meibomian Gland Dysfunction"
Incekalan, T. K., et al., *Ocular Immunology and Inflammation,* September 2019, 1345–1351.

"Clinical Results of Intraductal Meibomian Gland Probing Combined with Intense Pulsed Light in Treating Patients with Refractory Obstructive Meibomian Gland Dysfunction: A Randomized Controlled Trial"
Huang, X., et al., *BMC Ophthalmology,* October 28, 2019 (see sidebar 11.3).

"Efficacy of Intraductal Meibomian Gland Probing on Tear Function in Patients with Obstructive Meibomian Gland Dysfunction"
    Ma, Xiao, and Yan Lu, *Cornea,* June 2016, 725–730.

"Clinical Research on Intraductal Meibomian Gland Probing in the Treatment of Patients with Meibomian Gland Dysfunction"
    Dongju, Qin, Liu Hui, and Xu Jianjiang, *Chinese Journal of Optometry, Ophthalmology, and Visual Science* 16, no. 10 (2014), 615–621.

Sharing Knowledge

With expanded diagnostic capabilities, but still much to learn about Meibomian glands and MGD, I worked to quickly transform research findings and new understandings into therapies for my patients.

Believing patients anywhere in the world should have access to this same level of care, I disseminated my findings freely in studies published in peer-reviewed journals in an open-source format available to anyone with a computer and Internet access, in magazine articles, through interviews, in courses and posters presented at medical meetings, and in an ophthalmology textbook about MGD published in Japan, and in this book.

In 2019, over a decade after first probing Patient Zero, I established a translational research company, MGDinnovations, Inc. (MGDi), to make effective research-based and targeted treatments for MGD available to sufferers worldwide. MGDi (www.MGDi.com) conducts clinical research and provides training and support resources to doctors around the world seeking solutions for their MGD patients.

Here are chronological lists (most recent first) of my published works pertaining specifically to Meibomian glands, MGD, and associated ocular surface diseases (continues on p. 286).

Sidebar 11.2
Double-Blind Meibomian
Gland Probing Clinical Trial, 2020

An independent, prospective, double-blind, randomized control trial conducted at Massachusetts Eye and Ear Infirmary at Harvard University in 2014–2015, and presented as a poster in 2016 at the American Academy of Ophthalmology annual meeting, compared Meibomian gland probing with combination Blephamide® (a steroid-antibiotic ointment) treatment, and separately GenTeal® PM ointment, to sham probing with GenTeal PM ointment. The final study findings were published in October 2020. (Kheirkhah, Ahmad, et al., "A Randomized, Sham-Controlled Trial of Intraductal Meibomian Gland Probing with or Without Topical Antibiotic/Steroid for Obstructive Meibomian Gland Dysfunction," *The Ocular Surface*, October 2020, 852–856.)

Patients with refractory MGD for at least three months, who had tried traditional management with no success in resolving their clinical signs or symptoms, were included in the study, and only their upper lids were probed. Treatment that *included probing* improved symptoms to a statistically significant level that was not seen with sham probing, according to both the Ocular Surface Disease Index (OSDI) and the Symptom Assessment in Dry Eye (SANDE) survey (see glossary).

For the probing plus Blephamide group, post-probing OSDI and SANDE showed significant improvement, with p-values of 0.02 and 0.002, respectively. For probing plus GenTeal group, post-probing SANDE showed significant improvement, with a p-value of 0.01.

The investigators point out the limitations of their study, such as small sample size (only fourteen patients in each group) and no control group to assess the efficacy of probing alone versus probing with Blephamide or

GenTeal PM therapy. Here I have noted several additional limitations.

1. Probing was performed on upper lids only, but the clinical parameters—TBUT, Schirmer's test, fluorescein staining, lissamine green staining, OSDI, and SANDE—involve contributions from the Meibomian glands of *both* lids, which in turn affect the health of the *entire* ocular surface and related symptoms.

2. The lid tenderness quantitative assessment, asking patients to grade severity on a scale of 1 to 10, had the following limitations:

   - The lid tenderness assessments were done without using a topical anesthetic drop in the eye, so patients may have reported feeling lid tenderness but were, in fact, feeling discomfort from somewhere on the ocular surface other than the lid.

   - There was no controlling for variations in lid tenderness across an entire lid. Patients may have had level 10 pain in the area over only two glands and the rest of the lid may have had no tenderness. Or a patient may have had level 3 pain nasally, and level 10 temporally. But the study did not allow for these variations in tenderness in a single lid.

     My studies (and diagnoses) assess lid tenderness qualitatively as present or absent to avoid inconsistencies. Patients indicate if they experience tenderness across the entire lid, in a region, or in a single spot. If there is tenderness across at least one-third of the lid, it is designated as a "tender" lid. If there is tenderness across less than one-third of the

lid, focal tenderness is noted on the Meibomian Gland Classification Form, but the lid
is designated "not tender."

- The investigators injected lids that were to be
probed with anesthesia. The injection itself
can cause hemorrhage and edema, which can
persist for several weeks. Thus, at follow-up
appointments, when the patients' lids were
evaluated, tenderness was likely due to the
ongoing side effects of the injection, and *not*
because probing was ineffective.

3. Periductal scar tissue may be deep within the Meibomian glands, but only 1 and 2 millimeter probes
were used. (Glands vary in length, but glands in
upper lids are typically much longer than 2 millimeters.) Deeper scar tissue may not have been
reached by the shorter probes, therefore not released, and lid tenderness would have persisted.
Longer probes are available precisely because
periductal fibrosis can occur anywhere along the
gland's length. If patients experienced residual lid
tenderness after probing with the shorter probes,
their glands should have been probed with the
longer probes, which is part of my standard treatment protocol.

4. The study could have assessed signs and symptoms
not only at baseline and four weeks after probing,
but at additional points in time, that is, twenty-
four hours and one week later, to evaluate the
therapy before adverse effects from comorbidities
set in; as well as two to three months later, to
evaluate improvements in symptoms and signs
once ductal integrity and Meibomian gland function have been restored.

Sidebar 11.3
Meibomian Gland Probing and IPL

A 2019 randomized controlled trial compared Meibomian gland probing to IPL and to combination therapy of probing followed by IPL three weeks later (see chapter 10), with these results:

- Probing showed significant reduction in lid tenderness (p < 0.001) compared to IPL.
- After treatment, 93 percent of the probing-plus-IPL group, 37 percent of the probing group, and only 18 percent of the IPL group increased TBUT to greater than 5 seconds (p = 0.009).
- 64.29% of the probing-plus-IPL group, compared to 26.67% of the probing group, and only 14.29% of the IPL group showed a significant improvement (p = 0.02) in SPEED scores.
- 100 percent of the probing group and only 85.7 percent of the IPL group reported relief of symptoms.
- No patients in the probing-plus-IPL group needed repeat treatment after six months, compared to 35.7 percent who needed retreatment in the IPL group and only 20 percent in the probing group.

PAPERS PUBLISHED IN PEER-REVIEWED LITERATURE

"Meibography Guided Intraductal Meibomian Gland Probing Using Real-Time Infrared Video Feed"
Maskin, Steven L., and Sreevardhan Alluri, *British Journal of Ophthalmology*, December 2020, 1676–1682.

"Intraductal Meibomian Gland Probing: Background, Patient Selection, Procedure, and Perspectives"

Maskin, Steven L., and Sreevardhan Alluri, *Clinical Ophthalmology,* July 10, 2019, 1203–1223.

"Expressible Meibomian Glands Have Occult Fixed Obstructions: Findings from Meibomian Gland Probing to Restore Intraductal Integrity"
Maskin, Steven L., and Sreevardhan Alluri, *Cornea,* July 2019, 880–887.

"Infrared Video Meibography of Lower Lid Meibomian Glands Shows Easily Distorted Glands: Implications for Longitudinal Assessment of Atrophy or Growth Using Lower Lid Meibography"
Maskin, Steven L., and Whitney R. Testa, *Cornea,* October 2018, 1279–1286.

"Growth of Meibomian Gland Tissue After Intraductal Meibomian Gland Probing in Patients with Obstructive Meibomian Gland Dysfunction"
Maskin, Steven L., and Whitney R. Testa, *British Journal of Ophthalmology,* January 2018, 59–68.

"Intraductal Meibomian Gland Probing Relieves Symptoms of Obstructive Meibomian Gland Dysfunction"
Maskin, Steven L., *Cornea,* October 2010, 1145–1152.

"Effect of Ocular Surface Reconstruction by Using Amniotic Membrane Transplant for Symptomatic Conjunctivochalasis on Fluorescein Clearance Test Results"
Maskin, Steven L., *Cornea,* July 2008, 644–649.

"A Randomized, Double-Masked, Placebo-Controlled, Multicenter Comparison of Loteprednol Etabonate Ophthalmic Suspension, 0.5%, and Placebo for Treatment of Keratoconjunctivitis Sicca in Patients with Delayed Tear Clearance"
Pflugfelder, Stephen C., Steven L. Maskin, Bruce Anderson, James Chodosh, Edward J. Holland, Cintia S. De Paiva, Stephen P. Bartels, Teresa Micuda, Howard M. Proskin, and Roger Vogel, *American Journal of Ophthalmology,* September 2004, 444–457.

"Amniotic Membrane Transplantation for Symptomatic
Conjunctivochalasis Refractory to Medical Treatment"
Meller, Daniel, Steven L. Maskin, R.T.F. Pires, and Scheffer
C. G. Tseng, *Cornea,* November 2000, 796–803.

"Amniotic Membrane Transplantation for Symptomatic
Bullous Keratopathy"
Pires R.T. F., Scheffer C. G. Tseng, P. Prabhasaawat,
V. Puangsricharem, Steven L. Maskin, J.C. Kim, and D.T.H.
Tan, *Archives of Ophthalmology,* October 1999, 1291–1297.

"Regression of Limbal Epithelial Dysplasia with Topical
Interferon"
Maskin, Steven L., *Archives of Ophthalmology,* September
1994, 1145–1146 (also selected for publication in the
Chinese and Spanish editions).

"Clonal Growth and Differentiation of Rabbit Meibomian
Gland Epithelium in Serum-Free Culture"
Maskin, Steven L., and Scheffer C. G. Tseng, *Investigative
Ophthalmology & Visual Science,* January 1992, 205–217.

"Culture of Rabbit Meibomian Gland Using Collagen Gel"
Maskin, Steven L., and Scheffer C. G. Tseng, *Investigative
Ophthalmology & Visual Science,* January 1991, 214–223.

BOOK

*Reversing Dry Eye Syndrome: Practical Ways to Improve Your
Comfort, Vision, and Appearance*
Maskin, Steven L. New Haven, CT: Yale University Press,
2007.

BOOK CHAPTERS

"Intraductal Meibomian Gland Probing: A Paradigm Shift for
the Successful Treatment of Obstructive Meibomian Gland
Dysfunction"
Maskin, Steven L., in Tsubota, ed., *Diagnosis and Treatment
of MGD.* Tokyo: Kanehara, September 2016, chap. 17,
130–167.

"Classification of Conjunctival Surgeries for Corneal Disease Based on Stem Cell Concept"
Tseng, Scheffer C. G., J. J. Y. Chen, A. J. W. Huang, F. E. Kruse, Steven L. Maskin, and R. J. F. Tsai, in Sugar and Soong, eds., *Ophthalmology Clinics of North America*, vol. 3, no. 4. Philadelphia: Saunders, December 1990, 595–610.

PRESENTATIONS AND POSTERS

"Intraductal Meibomian Gland Probing (MGP) Leads to Ductal Epithelial Proliferation with Increased Duct Wall Thickness"
Maskin, Steven L., and Sreevardhan Alluri, poster presented at the annual meeting of the Association for Research in Vision and Ophthalmology, virtual meeting, March 2020. Abstract published in *Investigative Ophthalmology & Visual Science*, June 2020, 96.

"An Alternative Hypothesis of Atrophic Meibomian Gland Dysfunction Using Stem Cell Concept"
Maskin, Steven L., and Sreevardhan Alluri, poster presented at the annual meeting of the Association for Research in Vision and Ophthalmology, virtual meeting, March 2020. Abstract published in *Investigative Ophthalmology & Visual Science*, June 2020, 343.

"Real Time Infrared Video Feed Enables Visualization of Intraductal Meibomian Gland Probing"
Maskin, Steven L., and Sreevardhan Alluri, poster presented at the World Cornea Congress VIII, virtual meeting, March 2020.

"Infrared Video Meibography Feed Reveals Meibomian Gland Probing Restores and Confirms Central Duct Integrity in Areas of Whole Gland Atrophy"
Maskin, Steven L., and Sreevardhan Alluri, paper presented at the World Cornea Congress VIII, virtual meeting, March 2020.

"Real Time Infrared Video Meibography Feed Shows Intraductal Meibomian Gland Probing Confirms Presence of Duct and Restores Intraductal Integrity in Setting of Whole Gland Atrophy"

> Maskin, Steven L., and Sreevardhan Alluri, poster presented at the American Academy of Optometry, October 2019, Orlando, FL.

"Treatment of Obstructive Meibomian Gland Dysfunction Using Intraductal Probing: Emerging Importance of Restoring Ductal Integrity"

> Maskin, Steven L., presented at a course on New Treatments for Meibomian Gland Dysfunction at the annual meeting of the American Academy of Ophthalmology, October 2019, San Francisco.

"Visualization of Intraductal Meibomian Gland Probing Using Real Time Infrared Video Feed"

> Maskin, Steven L., and Sreevardhan Alluri, poster presented at the American Academy of Optometry, October 2019, Orlando, FL.

"Meibomian Gland Probing (MGP): Safely Providing Outflow Patency with Positive Physical Proof: Concepts, Literature Review and Results"

> Maskin, Steven L., presented at a course on New Treatments for Meibomian Gland Dysfunction at the annual meeting of the American Academy of Ophthalmology, October 2018, Chicago.

"Meibomian Gland Probing (MGP): Safely Providing Patency with Positive Physical Proof: Literature Review, Concepts and Results"

> Maskin, Steven L., presented at a course on New Treatments for Meibomian Gland Dysfunction at the annual meeting of the American Academy of Ophthalmology, November 2017, New Orleans, LA.

"Regrowth of Meibomian Gland Tissue After Intraductal Meibomian Gland Probing in Patients with Obstructive Meibomian Gland Dysfunction (O-MGD)"

Maskin, Steven L., and Whitney R. Testa, poster presented at the annual meeting of the Association for Research in Vision and Ophthalmology, May 2017, Baltimore, MD. Selected by ARVO Annual Program Committee as 2017 Hot Topic. Abstract published in *Investigative Ophthalmology & Visual Science,* June 2017, 4392.

"Meibomian Gland Probing (MGP): Safely Providing Patency to Glands Using Verifiable Physical Proof: Background, Technique and Results"

Maskin, Steven L., presented at a course on New Treatments for Meibomian Gland Dysfunction at the annual meeting of the American Academy of Ophthalmology, October 2016, Chicago.

"Meibomian Gland Probing (MGP): Safely Providing Patency to Glands Using Verifiable Physical Proof: Background, Technique and Results"

Maskin, Steven L., presented at a course on New Treatments for Meibomian Gland Dysfunction at the annual meeting of the American Academy of Ophthalmology, November 2015, Las Vegas, NV.

"Meibomian Gland Probing for Lid Tenderness and Non-Functioning Meibomian Glands in Meibomian Gland Dysfunction"

Maskin, Steven L., and Whitney Hethorn, poster presented at the annual meeting of the American Academy of Ophthalmology, November 2015, Las Vegas, NV.

"Meibomian Gland Probing Findings Suggest Fibrotic Obstruction Is a Major Cause of Obstructive Meibomian Gland Dysfunction (O-MGD)"

Maskin, Steven L., poster presented at the annual meeting of the Association for Research in Vision and Ophthalmology, May 2012, Fort Lauderdale, FL. Abstract published in *Investigative Ophthalmology & Visual Science,* March 2012, 605.

"Fantastic Voyage into the Meibomian Gland: Results of Intraductal Probing (MGP) and Successful Treatment of Meibomian Gland Dysfunction (MGD) from Within"
Maskin, Steven L., virtual presentation for the Japanese Dry Eye Research Society, 2011, Tokyo.

"Intraductal Meibomian Gland Probing to Restore Functionality for Obstructive Meibomian Gland Dysfunction"
Maskin, Steven L., and Kelly Kantor, poster presented at the annual meeting of the American Academy of Ophthalmology, October 2011, Orlando, FL.

"Intraductal Meibomian Gland Probing with Adjunctive Intraductal Microtube Steroid Injection (MGPs) for Meibomian Gland Dysfunction (MGD)"
Maskin, Steven L., and Kelly Kantor, poster presented at the annual meeting of the Association for Research in Vision and Ophthalmology, May 2011, Fort Lauderdale, FL. Abstract published in *Investigative Ophthalmology & Visual Science*, April 2011, 3817.

"Intraductal Meibomian Gland Probing for Meibomian Gland Dysfunction Using VAS Testing"
Maskin, Steven L., poster presented at the annual meeting of the American Academy of Ophthalmology, October 2010, Chicago.

"Long Term Safety and Retreatment Data After Intraductal Meibomian Gland Probing for Obstructive Meibomian Gland Dysfunction"
Maskin, Steven L., and Courtney Warsinski, poster presented at the annual meeting of the Association for Research in Vision and Ophthalmology, May 2010, Fort Lauderdale, FL. Abstract published in *Investigative Ophthalmology & Visual Science*, April 2010, 6283.

"Results of Intraductal Meibomian Gland Probing (MGP) for Symptoms of Inflammatory Meibomian Gland Dysfunction (MGD) Excluding Lid Tenderness"
Maskin, Steven L., poster presented at the annual meeting

of the American Society of Cornea and Refractive Surgery, April 2010, Boston.

"Intraductal Meibomian Gland Probing for Meibomian Gland Dysfunction Using VAS Testing"
Maskin, Steven L., poster presented at the World Cornea Congress VI, April 2010, Boston.

"Intraductal Meibomian Gland Probing Relieves Symptoms of Obstructive Meibomian Gland Dysfunction"
Maskin, Steven L., poster presented at the annual meeting of the Association for Research in Vision and Ophthalmology, May 2009, Fort Lauderdale, FL. Abstract published in *Investigative Ophthalmology & Visual Science*, April 2009, 4636.

"Loteprednol Etabonate 0.5% (Lotemax) Versus Vehicle in the Management of Patients with KCS and at Least Moderate Inflammation"
Maskin, Steven L., Bruce Anderson, James Chodosh, Edward J. Holland, Stephen C. Pflugfelder, Stephen P. Bartels, Teresa Micuda, and Roger Vogel, poster presented at the meeting of the Association for Research in Vision and Ophthalmology, May 2003, Fort Lauderdale, FL. Abstract published in *Investigative Ophthalmology & Visual Science*, May 2003, 686.

Expanded Understanding of Maskin® Probing and MGD

To further understand MGD and the effects of gland probing, I began using the Arita Meibom Pen® (Japan Focus, Tokyo, Japan) to collect infrared video meibography images. With the help of a research assistant, we analyzed meibography videos of fifty upper lids of twenty-eight patients with atrophic obstructive MGD, comparing the glands before and after probing. The retrospective comparison of images revealed more than 40 percent of lids showed increases in Meibomian gland tissue after probing. Changes included lengthening of the glands with reversal of proximal atrophy, partial restoration of faded glands with increases in density and improved definition, restoration of a continuous gland from discontinuous gland segments, and the appearance of new glands.

I now perform probing guided by video meibography using the Firefly Slit Lamp Imaging System. The system provides real-time visualization of the probing procedure, in the same way a radiologist uses CT-guided imaging to biopsy a vital organ. Meibography-guided probing has confirmed the safety of the procedure (the probe does not pierce through the duct wall nor damage acinar tissue). It enables whole or localized gland therapy and the collection of meibum specimens from deep within the gland, elegantly raising possibilities not only for future research, but also for therapeutic and regenerative treatments. For example, we are now able to study the lipid chemistry of uncontaminated meibum, rather than of expressed meibum collected from an orifice contaminated with surface lipids (see fig. 11.4).

Not only has meibography-guided probing confirmed the safety of probing, it has also revealed that periglandular tissue is spongy. It has also shown that when the probe enters the gland, the periglandular tissue compresses and reexpands, allowing the Meibomian glands to bend and flex the same way the veins and arteries bend and flex. (When you flex your wrist, your veins don't crack.) The flexible nature of periglandular tissue apparently prevents damage to the Meibomian glands in lids that are often rubbed, pulled, pushed, or tugged in different directions (see fig. 3.2). Meibography-guided probing has also shown that areas of whole gland dropout or atrophy maintain a central duct as long as a gland's orifice is intact (see fig. 11.1, D). Furthermore, in cases of whole gland atrophy, it has shown that probing restored central duct integrity in over 75 percent of atrophic glands that had fixed periductal fibrosis.

Indications for Probing

Intraductal probing of the Meibomian glands, because it confirms or restores ductal integrity, is used for both diagnostic evaluation and therapeutic intervention for patients with MGD.

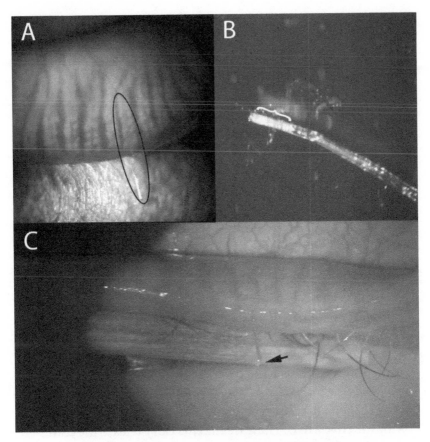

Fig. 11.4. Retrieving Meibum from a Gland with a Maskin® MicroStent, Seen with Infrared Meibography

A. A sterile Maskin MicroStent within the duct of a gland as it retrieves a meibum specimen (oval)

B. The tip of the Maskin MicroStent, after its removal from the gland, filled with the specimen of meibum (bracket)

C. A drop of uncontaminated meibum (arrow), retrieved from within the gland, as it oozes out of a Maskin MicroStent partially positioned within the central duct.

Sources: A and B: Reproduced from Steven L. Maskin and Sreevardhan Alluri, "Meibography Guided Intraductal Meibomian Gland Probing Using Real-Time Infrared Video Feed," *British Journal of Ophthalmology* 104, no. 12 (2020), 1676–1682, with permission from BMJ Publishing Group Ltd.; C: Courtesy of Steven L. Maskin, MD.

Sidebar 11.4
Similar Medical Procedures

The human body has many tubes that can become blocked: veins, arteries, intestines, ureter, urethra, birth canal, esophagus, fallopian tubes, tear ducts, and more. Blockage of these tubes can be painful and cause inflammation and scarring. In some cases, blockage can be fatal.

Clearing the blockage restores normal function, allowing the contents of the tube to flow, like unblocking the drain of a kitchen sink with a plumbing snake. Imagine clearing blockages in the circulatory system with angioplasty, or dilating a strictured esophagus. Because these blockages are mechanical, they require a mechanical solution, which often involves a device pushing against the blockage or releasing it. If the blockage is a ring of tissue that constricts and invades the tube, a probe directed into the tube can release the blockage from within.

This is why heat, massage, expression, blinking, or even topical medications are ineffective treatments for fixed obstructive MGD. These treatments can't release the constricting and invading fixed blockage of scar tissue that occurs at different depths in over 90 percent of glands with MGD. Instead, if ductal integrity is not first restored, these treatments can exacerbate the disease, increasing intraductal pressure and likely enabling progressive stem cell loss from progressive unreleased and unresolved invasive periductal fibrosis.

Diagnostic Evaluation

Diagnostic probing reveals occult disease. It finds obstructed glands when the probe encounters resistance, and it indicates the nature of the resistance. If the resistance is fixed, firm, focal, and unyielding

(FFFUR), the obstructions are fibrotic. Resistance that is nonfixed, nonfocal, and easily yielding suggests an altered duct or duct contents. Probing also finds the location of the resistance—distal, near the orifice; or proximal, deeper within the lid.

Probing is essential for confirming the asymptomatic patient's occult subclinical fixed obstructive MGD when the disease is only suspected after a slit-lamp examination or meibography. For these patients, despite having normal expressible glands and no common MGD symptoms, only probing can definitively rule out the presence of occult fixed fibrotic constrictions. These constrictions can lead to severe pain (the kind reported by patients diagnosed with neuropathic eye pain) and gland atrophy.

Therapeutic Intervention

In my practice, I perform intraductal Meibomian gland probing for all patients with MGD. Probing releases the tight bands of periductal fibrosis that invade and contract around the external duct walls constricting the duct lumen. With unequivocal positive physical proof, probing eliminates this intraductal resistance while restoring or confirming the integrity of the duct. With the release of resistance, intraductal pressure equilibrates and the flow of meibum resumes. Follow-up annual probing (like biannual teeth cleaning) maintains ductal integrity by preventing or releasing recurrent obstructions. Because probing targets the proximate cause of obstructive MGD, it resolves lid tenderness and improves ocular comfort dramatically.

Furthermore, as previously noted, treatment with probing resolves not only primary complaints and symptoms, but also symptoms patients hadn't been fully aware of (see fig. 11.2).

We even have evidence that probing is associated with increased gland tissue and may lead to gland regeneration. A 2018 retrospective study I published in the *British Journal of Ophthalmology* showed over 40 percent of upper eyelids with signs of gland growth after probing. These findings are supported by a 2019 study of mouse Meibomian glands with MGD showing that ductal integrity (confirmed or established with probing in humans) plays a necessary role in regenerating acinar-ductular units and reestablishing gland function.

Sidebar 11.5
Cataract Surgery and MGD

Patients undergoing elective cataract extraction surgery all too often develop postoperative, painful MGD symptoms and are unhappy with their surgery results. Sometimes these cataract patients have asymptomatic, occult, undiagnosed MGD so their doctors do not initiate therapy before surgery. But postoperatively, inflammation, toxicity or sensitivity to topical medications, and ATD can exacerbate asymptomatic MGD, converting it to symptomatic MGD.

The high rate of unhappy postsurgery cataract patients may be explained by a recent study examining patients for MGD during their preoperative visit for cataract surgery. Fifty-two percent of patients had untreated MGD. Half of the patients with MGD had no symptoms, even though 56 percent showed Meibomian gland atrophy.

If MGD were diagnosed and treated prior to cataract surgery, I expect patients would be much happier after surgery. I base this opinion on my experience treating MGD patients with probing before cataract surgery. They all seemed to do very well postoperatively versus the many patients who sought my help after their surgeries because they were unhappy with the results.

Consequently, I recommend patients planning elective cataract surgery first undergo an evaluation for Dry Eye and MGD. Based on the slit-lamp exam or meibography, if I suspect the patient has MGD, whether they are symptomatic or asymptomatic, I recommend probing the glands prior to surgery. These patients may also benefit from preoperative topical corticosteroid therapy and increased postoperative dosing or other pre- and postoperative treatments, depending on their comorbid ocular surface diseases.

My studies also suggest probing leads to stem cell activation as indicated by the proliferation of ductal epithelial cells with a thickening of duct walls. We reviewed confocal microscopy images of the orifice duct wall to assess the impact of probing. Without a marker system and relying on landmarks alone, we were able to successfully identify ten cases of the identical gland before and after probing. In each case we noted a consistent increase in duct wall epithelial cell proliferation. In five cases with a follow-up of less than one year, we found an average of 20 percent increase in duct wall thickness (with increase ranging from 8.4 to 38.3 percent) at an average of 4.5 months after probing (ranging from 3 weeks to 9.2 months after probing). The increase in duct wall thickness suggests probing activated stem cells (see fig. 11.5, C and D). Through the release of periductal fibrosis, probing may also prevent or minimize further stem cell loss or structural gland changes.

SYMPTOMATIC PATIENTS WITH MGD

Many patients benefit from therapeutic intervention with probing, including those with the following signs and symptoms of mild to severe MGD:

- Lid tenderness and soreness (whether reported by the patient or elicited during the exam), which suggest elevated intraductal pressure behind an obstruction
- Meibum deficiency
- Nonexpressible and expressible glands, each with signs of MGD visible at the slit lamp, including lid margin or tarsal hyperemia; lid margin telangiectasia, thickening or irregularity; orifice metaplasia; anterior migration of the mucocutaneous junction
- Nonobvious MGD (NOMGD) with minimal to no signs of MGD visible at the slit lamp except reduced numbers of expressible glands (see chapter 4)
- Early hordeolum or chalazion (These patients may also benefit from adjunctive intraductal microtube steroid injection along with Meibomian gland probing.)

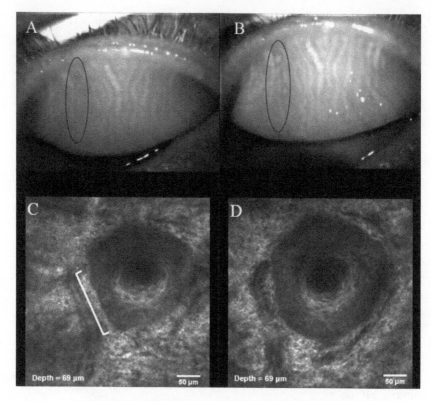

**Fig. 11.5. Gland Tissue Appears to Increase with
Stem Cell Activation After Maskin® Probing**

A and B: Examples of infrared video meibography images showing growth of
gland tissue in an upper lid after probing.

A. Before probing, an area of atrophy with few visible acinar-ductular units
(oval).

B. After probing, a statistically significant increase in glandular tissue and greater
overall definition and density of acinar-ductular units (oval). Analysis revealed
an approximately 21 percent increase in glandular tissue ($p = 0.03$).

C and D: Examples of confocal microscopy images showing an increase in duct
wall thickness (dark donut-shaped ring in images) after probing. The solid black
circular shape in the center is the lumen (see fig. 4.1, A).

C. Before probing. Note the flat edge of the external duct wall (bracket), suggestive of periductal fibrosis.

D. About 6.5 months after probing. Note the increased duct wall thickness
from a proliferation of healthy duct wall epithelial cells. Statistical analysis revealed a 38.3 percent increase in the duct wall thickness.

Sources: A and B: Adapted by permission from BMJ Publishing Group Limited. From Steven L.
Maskin and Whitney R. Testa, "Growth of Meibomian Gland Tissue After Intraductal Meibomian Gland Probing in Patients with Obstructive Meibomian Gland Dysfunction," *British Journal of Ophthalmology* 102, no. 1 (2018), 59–68. C and D: Courtesy of Steven L. Maskin, MD.

Sidebar 11.6
The Need for Early Intervention

Halting the progress of virtually any disease is often achieved proactively with early or preventative interventions. So even if you brush and floss your teeth at home regularly, dentists recommend a professional cleaning twice a year to remove the buildup of plaque and tartar, which causes tooth decay and gum disease. Similarly, probing the Meibomian glands annually releases invasive intraductal fibrosis, establishing and maintaining ductal integrity while preventing the building-up of intraductal pressure (IDP), which can lead to whole gland atrophy (WGA) or partial gland atrophy.

In a 2020 peer-reviewed paper published in the *British Journal of Ophthalmology,* we explained the importance of early intervention with probing as follows:

> Also interesting is the observation that 73% of non-WGA [glands without complete whole gland atrophy] cases showed fixed obstruction suggesting that [fixed obstruction] is a common probe finding in Meibomian gland dysfunction, indicating a risk for future gland atrophy. This risk for future gland atrophy, from elevated IDP or possibly stem cell loss within the ductal epithelium, suggests the need to be pro-active and restore ductal integrity in patients with MGD, a disease well known to progress in a subclinical manner. For these reasons and from the lack of adverse sequelae reported in the published peer reviewed literature as well as after personally probing more than 100,000 glands, I have developed an initial therapeutic approach toward obstructive MGD focusing on *early intervention with gland prob-*

ing. This early intervention would serve to confirm or restore ductal integrity through the release of fixed obstructions from periductal fibrotic bands. Indications include MGD patients who are symptomatic as well as those who are asymptomatic with sub-clinical disease but with signs of MGD at the slit lamp or on IR (infrared) meibography. Lids showing minimal disease such as non-obvious MGD as well as more moderate and severe disease are all probed to release periductal fibrosis and confirm or restore ductal integrity.

Glands are probed annually to maintain intra-ductal integrity. Patients to consider earlier for re-probing are those with MGD presenting for cataract or refractive surgery as well as those with significant comorbidities, which increase the incidence and severity of obstructive MGD with fixed resistance. Additional MGD patients in whom to consider earlier re-probing include those with delayed tear clearance, a history of exposure to particulate matter, long-term use of eye cosmetics, chronic topical glaucoma therapy and those with tarsal inflammation such as from [graft-versus-host] disease, chemical and thermal injury and systemic autoimmune disease.

Source: Reproduced with permission from BMJ Publishing Group Ltd. From Steven L. Maskin and Sreevardhan Alluri, "Meibography Guided Intraductal Meibomian Gland Probing Using Real-Time Infrared Video Feed," *British Journal of Ophthalmology* 104, no. 12 (2020), 1676–1682.

- Lids showing signs of Meibomian gland obstruction on infrared meibography or transillumination, including dilated ducts and cystic acini as well as atrophic changes
- Patients diagnosed with "neuropathic" eye pain, as a high

percentage of these glands have been found to have occult fixed obstruction

(List adapted from Steven L. Maskin and Sreevardhan Alluri, "Intraductal Meibomian Gland Probing: Background, Patient Selection, Procedure, and Perspectives," *Clinical Ophthalmology*, July 10, 2019, 1203–1223.)

SUBCLINICAL (ASYMPTOMATIC) PATIENTS

In lids with MGD, periductal fibrosis occurs in over 90 percent of glands, and at the same frequency in both expressible and nonexpressible glands. It often develops subclinically without symptoms. Doing nothing for patients with subclinical MGD may result in ductal stem cell loss as periductal fibrosis invades the external duct wall. The invasion may not initially cause obstruction, elevated intraductal pressure, or lid tenderness—common signs and symptoms of MGD. Instead, the invasion and subsequent stem cell loss may lead to gland atrophy and meibum deficiency, with symptoms such as burning and photophobia but excluding lid tenderness (because the gland's duct is not obstructed).

Therefore, early intervention with probing is indicated for asymptomatic patients with the following signs:

- Nonexpressible glands and expressible glands, each with signs of MGD visible at the slit lamp
- Nonobvious MGD (NOMGD) with minimal to no signs of MGD visible at the slit lamp except reduced numbers of expressible glands (see chapter 4)
- Lids showing signs of Meibomian gland obstruction on infrared meibography or transillumination, including dilated ducts and cystic acini as well as atrophic changes

(List adapted from Steven L. Maskin and Sreevardhan Alluri, "Intraductal Meibomian Gland Probing: Background, Patient Selection, Procedure, and Perspectives," *Clinical Ophthalmology*, July 10, 2019, 1203–1223.)

Patients with MGD and a range of ocular surface comorbidities, such as ATD, anterior blepharitis, and allergies among many others, benefit from therapeutic Meibomian gland probing, as do patients with a wide range of other risk factors, such as planned cataract and refractive surgeries. Glaucoma surgery, glaucoma-related drainage devices, scleral lenses, and other types of contact lenses can all lead to friction-induced MGD. Untreated ocular surface comorbidities and these risk factors reduce the duration of probing's therapeutic benefits. Consequently, in these settings, initial or repeated maintenance probing may be indicated after satisfactory treatment of comorbidities.

PART II: THE MASKIN® PROBING PROTOCOL

Six Steps of Intraductal Meibomian Gland Probing

Intraductal Meibomian gland probing is a simple procedure that can be performed in the office. The entire six-step procedure, probing all glands in both lids of one eye, takes less than one hour, including the time for the topical anesthetic to take effect. Steps 3 through 5 are optional, depending solely on the patient's comorbidities.

Step 1: Applying anesthetic
Step 2: Probing glands
Step 3: Dilating glands
Step 4: Gently expressing glands
Step 5: Injecting with steroid or other therapeutics, and lavage
Step 6: Irrigating

Step 1. Applying Anesthesia

With the patient seated comfortably in a reclined position, an anesthetic drop is placed in the fornix of the eye. Once numb, a bandage contact lens is placed over the eye to protect the cornea from the strong topical anesthetic.

Next, a generous amount of proprietary jojoba ophthalmic an-

Sidebar 11.7
Treating "Neuropathic" Pain with Maskin® Probing

With probing I have found firm, fixed, focal, unyielding resistance (FFFUR) within the intraductal space in dozens of patients who were previously diagnosed with neuropathic pain but showed no significant commensurate signs of ocular surface diseases at the slit lamp or with infrared meibography. These patients had an adequate number of expressible glands and minimal to no lid tenderness. While probing, I found over 92 percent of their glands had FFFUR within 1 millimeter of the orifice. Probing both detected the underlying occult disease and released the obstruction. Along with additional treatments for ATD and other comorbidities, probing quickly reversed these misidentified "neuropathic" symptoms.

Fig. 11.6 shows the Probe Findings form of a patient who came to me with a diagnosis of ocular neuropathic pain. She was in severe pain when she arrived in my office. I diagnosed MGD and a number of comorbidities. I then initiated targeted treatment, beginning by probing her glands with a 1 millimeter probe. (In fig. 11.6, gland number 1 is the gland at the outer corner of the left eye.) The results are summarized here:

LEFT EYE, 1 MILLIMETER PROBE (SHOWN)

Upper lid
- Total glands probed: 34
- Firm resistance: 29 (85.3%)
  - Firm pop: 28 (96.6%)
  - Firm gritty: 1 (3.4%)
- Soft resistance: 3 (8.8%)
- No resistance: 2 (5.9%)

Lower lid
- Total glands probed: 27
- Firm resistance: 26 (96.3%)
  - Firm pop: 19 (73.1%)
  - Firm gritty: 7 (26.9%)
- Soft resistance: 1 (3.7%)
- No resistance: 0 (0%)

Note the high percentage of glands with fixed resistance within a depth of 1 millimeter in both upper and lower lids:

→ 85.3 percent in the upper lid
→ 96.3 percent in the lower lid

Because the patient had residual tenderness in parts of the lids, I reprobed those glands with a longer 2 millimeter probe.

LEFT EYE, 2 MILLIMETER PROBE (NOT SHOWN)

Upper lid
- Total glands probed: 21
- Firm resistance: 10 (47.6%)
  - Firm pop: 4 (40%)
  - Firm gritty: 6 (60%)
- Soft resistance: 11 (52.4%)
- No resistance: 0 (0%)

Lower lid
- Total glands probed: 15
- Firm resistance: 12 (80%)
  - Firm pop: 5 (41.7%)
  - Firm gritty: 7 (58.3%)
- Soft resistance: 2 (13.3%)
- No resistance: 1 (6.7%)

Note the high percentage of glands with residual fixed resistance deeper in the glands, within 2 millimeters in both upper and lower lids:

→ 47.6 percent in the upper lid
→ 80 percent in the lower lid

Also note the higher percentage of firm gritty encountered by the longer 2 millimeter probe. This suggests the presence of more bands of scar tissue deeper in the glands.

→ Upper lid: 60 percent with the 2 millimeter probe, compared to 3.4 percent with the 1 millimeter probe
→ Lower lid: 58.3 percent with the 2 millimeter probe, compared to 26.9 percent with the 1 millimeter probe

After probing with the 2 millimeter probe, lid tenderness resolved. Additional deeper probing with the longer 4 millimeter probes was not necessary.

Probe findings were similar in the patient's right eye.

esthetic ointment (JAO)—a refrigerated 8% lidocaine in a petrolatum base ointment containing 25% jojoba prepared by O'Brien Pharmacy in Mission, Kansas—is applied to the lower lid margin with a sterile cotton swab. Jojoba is thought to chaperone the lidocaine anesthetic into the lid and Meibomian gland tissues, preempting the need for infiltrative (injected) anesthetic in most cases.

Any stinging will dissipate in about sixty seconds. The patient then keeps the eyes closed for ten minutes.

After ten minutes, patients with chronic, long-standing inflammation receive a second dose of JAO, followed five minutes later by another anesthetic drop.

Sidebar 11.8
Ensuring Patient Comfort During Probing

For the best outcomes and to ensure patients are comfortable during the probing procedure, the eyelid is anesthetized. Patients also must be relaxed. If they express anxiety, I advise them to avoid caffeine for a few days prior to probing and/or take an oral anxiolytic, for example, Xanax® or Valium®. A second round of jojoba ophthalmic anesthetic (JAO) and anesthetic drops can boost comfort. (The JAO must be fresh and kept refrigerated. Refrigerated, JAO loses potency in approximately two months, and unrefrigerated, in just two weeks.) Less than 5 percent of my patients have needed a deeper level of anesthetic. For these patients, I inject 2% lidocaine with epinephrine into the lid, the same anesthetic commonly used for cosmetic lid procedures.

If the patient has significant comorbid anterior blepharitis, I will likely delay probing and treat first with antibiotic ophthalmic ointment and lid hygiene to reduce overall lid sensitivity.

As of this writing, I have been evaluating an alternative approach to anesthesia for patients with severely sensitive lids. This approach, used in anesthetic facial procedures, uses an injection of anesthetic that blocks the nerve that supplies sensation to the upper as well as lower lid. Using this technique, these patients have reported experiencing no pain during the entire procedure, from initial probing to intraductal lavage with corticosteroid.

Step 2. Probing Glands

With the chair in an upright position at the slit lamp, the patient rests their forehead against the band and their chin in the chin cup.

A technician cradles the patient's head, gently pressing their hand to the back of the head while recording the probe finding data.

To minimize disturbances to the Meibomian gland tissues, I developed fine probes only 76 microns in diameter, intentionally designed with nonsharp tips that allow the operator to detect and release fixed obstructions rather than slice or pierce through them the way a sharp tip would. The probes are available in 1-, 2-, and 4-millimeter lengths.

Probing begins with the 1-millimeter probe. This is the stiffest and shortest probe and is best suited for finding the correct angle of entry into the orifice and distal duct. The probe's tip is placed on the gland's orifice, then, with a quick motion akin to throwing a dart, advanced into the gland. If the probe does not enter the orifice, the angle and placement of the probe is adjusted to locate the correct angle and point of entry.

When the probe encounters resistance, within the orifice or deeper within the gland, added mild force advances the probe through the constriction, releasing the periductal fibrotic band.

As the probe releases the constriction, it typically makes an audible *pop* sound. Several consecutive bands of constriction feel gritty and make a sound like nails on a washboard.

Longer probes should be used if lid tenderness persists after probing with the 1-millimeter probe, suggesting deeper obstruction. After I finish probing the glands in one lid, I apply moderate pressure to that lid and ask patients if there is residual tenderness. If there is, I reprobe the area of tenderness with the longer probes.

I record results on a Probe Findings form, available on MGDi .com. Each gland in the upper and lower lids is numbered. (We always record probe findings beginning with number 1 on the form, and I always probe from my right to my left. With the left eye, I start probing temporally and move nasally. With the right eye, I start nasally and move temporally.) An assistant fills out the form as I call out the resistance encountered by the probe in each gland. The upper row of the form is for the upper lid; the lower row is for the lower lid. The table in the center of the form is for tabulating findings (see fig. 11.6).

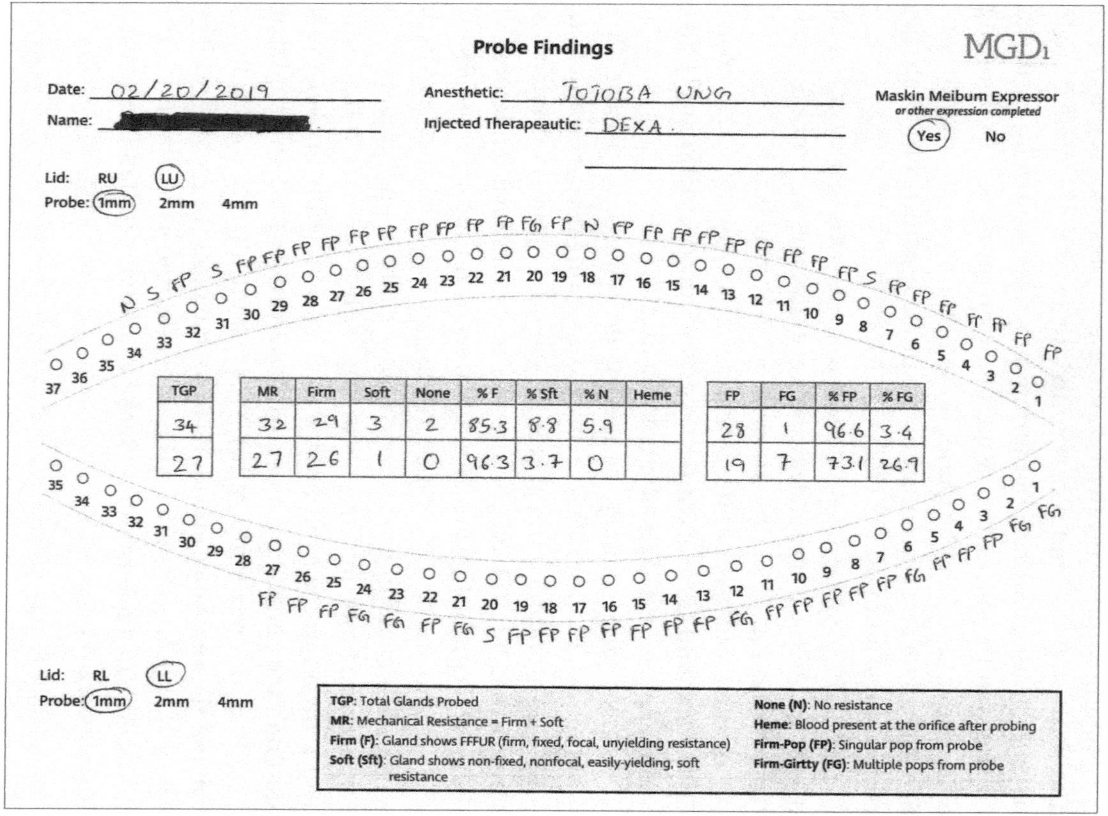

Fig. 11.6.
Probe Findings Form of a Patient Who Had Been Misdiagnosed with Ocular Neuropathic Pain

Shown here is the Probe Findings form, using a 1 millimeter probe, of a patient whose doctors had diagnosed and treated her unsuccessfully for ocular neuropathic pain. She was in severe pain when she arrived in my office, but symptoms subsided immediately after targeted treatment that included Meibomian gland probing (see sidebar 11.7).

Source: Courtesy of Steven L. Maskin, MD.

Step 3: Dilating Glands

After probing the glands, a solid dilator probe, 150 microns in diameter, may be used in one or more glands to expand the orifice and distal duct and prepare the glands for a therapeutic injection of a small particle suspension, such as Celestone®, a corticosteroid, if indicated.

Step 4: Gently Expressing Glands

Expression can accelerate the evacuation of any stagnant material inside the glands. Because probing has either confirmed or restored a clear unobstructed outflow path, mild pressure applied to the lids at this point is both therapeutic and safe.

For this step I developed the Maskin® Meibum Expressor, an instrument that gently compresses the lids and expresses the glands with a rolling motion. The rolling motion from the back of the lid to the front helps direct meibum and any stagnant material toward gland orifices.

Step 5: Injecting with Steroid or Other Therapeutics, and Lavage

If the Meibomian glands are severely inflamed with significant co-morbidities, intraductal corticosteroid injection may be administered to help reduce inflammation and improve the quality of meibum. Using a Maskin® MicroTube, 5–8 microliters of the corticosteroid are injected slowly and steadily into each gland, taking about five seconds per gland. Additional volume may be used to lavage, or wash out, the gland.

For glands that weren't dilated, a 110 (outer diameter) micron Maskin MicroTube may be used to inject therapeutic steroid solutions such as dexamethasone, as well as autologous serum to reduce recurrence of FFFUR. A larger 150 (outer diameter) micron tube can be used to deliver particulate-containing therapeutics as described in step 3.

Step 6: Irrigating

When the procedure is completed, the bandage contact lens is removed and the eye is copiously rinsed with a sterile, preservative-free, 0.9% saline solution. This removes anesthetic and debris released into the eye from the Meibomian glands. A sterile cotton swab is used to remove any residual anesthetic from the lashes and lid margins.

Preservative-free lubricating drops can be used hourly by the patient if needed until bedtime to help lubricate the ocular surface for the remainder of the day.

Additional Considerations

Which Glands Should Be Treated?

Generally, all glands in lids with MGD should be treated with intraductal probing. Sometimes patients need one lid or one section of a lid reprobed early if persistent or new comorbidities cause inflammation and exacerbate periductal fibrosis leading to recurrent constriction and loss of ductal integrity. This depends entirely on the patient, symptoms, and comorbidities.

When to Reprobe

I like to use the dental analogy when explaining the importance of periodic maintenance probing. Most people brush their teeth twice a day, but dentists also recommend professional cleaning by a dental hygienist at least twice a year. Similarly, probing should be done at least once a year for maintenance to ensure Meibomian glands are clear of obstructions and able to synthesize and secrete meibum.

Variations or Modifications to the Protocol

Doctors sometimes adopt different techniques when they probe Meibomian glands. Some routinely inject lidocaine anesthetic into the eyelid tissue of all patients, as they would for a cosmetic lid surgery. Some doctors have patients lie down in a procedure room, rather than sit at a slit lamp. Some doctors prefer to hold the lid with forceps while advancing the probe with the other hand. There are other perfectly acceptable variations, all of which lead to positive outcomes. On the other hand, for studies or clinical trials, I recommend

Sidebar 11.9
With MGD, Even Expressible
Glands Can Be Obstructed

In a 2019 study published in the journal *Cornea,* we reported that even when glands are expressible and appear healthy, probes often encounter fibrosis and scarring deeper inside, indicating fixed, firm, focal, unyielding resistance in patients with MGD. At a depth of 1 millimeter, probing revealed 67 percent of all glands displayed FFFUR, and at 2 millimeters, over 90 percent of all glands displayed FFFUR. There was no statistical difference in frequency of FFFUR between expressible and nonexpressible glands, suggesting that expressible glands only *seem* healthy. Most unprobed glands are obstructed with periductal fibrosis somewhere along their length, even if the glands can express oil.

using my published protocol unless the study expressly aims to compare one probing protocol to another.

I also highly recommend using Maskin Probes and MicroTubes, designed and sized specifically for Meibomian glands (the probes and microtubes are 76 microns and 110 microns in diameter, respectively), rather than devices retrofitted for Meibomian gland probing. In the randomized controlled trial comparing IPL and probing discussed in chapter 10, for example, researchers used much larger probes measuring 120 and 160 microns, respectively. The larger diameter would have caused patients more discomfort.

Plus, it is very important to start with a short, stiff 1-millimeter probe to find the angle of entry, then switch to longer probes if there is persistent lid tenderness suggesting deeper obstruction and elevated intraductal pressure. If the longer probes aren't used when indicated, deep fixed obstructions will remain intact.

Sidebar 11.10
Clinical Pearl

Clinical pearls are important pieces of relevant information based on a doctor's clinical experience and observations. Sometimes these observations are formally studied, and sometimes not. I offer this clinical pearl.

Treatments for MGD that do not include probing to restore ductal integrity may appear to increase the volume of meibum in the tear film effectively, when in fact there may be only one distal acinus near the orifice producing expressible meibum. Just beyond that single functioning acinus, occult bands of periductal fibrosis may be lurking deeper within, constricting and invading the gland and causing damage.

Without probing, periductal fibrosis may progress unchecked, eventually causing focal or whole gland atrophy, or gland truncation.

Effectiveness of Intraductal Meibomian Gland Probing

In clinical studies, intraductal Meibomian gland probing has shown to be a safe and very effective therapy for obstructive MGD. In one study, both lids with more and less advanced atrophy, as seen with meibography, showed the following statistically significant results:

- Improvements in lid tenderness
- Increase in the number of expressible glands
- Increase in meibum-secreting lid functionality (MSLF), defined as five or more expressible glands per lid

Although there was no statistically significant difference between advanced and less advanced atrophy, lids with less advanced atrophy had better results at each point in time.

Table 11.1
Maskin® Probing Reduces Lid Tenderness
(N = 541 lids)

Time Frame	Lids Evaluated	% Nontender Lids	% Tender Lids
Preprobing	541	0%	100%
1 Week Follow-up	144	86.1%	13.9%
3–6 Months Follow-up	215	82.3%	17.7%
1 Year Follow-up	113	58.4%	41.6%

Source: Adapted by permission from BMJ Publishing Group Limited. From Steven L. Maskin and Whitney R. Testa, "Growth of Meibomian Gland Tissue After Intraductal Meibomian Gland Probing in Patients with Obstructive Meibomian Gland Dysfunction," *British Journal of Ophthalmology* 102, no. 1 (2018), 59–68.

In this study, a total of 541 tender lids were probed. At one week, three to six months, and one year after probing, 86.1 percent of 144 evaluated lids, 82.3 percent of 215 evaluated lids, and 58.4 percent of 113 evaluated lids were nontender, respectively (see table 11.1).

In another study, a total of 271 nonfunctioning lids (having four or fewer expressible glands per lid) were probed. At one week, three to six months, and one year after probing, 93.8 percent of 64 evaluated lids, 92.2 percent of 102 evaluated lids, and 73.9 percent of 46 evaluated lids achieved, respectively, meibum-secreting lid functionality (MSLF), defined as five or more expressible glands per lid (see table 11.2).

This study included a cohort of nonfunctioning lids (see table 11.3) whose preprobing average of expressible glands was 2.3 ±1.5 per lid (*counting only up to ten expressible glands per lid*). At one week, three to six months, and one year after probing, the number of expressible glands per lid increased markedly to 8.7 ±2.1 (264% increase, p < 0.0001), 8.5 ±2.2 (253 percent increase, p < 0.0001) and 7.0 ±3.0 (193 percent increase, p < 0.0001), respectively. A third study looked at the total number of expressible glands counted before and after probing, and did not stop at ten expressible glands (see table 11.4). (Note: p-value, short for "probability value," indicates if

Table 11.2
Maskin® Probing Restores Meibum Secreting Lid Functionality (MSLF)
(N = 271 lids)

Time Frame	Lids Evaluated	% Lids with MSLF (≥ 5 Expressible Glands)	% Nonfunctioning Lids (≤ 4 Expressible Glands)
Preprobing	271	0%	100%
1 Week Follow-up	64	93.8%	6.2%
3–6 Months Follow-up	102	92.2%	7.8%
1 Year Follow-up	46	73.9%	26.1%

Source: Adapted by permission from BMJ Publishing Group Limited. From Steven L. Maskin and Whitney R. Testa, "Growth of Meibomian Gland Tissue After Intraductal Meibomian Gland Probing in Patients with Obstructive Meibomian Gland Dysfunction," *British Journal of Ophthalmology* 102, no. 1 (2018), 59–68.

Table 11.3
Maskin® Probing Increases Expressible Glands Per Lid
(N = 271 lids)
Limiting count of expressible glands to a maximum of 10

Time Frame	Mean Expressible Glands/Lid (±SD)	% Increase (p-value)
Preprobing	2.3 (±1.5)	NA
1 Week Follow-up	8.7 (±2.1)	264% (p < 0.0001)
3–6 Months Follow-up	8.5 (±2.2)	253% (p < 0.0001)
1 Year Follow-up	7.0 (±3)	193% (p < 0.0001)

Source: Adapted by permission from BMJ Publishing Group Limited. From Steven L. Maskin and Whitney R. Testa, "Growth of Meibomian Gland Tissue After Intraductal Meibomian Gland Probing in Patients with Obstructive Meibomian Gland Dysfunction," *British Journal of Ophthalmology* 102, no. 1 (2018), 59–68.

Table 11.4

Maskin® Probing Increases Expressible Glands Per Lid

(N = 25 lids)

Counting all expressible glands without limitation

Time Frame	Mean Expressible Glands per Lid	% Increase (p-value)
Preprobing	2.8 (±1.1)	NA
2.4 Months Follow-up	14.4 (±6.4)	412% (p < 0.0001)

Source: Adapted by permission from BMJ Publishing Group Limited. From Steven L. Maskin and Whitney R. Testa, "Growth of Meibomian Gland Tissue After Intraductal Meibomian Gland Probing in Patients with Obstructive Meibomian Gland Dysfunction," *British Journal of Ophthalmology* 102, no. 1 (2018), 59–68.

data is statistically significant or not. A p-value less than or equal to 0.05 is considered statistically significant.)

In this third study (see table 11.4) of a cohort of 25 nonfunctioning lids, *counting all expressible glands without stopping at ten,* the average number of expressible glands was 2.8 ±1.1 glands per lid before probing. At 2.4 months after probing, the number of expressible glands per lid had increased dramatically to 14.4 ±6.4 (a 412 percent increase, p < 0.0001). (Note: A p-value less than or equal to 0.05 is considered statistically significant.)

Summary

Maskin Probing directly targets the underlying proximate cause of obstructive Meibomian gland dysfunction. While we continue to study how probing benefits our patients, from the mid-2000s and Patient Zero to this day, probing has proven to be a safe and effective treatment.

Probing Releases Constricting Fibrotic Tissue,
Confirms and Restores Ductal Integrity

Probing releases constricting fibrotic tissue and restores ductal integrity of the glands, necessary steps for future acinar regeneration.

Where Conventional Treatments Fail, Maskin® Probing Succeeds

This case study illustrates how quickly and effectively Maskin Probing can increase the number of functioning glands, improve the symptoms of obstructive MGD, and stimulate the growth of gland tissue. Over time, with fibrotic obstructions released, Meibomian glands can be restored.

A middle-aged man was referred to [my] practice with a 5-year history of severe, excruciating pain, like firecrackers exploding in his eyes accompanied by symptoms described as gritty, sandy, scratchy and foreign body sensation with lid swelling, which began 5 years after LASIK. His symptoms were "greater than 10 out of 10" on a severity scale of 0–10 and were refractory to warm compresses with lid hygiene, preservative-free artificial tears, omega 3 fatty acids, punctal plugs, steroid drops, Restasis, Azasite, autologous serum, kineret, minocycline, LipiFlow and PROSE (prosthetic replacement of the ocular ecosystem [scleral, PROSE, lenses]). He was diagnosed with post-LASIK corneal neuropathic pain, put on Prozac, and wore goggles while awake.

[My] examination led to additional therapies, including antibiotic ointment to lash roots, tea tree oil treatment for Demodex, topical antihistamine, punctal occlusion using thermocautery, oral cholinergic agents and ocular surface reconstruction with amniotic membrane for conjunctivochalasis. His lids showed obstructive MGD and were tender over the glands in each eye. He had expressible glands of 6 in the right upper lid (RU) and 3 in the left upper lid

(LU). The right lower (RL) and left lower (LL) lids each showed 10. Preprobing meibography of the right upper lid showed . . . proximal atrophy and shortened, truncated glands. [Meibomian gland probing] of all orifices was performed on all four lids.

Within 1 week after probing upper and lower lids, the lids were no longer tender and by 1 month expressible glands had increased to 10 (RU) and 17 (LU). The left lower lid increased to 16. Symptoms improved, and over the course of the next 2 years he has done progressively well overall with occasional irritation from episodes of anterior blepharitis, distichiasis, cellulose residue on lashes from artificial tears and stopping the use of topical antihistamine. He has been able to go to and enjoy the beach, and not wear his goggles for 4 hours per day. His Prozac dosage has been cut in half. His lids remained nontender and expressible glands further increased to 17 (RU), 18 (LU), 21 (RL) and 19 (LL). Postprobing meibography showed statistically significant lengthening of glands.

Source: Reproduced with permission from BMJ Publishing Group Ltd. From Steven L. Maskin and Whitney R. Testa, "Growth of Meibomian Gland Tissue After Intraductal Meibomian Gland Probing in Patients with Obstructive Meibomian Gland Dysfunction," *British Journal of Ophthalmology* 102, no. 1 (2018), 59–68.

Meibum can flow, promoting the natural evacuation of any remaining debris or sludgy material, and glands can heal. Intraductal lavage (washing out) can be administered to remove stubborn material. Corticosteroid or other therapeutics can be injected directly into the duct to treat inflamed or otherwise unhealthy tissues. With ductal integrity restored and confirmed, applying heat to thin and liquefy meibum and mild expression to evacuate gland contents can be safe adjunctive therapies.

During probing, sounds and visual cues indicate the release of periductal fibrotic vascularized scar tissue. The sounds—a single *pop*, like the sound of a rubber band snapping, or a series of *pops* in quick succession creating a gritty nails-on-a-washboard noise—occurs when the fibrosis is released. One visual cue is the release of sequestered meibum along the wire probe through the restored duct and out through the orifice. Sometimes a drop of blood that is self-limiting is seen at the orifice or in the periglandular tissue. This drop of blood comes from blood vessels within the periductal and invasive scar tissue (imagine if the snapped rubber band could bleed) and not from healthy Meibomian gland tissue. Once the scar tissue is released, stem cells can activate, leading to a proliferation of Meibomian gland ductal epithelium and a restoration of normal function.

Probing Relieves and Equilibrates Intraductal Pressure

Probing relieves and equilibrates elevated pressure inside the gland immediately and dramatically, decreasing lid tenderness. Once the outflow channel is reestablished, intraductal pressure reaches a state of equilibrium, reducing the tension on the glandular epithelial cells. Our latest research using confocal microscopy shows, after probing, a proliferation of ductal epithelial cells with a thickening of duct walls, suggesting stem cell activation.

Probing Improves Symptoms

As indicated earlier, patients overwhelmingly report their symptoms improve after probing. Eyes are more comfortable and even vision can improve.

Probing Promotes Regrowth of Glands

Releasing periductal fibrosis and duct constrictions may activate stem cells, leading to a proliferation of ductal epithelial cells with a thickening of duct walls of up to 38 percent. This finding may explain an earlier study that showed, with meibography, the following results after probing:

- Truncated glands lengthened, that is, new acinar-ductular units were visible at the proximal end of the duct.
- The sections of glands with discontinuous acinar-ductular units showed growth of acinar-ductular units.
- Completely atrophic glands grew acinar-ductular units.
- Acinar-ductular units became denser and more defined.

In this retrospective study published in the *British Journal of Ophthalmology* in 2018, we found signs of growth of Meibomian gland tissue after probing in 40 percent of lids.

Probing Is Safe

With virtually no adverse outcomes reported by my patients, and over one hundred thousand glands probed by me alone over the span of ten years, probing has emerged as a safe and effective treatment and preventative therapy for obstructive MGD. Its safety has been underscored since 2012 in many peer-reviewed studies by eye doctors around the world. None have reported immediate adverse effects or long-term adverse consequence. As we reported in 2020 in the *British Journal of Ophthalmology,* meibography-guided real-time visualization has confirmed the safety of intraductal Meibomian gland probing.

12

Guidelines for Managing
Your Life with Meibomian
Gland Dysfunction

Myth
Over a lifetime, if left alone,
Meibomian glands will not cause trouble.
Fact
The best defense is a good offense. Do whatever you can to
keep your Meibomian glands healthy. Your eyes will thank you.

Maskin® Probing can release the fibrotic tissue that constricts
and invades the Meibomian gland. Other treatments your
doctor may recommend or prescribe can reverse comorbidities of
the ocular surface. These are critical steps to recovery for patients
with MGD. However, patients should also take whatever measures
they themselves can to defend their Meibomian glands against the
recurrence of disease and debilitating symptoms.

Some measures may be simple, others may require more effort.
Some may support Meibomian glands directly, some indirectly.

GUIDELINES FOR SUCCESSFULLY
MANAGING YOUR LIFE WITH MGD

1. Don't give up hope.
2. Find the right doctor.
3. Understand your disease.
4. Describe your symptoms precisely.
5. Embrace the importance of Meibomian glands.
6. Seek proper treatment.
7. Don't expect improvement unless the treatment targets the root cause of the problem.
8. For best results, address each comorbidity.
9. Ease pain temporarily.
10. Practice good eyelid hygiene.
11. Take care of your eyes and protect them.
12. Optimize your lifestyle.

1. DON'T GIVE UP HOPE

Don't give up hope is the single most important message I offer. For patients, not giving up hope may demand tremendous reserves of inner strength. For their doctors, restoring hope begins with an accurate diagnosis.

Sometimes patients are demoralized believing they've exhausted all possibilities, particularly when they've already seen many doctors and tried a variety of treatments without success. In my experience, there are additional diagnoses and treatment options that can help even those patients incapacitated by severe, unrelenting pain.

For example, my research has led to breakthroughs in understanding what happens inside a gland with obstructive MGD and has laid the foundation for Maskin Probing as a treatment that can restore comfort to eyes and stimulate the growth of gland tissue. Now we can manage the disease with targeted treatment that gets at the root of the problem—periductal fibrosis constricting and invading the glands. Similarly, with precise diagnostic protocols, doctors can find and treat other comorbidities.

There's no reason for patients to suffer while their glands deteriorate and ocular surface comorbidities advance, nor for doctors to say they've tried everything. Based on my experience, we can always do more.

2. FIND THE RIGHT DOCTOR

Effectively managing MGD, like many other diseases, requires a partnership between the doctor and the patient. The doctor applies his or her expertise to diagnose accurately and prescribe treatments. The patient submits to exams, participates in treatment, and keeps the doctor informed of their progress. This doctor-patient relationship is among the most intimate human relationships, one built on trust and shared goals. Here, the goal is a healthier patient. Therefore, finding the right eye doctor is a critical step in the treatment of MGD.

There are two kinds of eye-care professionals who diagnose and treat diseases of the eye: ophthalmologists and optometrists. Some ophthalmologists and optometrists advertise themselves as Dry Eye specialists. Because Dry Eye and MGD are so prevalent, most have seen patients with these diseases. However, if you've been seeing a doctor for some time but your symptoms aren't improving, you may need to find a new doctor.

Ophthalmologists

An ophthalmologist is a medical doctor with extensive training, including a four-year college degree, a four-year medical degree, a one-year internship, and a three-year residency in ophthalmology (the study and care of eyes). After that, training often includes a one- to three-year postgraduate fellowship in a specific subspecialty of ophthalmology diseases and surgery, such as cataracts, glaucoma, refractive, retina, pediatric, oculoplastic, or cornea and external (my specialty).

All ophthalmologists are surgeons, trained and licensed to perform invasive procedures. They look for disorders and diseases of the eye as well as systemic diseases and other medical conditions, because, like all medical doctors, they trained in internal medicine. They prescribe medications and perform surgeries but also may prescribe glasses and contact lenses.

Cornea and external disease specialists are the ones usually most familiar with the diagnosis and treatment of MGD and other ocular surface diseases. However, many cornea and external disease specialists now focus exclusively on refractive (such as LASIK and PRK) and cataract surgeries, and don't focus on Dry Eye and MGD.

Optometrists

Optometrists are health-care professionals trained to assess the quality of vision and prescribe glasses or contact lenses if needed. Some are very adept at fitting scleral contact lenses. They have four-year college degrees and four-year degrees from a college of optometry, earning a doctor of optometry (OD) degree. Some may have a residency in a specific area of optometry.

Optometrists can diagnose, treat, and manage eye diseases or injuries, including Dry Eye and MGD. In some states they are allowed to perform Meibomian gland probing. Because they aren't medical doctors or surgeons, they are not as experienced in diagnosing systemic conditions and may not prescribe certain medications or perform surgeries. Optometrists refer patients to ophthalmologists when needed.

Finding a Doctor

Cornea and external disease specialists can be found with these steps:

- Check online.
  - Enter the term "Cornea and External Disease" in your search engine.
  - The American Academy of Ophthalmology (AAO) maintains lists of licensed ophthalmologists by specialty on their website, aao.org. Follow directions to navigate to the "Find an Ophthalmologist" page. Once there, select Cornea/External Disease in the subspecialty drop-down menu.
- Call your health insurance company and ask for a list of cornea and external disease specialists in your area.

Finding an optometrist who treats MGD may be as simple as entering the terms "optometrist Dry Eye" or "optometrist MGD" in your search engine, calling your insurance company for a list of optometrists, or even asking a friend for a recommendation. Once you have a list of names of local ophthalmologists and/or optometrists, contact the office and ask if the doctor treats MGD with intraductal Meibomian gland probing. If the answer is no, you should keep looking.

If you see a doctor who tells you the pain is all in your head, look for another doctor. If the doctor has convinced your loved ones that the pain is all in your head, share this book with your loved ones and ask them to take the steps I've listed to help you find another doctor.

3. UNDERSTAND YOUR DISEASE

Think constructively about what is happening each day and how that might affect your Meibomian glands and symptoms. Learn the terminology of MGD. Remember, with MGD, complexity rules; there can be many comorbidities, for example, MGD plus x, plus y, plus z, or more. Learn which comorbidities you have, how your behavior and environment affect them, and how to manage them so you can minimize your symptoms.

The therapeutic process—diagnosis and treatment—will advance along with your learning process. As your condition improves and your symptoms abate, you will develop the capacity to respond to temporary fluctuations in your symptoms and resolve many of them yourself because of what you've learned along the way. At other times, you may need your eye doctor's help.

These fluctuations in symptoms are normal. (Even people without MGD will experience transient eye discomfort during their lives.) Understanding your disease and your comorbidities, knowing what triggers your symptoms and how you can resolve them will put you in control of your life.

4. DESCRIBE YOUR SYMPTOMS PRECISELY

Describing symptoms accurately, specifically, and with the right amount of detail helps doctors—in-person or remotely—diagnose and prescribe effective treatments. Begin by seating yourself comfortably and taking a few breaths. Try to relax and focus on the specifics of the pain by asking yourself these questions:

- What exact sensation(s) are you feeling, for example, pain, burning, foreign body. Are you feeling more than one? Review the symptoms described in chapter 6 if you are having a hard time finding the words to describe the sensation. Determine which symptom is worst, that is, your "primary complaint."
- Is the pain focal, global, or diffuse, that is, felt in a specific spot, across the entire eye, or in a smaller region?
- Does something make the pain better or worse, for example, opening or closing the eyes, blinking, looking up, down, or sideways?
- When does the pain occur? For example, in the morning when you wake up, or whenever you go outside?
- As the day progresses, does the pain get better or worse?
- How bad is the pain on a scale of 0 to 10?
- Is the pain constant or intermittent?
- Is the pain worse if you touch your eyelid?

Consider the questions pertinent to you. Think carefully how you would answer them, so you can better communicate with your doctor.

5. EMBRACE THE IMPORTANCE OF MEIBOMIAN GLANDS

Without healthy functioning Meibomian glands, a lot can go wrong on the surface of the eye that can contribute to painful symptoms. Ductal integrity is the key. If MGD progresses, the glands' ducts can lose their integrity. Scar tissue will invade and strangulate the duct wall, leading to stem cell deficiency and increased intraductal pressure that together can cause gland atrophy.

6. SEEK PROPER TREATMENT

For best results, seek proper treatment for all your ocular comorbidities so you and your doctors can effectively resolve or manage them as quickly as possible. But even if MGD and comorbidities have festered for years, within two or three months of starting targeted treatment, or as little as just one day, symptoms can improve dramatically. With Meibomian gland probing, relief of lid tenderness, due to fibrotic obstruction and elevated intraductal pressure, can be instantaneous. Burning and photophobia can take up to two months to resolve while glands resume their normal function.

Remember, proper treatment begins with an accurate diagnosis, and don't neglect systemic comorbidities (see the later section "Address Systemic Diseases.")

7. DON'T EXPECT IMPROVEMENT UNLESS THE TREATMENT TARGETS THE ROOT CAUSE OF THE PROBLEM

All too often doctors prescribe treatments for MGD or Dry Eye, but patients don't feel better afterward. This happens when the treatment doesn't target the root cause of the problem, so the problem persists, as do symptoms. For example, a doctor may express your Meibomian glands, but without first releasing the underlying periductal fibrosis to optimize treatment, symptoms may not improve. If your eyes burn but the doctor doesn't identify, treat, and manage an existing allergy, MGD, or an infection, don't expect to feel better. If your eyes are sandy or gritty and you have ATD, you won't feel better unless your doctor treats aqueous tear deficiency effectively. If your doctor treats flare-ups with topical steroids but doesn't address the specific cause of the flare-up, your symptoms will eventually return.

8. FOR BEST RESULTS, ADDRESS EACH COMORBIDITY

Not addressing each comorbidity is just like not prescribing the right treatment. The untreated comorbidity and related symptoms will advance unchecked, plus prescribed treatments won't reach their full potential.

So be mindful of improvement, or the lack of it. First, give your doctor feedback. If your doctor doesn't take another approach or prescribe other treatments, it may be time to find another doctor.

9. EASE PAIN TEMPORARILY

Managing eye pain can be difficult, especially if you are still looking for a doctor to diagnose and treat your condition. These tips may help you ease pain, but they are not a substitute for a doctor's care.

Locating the Source of Pain

Figuring out the location of the pain is sometimes half the battle. Is it in the lid? In the eyeball? In the tear film? Where it is determines how you treat it. For instance, if the pain is due to something floating in the tear film, you can try irrigating the eye with a few squirts from a vial of 0.9% sterile preservative-free saline. Be careful not to touch the tip of the vial to the eye. If the pain is in the lid, applying the rolled-up corner of a warm damp washcloth directly to the closed lid in the spot of pain may help. If the pain is in the eyeball, you can try irrigating, but it may be best to see a doctor.

As a very rough general test to determine where the pain is, pull the lid away from the eyeball slightly and very gently. If you still feel the pain, it's probably coming from the eyeball. If the pain moves around, there's probably something in the tear film. If the pain stops, it's most likely associated with the eyelid rubbing against the eyeball. There could be an aberrant eyelash poking the eye, a congested Meibomian gland at the lid margin, or possibly a corneal abrasion.

Temporarily Easing the Pain

Sometimes you just need immediate relief while waiting to see your doctor. In those cases, you can try these methods for easing pain without resorting to pain medication:

- Place an ice cube for a few seconds on your brow or cheekbone. The cold sensation should take focus away from the pain. You can do this intermittently throughout the day, but be careful not to let the water from the ice cube drip into your eye. Do not put the ice cube on your eyelids.
- Eat something. Eating can direct focus away from your eyes. One of my patients swears by crunchy foods like celery.

- Stay calm and consider where your pain severity would be on a 0–10 scale, where 10 is the most severe and incompatible with life, while 0 is the most comfortable. Staying calm and not panicking can help to minimize the trauma of pain, even if the pain is still there. Deep breathing may help you stay calm and reduce the perception of pain.
- Analyze the pain and imagine describing it to your doctor. Thinking about the pain objectively can give you perspective (see "4. Describe Your Symptoms Precisely").
- Distract yourself. Sometimes listening to the radio or a podcast can distract from pain. Listen to TV rather than watch it, so you can keep your eyes closed, which sometimes helps, too. Natalia listened to comedies with her eyes closed. They kept her mind off her pain and lifted her spirits.

10. PRACTICE GOOD EYELID HYGIENE

I cannot stress enough the importance of good lid hygiene in the management and prevention of MGD. This includes the right ways to wash your eyelids and to apply warm compresses.

To clean your eyelids and face properly, follow these guidelines (also see chapter 10):

- Wash your face twice a day.
- Wash eyelids, the area around the eyes, and the roots of the lashes twice a day. (Washing the roots of the lashes will also cleanse the lid margins.)
- Use a mild soap on both your face and eyelids. Using only water or something that doesn't lather does not remove the organic material that builds up each day. Dove Sensitive Skin Beauty Bar, an unscented soap, is a favorite of some of my patients. Another is Stone Crop Gel Wash, by Éminence Organic Skin Care, an organic cleanser.
- Make a good lather in your hands. Close your eyes and gently wash your eyelids and the skin around the lids.
- Don't hover too long, to avoid getting soap in the eyes or drying out the lid margin and skin.
- Rinse thoroughly with warm, not hot, water.

Follow these guidelines if your doctor recommends warm compresses for your Meibomian glands.

- Always begin by washing your hands.
- Use a clean cloth. Avoid using cloths washed with scented detergents or dried with scented dryer sheets, as the scents can be irritating.
- Generally, warm damp compresses are best for Meibomian glands. You can warm the cloth in a microwave or even a regular oven or toaster oven, just be sure it doesn't burn.
- The cloth should be warm, not hot.
- Place the cloth over your closed eyes without applying pressure. Leave it there as long as your doctor has prescribed.

Follow these guidelines for applying a warm compress if you have focal pain in an eyelid from a few blocked glands or a muscle spasm. First, check for a foreign body, like an eyelash in the eye.

- Roll up a corner of a clean washcloth.
- Run the corner under warm water and wring it out.
- With the eye closed, place the warm, damp corner of the washcloth directly over the site of the pain.
- You can do this for five minutes.
- Repeat the application two more times with a gap of five minutes between each.

11. TAKE CARE OF YOUR EYES AND PROTECT THEM

Do whatever you can within reason to protect your eyes all day, every day. Protecting your eyes during waking hours—while at work, driving, reading, using a computer or handheld device, walking, running, and so forth—is as important as protecting them during sleep.

Contact Lenses

- Use daily disposable lenses if possible.
- Remove your contact lenses before going to sleep so your

corneas can get the oxygen they need and your eyes can recover from daily "wear and tear."

Crying

- Try to limit crying emotional tears, if possible. They can be irritating. If you can, avoid tearjerkers or situations that might evoke emotional tears.

Eye and Lid Hygiene

- Never touch your eyes unless your hands are clean and just washed to avoid introducing microbes into your eyes.
- Practice good face and eyelid hygiene. (See "10. Practice Good Eyelid Hygiene" and chapter 10 for more information.)

Lighting and Sunshine

- Always wear UV blocking sunglasses outdoors in daylight.
- Use direct task lighting in your home or office and adjust lights so you can see clearly and without squinting.
- Wear glasses that increase their tint automatically when lights become brighter.
- Reduce the wattage of light bulbs and use lubricating drops if lights are irritating.

Lubricating Eye Drops

- Use lubricating drops as little as possible, but use them when necessary.
- Use only preservative-free drops.
- When using eyedrops, make sure the bottle is completely inverted and vertical, to prevent air flow into the bottle which can lead to air within the drop itself, reducing the dose of medication delivered to the eye.

Makeup

Be mindful of how you apply and remove makeup and which cosmetics you use:

- Use clean applicators.
- Be careful when applying makeup so it doesn't get in the eye or onto the eyelid margin, where it can block or enter Meibomian glands, infiltrate mucosal tissue, or cause lid-margin inflammation.
- Beware of lash cosmetics such as lash glue, magnets, and other artificial-lash-extension materials plus eyelid tattooing, lash tinting, and growth serums, all of which may cause lid-margin inflammation and exacerbate MGD. One of my patients had used a superhold hair spray on her eyelashes to make them look longer and point upward, which led to MGD with extensive distal atrophy of the acinar-ductular units near the orifice (see fig. 9.3, B).
- Watch out for eyeshadow powder or glitter, which can migrate to the lid margin and Meibomian gland orifices.
- Avoid blepharopigmentation, also known as permanent eyeliner, which has been associated with an increased risk of MGD.
- Replace your makeup often. Bacteria that accumulate in the containers can transfer to your eyes.
- Always remove makeup at bedtime.

Reading

- Blink often and completely.
- Before reading, blink quickly ten times, rest for one minute, then repeat. This exercise helps with meibum secretion and spreading tear film across the entire ocular surface.
- Take breaks when reading, using electronic devices, or during any gazing activities. Every twenty minutes stop what you're doing, look away, and blink completely to redistribute tear film and stimulate meibum secretion. Some of my patients use Eyeblink, an app from Blinking Matters, which improves blinking. You can download it at blinkingmatters.com.

Removing a Foreign Body

- Use preservative-free irrigation solution to remove a foreign body, like a loose eyelash, from the eye.
- Irrigate your eyes with a preservative-free irrigation solution if they come in contact with irritants, like smoke from a candle, tobacco, or fire, or a sudden burst of particulate matter from a vacuum cleaner bag or bus exhaust.
- Always carry a preservative-free irrigation solution and a 10× (or stronger) magnifying mirror. You never know when you might need them.

Temperature and Humidity

- Keep the humidity level in your home and office between 50 and 55 percent to prevent excessive aqueous tear evaporation.
- Apply warm compresses more frequently in low temperatures because meibum becomes more brittle when temperatures drop, affecting the normal spreading of tear film.

Touching Eyes

- Avoid putting too much physical pressure on your Meibomian glands, and never rub your eyes.
- If you apply warm compresses daily, don't push too hard on your eyes. Just place the warm compress over your closed eyes.
- When you need to remove excess tears, close your eyes and blot gently against the closed upper lid only. Never blot from below, to avoid touching the mucosal surface. Don't rub or wipe from side to side.

Wind and Drafts

- Keep wind and drafts away from your face and eyes. Overhead vents in offices can disturb tear film, as can vents in cars directed at the face, ceiling fans in restaurants, a loose-fitting face mask, or the wind.

- Wear wraparound glasses, with wide sidepieces to minimize tear film disruption and protect the eyes.

12. OPTIMIZE YOUR LIFESTYLE

The best defense is a great offense. Do whatever you can to stay healthy in defense of your Meibomian glands. Here are a few tips to help you make healthy lifestyle choices:

Consume a Healthy Diet

Eat a variety of healthy foods so your Meibomian glands get the nutrition they need. Take good quality supplements if you need to. Eliminate or limit foods low in nutrition like sweets and sugary drinks. Avoid binge eating that can increase blood sugar, putting Meibomian glands into a dormant state or even be toxic to Meibomian gland epithelial cells. Minimize alcohol consumption.

Include Omega Fatty Acids in Your Diet

Omega fatty acids are essential nutrients that can reduce inflammation. If your diet does not include healthy omega fatty acids, consider taking a supplement. (See the section "Oral Omega Fatty Acid Supplements" under "C. Conventional Therapy: Anti-Inflammatory Medications" in chapter 10.)

Stay Hydrated

The eyes, like other bodily tissues, need to be hydrated for healthy functioning, which includes the production of aqueous tears. Drink at least eight glasses of water a day. One of my patients keeps a glass of water on the kitchen counter to remind herself to drink. Others carry water bottles wherever they go and sip throughout the day. Do whatever works for you and try to stick to it. If you live in areas where the climate is dry or hot or you sweat a lot, you may need to drink even more water.

You can gauge if you're drinking enough water by the color of your urine. It should be a clear, pale yellow, not a deep yellow.

Cut Out, or At Least Limit, Caffeine

Because it's a diuretic, caffeine can dehydrate ocular tissue. Because it's a stimulant, caffeine can increase the palpebral fissure, the distance between the upper and lower eyelids. An increased distance between the lids thins out the tear film between blinks. Blinks may be partial. Caffeine use may increase epinephrine in the bloodstream and tear film. Increased epinephrine in the tear film has been associated with MGD in an animal model. Caffeine can also increase the size of the pupil. A dilated pupil may cause photophobia and play a role in blepharospasm.

Try not to consume foods containing caffeine, for example, coffee, tea, soda, chocolate, and energy drinks. It can take up to two weeks for the body to completely eliminate caffeine after it's cut from the diet. So you may not see immediate results. Eliminating caffeine can cause mild to severe withdrawal headaches, so consider a gradual tapering off.

Get Plenty of Sleep

Sleep is as important as food and water to sustaining life. You spend about one third of your life sleeping, so getting it right is important. Sleep affects virtually every system of the body.

The eyes require sleep because when the eyes are closed, the surface tissues, such as the epithelial cells of the cornea, have time to regenerate. During sleep a reserve of meibum builds up in the Meibomian gland and on the lid margin.

Research has shown that the quality of sleep influences tear secretion and tear film stability. Poor sleep may aggravate anxiety and depression, which can exacerbate the sensation of symptoms.

Altered quality of sleep can affect the health of Meibomian glands. In patients with severe obstructive sleep apnea syndrome (OSAS; during sleep the throat muscles relax intermittently and block the airways), significant morphological changes have been observed, including duct distortion, thinning, dilation, and Meibomian gland dropout. If you have OSAS, your eye doctor should evaluate you for Dry Eye, floppy lid, and MGD. In the meantime, if you have symptoms, you can wear a sleep mask or shield over your eyes when you sleep. The Onyix™ Hydrating Sleep Mask by Eye Eco may work well for you.

Exercise

Exercise naturally strengthens the immune system and enhances the circulatory system and blood flow, improving mental status and the way the body responds to disease. Since your eyes and Meibomian glands are always "under attack" from the environment, microbes, particulate matter, UV rays, and the list goes on and on, it's best to have a good natural system of defense.

Experts don't know exactly how or why exercise strengthens the immune system, but if you exercise moderately and regularly, you boost your immune system and improve your health. (Always see your doctor before beginning any regular exercise program.)

Address Systemic Diseases

Many systemic diseases can affect the Meibomian glands. It's always best to have these diagnosed and treated promptly. When treatable diseases are neglected, complications that could have been avoided can arise.

Address Allergies

Allergies are very common and can cause inflammation of the ocular surface and Meibomian glands. Eliminating allergens can help tremendously with ocular symptoms.

- Get tested for allergies so you can avoid known allergens, but keep in mind that no allergy test covers every allergen. If you travel, you may need a patch test that includes that locale's native plants and trees.
- If you are allergic to animals and your condition is severe or more than you can handle, avoid them completely. If your beloved pet is the source of allergens, consider sequestering your pet to one part of the house. At a minimum, keep your pet off your bed and out of your bedroom. However, these

steps will not stop your exposure to their dander completely. (Pet dander, even in the absence of allergies, can cause ocular inflammation and irritation.)

- Change into indoor clothes when you come inside, and leave your shoes at the door or in the mudroom so you don't spread allergens throughout your house.
- Take a shower and wash your hair at night to wash off any allergens that may have accumulated during the day and before your head lands on the pillow, where these allergens can transfer.
- Remove carpeting, which collects dust, dust mites, dander, and other allergens, and replace with hard flooring.
- Consider immunotherapy to reduce the severity of your allergic reaction.

Quit Smoking or Vaping

Smoking or vaping tobacco or other products can be harmful to your overall health and the health of your Meibomian glands. The smoke can irritate and cause ocular surface inflammation. It's best to quit smoking and vaping.

Don't Give Up Hope

Remember, even if you think you've tried every treatment and seen every doctor, there's virtually always something more that can be done (see guideline 1 at the beginning of the chapter). So don't give up hope.

GLOSSARY

Note: All terms are defined here as they relate to Meibomian gland dysfunction and Dry Eye.

Adapted from Steven L. Maskin, Reversing Dry Eye Syndrome: Practical Ways to Improve Your Comfort, Vision, and Appearance *(New Haven, CT: Yale University Press, 2007).*

ABSORPTION The process by which tear components are taken back into or used by the body.

ACINAR-DUCTULAR UNIT A Meibomian gland ductule and all of the acini attached to it.

ACINI Plural of acinus; illuminated with meibography, acini reveal the outline of the Meibomian gland.

ACINUS One of the grape- or berry-like clusters of cells surrounding the Meibomian gland central duct, which synthesize meibum.

ADJUNCTIVE THERAPY Therapy that is administered in addition to a primary therapy to either support the treatment of the primary condition or to treat comorbidities that may affect the primary condition.

ALLERGEN A substance that when introduced into the body stimulates an allergic reaction.

ALLERGIC REACTION A complicated chemical response to the presence of an allergen in the body.

ALLERGY An acquired sensitivity to certain substances, such as plants, pollens, or drugs, that may include such symptoms as sneezing, runny nose, red or inflamed eyes, and rash.

AMNIOTIC MEMBRANE A layer of human placenta tissue used as a graft or therapeutic dressing in many different fields of medicine.

ANDROGEN A steroid hormone that controls the development and maintenance of masculine characteristics, such as facial and body hair and the development of the penis. Androgens also support various glands, including the tear glands. In women, the ovaries secrete small amounts of androgens that typically decrease with menopause.

ANTERIOR Situated in the front.

ANTERIOR BLEPHARITIS Inflammation of the anterior section of the lid margin, usually from a bacterial infection or due to demodex mites, with discharge around the lash root. See also **blepharitis.**

ANTERIOR CHAMBER The space between the cornea and the iris, filled with a fluid that nourishes eye cells.

ANTERIOR LAMELLA The outer layer of the eyelid; includes the skin and orbicularis muscles that close the lids.

ANTIANDROGEN (also called androgen antagonist, testosterone blockers) Drugs that prevent the production of androgens or block androgen receptor signaling.

ANTIBODY A protein substance produced in the tissues of the body in response to the presence of an antigen (a toxin, for example), destroying or weakening it and thus creating the basis for immunity.

ANTICHOLINERGIC A type of drug that blocks nerve impulses.

ANTICONVULSANT A drug used to treat epileptic and other seizure disorders.

ANTIDEPRESSANT A drug used to prevent or relieve depression.

ANTIGEN A substance such as a bacterium, toxin, or microbe that when introduced into the body stimulates the production of antibodies.

ANTIHISTAMINE One of several drugs used to counteract the physiological effects of histamine.

ANTIHYPERTENSIVE A drug that treats high blood pressure.

ANTI-PARKINSON'S DRUG A drug used to counteract the effects of Parkinson's disease.

ANTIPSYCHOTICS Also called major tranquilizers or neuroleptics; drugs used for managing psychosis, schizophrenia, and bipolar disorder.

ANXIOLYTICS, ANTIANXIETY DRUGS Drugs used to relieve anxiety and aid sleep.

APPOSING In juxtaposition to each other, such as the upper and lower lid margins.

AQUEOUS HUMOR The transparent fluid within the anterior chamber of the eye that nourishes the cells inside the eye, controlling eye cell growth and maturation.

AQUEOUS TEAR DEFICIENT DRY EYE A form of Dry Eye that occurs when the lacrimal glands fail to produce watery tears.

AQUEOUS TEAR LAYER The middle, watery layer of the tear film; composed mostly of various proteins, electrolytes, sugars, and water, and secreted primarily by the lacrimal gland.

ARTIFICIAL TEARS A fluid prepared to supplement inadequate tear production in aqueous tear deficient Dry Eye patients. May also be used to relieve mild discomfort caused by drying irritants such as wind, smoke, or dust. Also called lubricating eye drops.

ASTHMA A condition in which the airways (mouth, throat, windpipe, lungs) are swollen and narrowed because of hypersensitivity to certain stimuli, including pollen, smoke, or even cold air.

ASTIGMATISM A defect of vision usually due to an irregularly shaped cornea.

ASYMPTOMATIC Experiencing no symptoms. The opposite of symptomatic.

ATOPIC KERATOCONJUNCTIVITIS A chronic, severe allergic reaction to pollen, animal dander, and other substances usually affecting middle-aged men. If advanced, can cause scarring of the cornea and even blindness.

ATROPHY The gradual degradation of tissue.

AUTOLOGOUS SERUM A patient's own blood.

AUTOLOGOUS SERUM EYE DROPS, AUTOLOGOUS SERUM TEARS Eye drops derived from the patient's own blood.

BANDAGE CONTACT LENS A contact lens used to protect the corneal surface and/or promote healing.

BELL'S PALSY Paralysis or weakness of the facial muscles due to a malfunction of cranial or facial nerves.

BENIGN ESSENTIAL BLEPHAROSPASM (BEB) A non–life-threatening involuntary neurologic disorder of unknown origin wherein the eyelids and sometimes the facial muscles spasm.

BETA-BLOCKER A drug that typically decreases blood flow and consequently blood pressure.

BLEPHARA Greek for eyelid.

BLEPHARITIS An inflammatory condition that affects the eyelids. There are two variants: anterior blepharitis and posterior blepharitis.

BLEPHAROPLASTY Surgery to remove excess skin of the eyelid.

BLEPHAROSPASM A spasm of the eyelid. See also **benign essential blepharospasm** and **secondary blepharospasm.**

BLINK A usually involuntary movement of the eyelid that distributes the tear film over the surface of the eye and creates negative pressure, drawing tear film out through the puncta and into the nose. May also be voluntary (blinking on purpose) or reflexive (blinking if the eye detects a foreign body or substance).

BLINK RATE The frequency of blinking. In adults, this should be approximately every five to seven seconds.

BOTULINUM TOXIN, TYPE A (also called BOTOX®) A neurotoxic protein (a protein that prevents the release of chemical signals from nerves leading to the relaxation of muscles) used for cosmetic purposes; also used to treat essential blepharospasm.

BRAIN STEM Controls messages between the brain and the rest of the body; responsible for many autonomous bodily functions.

BULBAR CONJUNCTIVA The conjunctiva that covers the sclera, the white part of the eye.

CANTHAL Pertaining to the canthus, a corner of the eye.

CANTHAL TENDONS Extensions of the orbicularis muscle; attached to the bones of the eye socket near the corners of the eyes. The lateral canthal tendon is the portion attached to the outer corner of the eye. The medial canthal tendon is attached at the inner corner of the eye.

CANTHUS The corner of the eye. The lateral canthus is the outer corner of the eye. The medial canthus is the inner corner of the eye.

CARUNCLE, see **lacrimal caruncle.**

CATARACT A clouding of the eye's lens, the part of the eye responsible for focusing light on the retina.

CAUSATIVE FACTOR A factor that, if eliminated, will stop the occurrence of disease. For example, periductal fibrosis is a causative factor in Meibomian gland dysfunction. See also **contributing factor.**

CELLULOSE COMPOUND A type of polysaccharide that swells in water in order to retain moisture; used in artificial tears in varying amounts, resulting in different degrees of viscosity.

CENTRAL DUCT The tube, or lumen, that gives a Meibomian gland its shape and through which meibum flows on its way to the orifice at the lid margin.

CHALAZION A variably sized bump in the eyelid caused by chronic obstruction and inflammation of the Meibomian gland.

CHEMICAL BURN Inflammation of the ocular surface and front of the eye of varying severity, caused by exposure to a chemical (acid or lye, for instance).

CHEMOTHERAPY Drugs that treat various cancers.

CICATRIZING, CICATRICIAL Causes scarring, characterized by scarring.

COMORBIDITY Disease that occurs at the same time as another disease.

COMPLETE DISTAL OBSTRUCTION (CDO) A classification assigned to a lid with obstructive MGD based on the predominant condition of the glands. Glands have periductal fibrosis leading to a loss of ductal integrity with stricture formation and a compromised lumen. The fixed, firm, focal obstruction is located between the orifice and the first acinus. Four or fewer glands are expressible. Lid tenderness is present due to increased intraductal pressure. Can lead to complete distal obstruction–nonfunctional (CDO-NF).

COMPLETE DISTAL OBSTRUCTION–NONFUNCTIONAL (CDO-NF) A classification assigned to a lid with obstructive MGD based on the predominant condition of the glands. Develops from chronic complete distal obstruction (CDO) when glands stop synthesizing meibum. Because there is no buildup of meibum, pressure is not increased and the lid is typically not tender. May lead to whole gland atrophy. When pressure is applied to the lid, the glands do not secrete meibum.

COMPLETE PROXIMAL OBSTRUCTION (CPO) A classification assigned to a lid with obstructive MGD based on the predominant condition of the glands. Glands have periductal fibrosis, leading to a loss of ductal integrity with stricture formation and a compromised lumen. The fixed, firm, focal obstruction is located proximal to at least one acinus. Five or more glands are expressible. Lid tenderness is present due to increased intraductal pressure. Can lead to complete proximal obstruction–partial atrophy (CPO-PA).

COMPLETE PROXIMAL OBSTRUCTION–PARTIAL ATROPHY (CPO-PA) A classification assigned to a lid with obstructive MGD based on the predominant condition of the glands. Glands have periductal fibrosis leading to a loss of ductal integrity with stricture formation and a compromised lumen. The fixed, firm, focal obstruction is located proximal to at least one acinus. Five or more glands are expressible. Lid tenderness is gradually lost due to reduced meibum production and progressive atrophy proximal to the band of periductal fibrosis and lumen stricture.

CONCOMITANT Naturally accompanying or associated with.

CONFOCAL MISCROSCOPE, CONFOCAL MICROSCOPY A device used to evaluate tissue in vivo at a cellular level; the high-resolution analysis of such tissue.

CONJUNCTIVA The transparent membrane that covers the inner lining of the eyelid and the white part of the eyeball (the sclera). The conjunctiva starts at the limbus, extends over the sclera, continues toward the back of the eye where it forms a loose pouch called the fornix, then turns and covers the inner lining of the eyelids and the posterior lid margin, and ends at the mucocutaneous junction on the lid margin, forming one continuous blanket of mucosal tissue.

CONJUNCTIVITIS (also called pink eye) An inflammation of the conjunctiva, the outermost layer of the eye that covers the sclera, characterized by redness and sometimes accompanied by a discharge.

CONJUNCTIVOCHALASIS (also called conjunctival chalasis) A common disorder in which the conjunctiva loses its elasticity, becomes wrinkled or pleated, droops over the lid margin, and becomes pinched between the lid and the eyeball, causing pain and other discomfort.

CONSTRICTION A narrowing or strangulation.

CONTACT CONJUNCTIVITIS A common allergic response to an allergen that has been introduced directly onto the eye, such as an eye drop or a cosmetic like eyeliner.

CONTACT LENS A plastic or polymer disk that is placed directly onto the eye to correct refractive vision disorders (nearsightedness, farsightedness, astigmatism).

CONTRAINDICATION A reason why a treatment should not be administered; the opposite of indication.

CONTRIBUTING FACTOR, COFACTOR A factor that, if eliminated, may reduce the symptoms of disease. For example, reversing a contributing factor to Meibomian gland dysfunction may slow its advancement but will not stop the occurrence of disease unless the causative factor (periductal fibrosis) is also eliminated. See also **causative factor.**

CORNEA The transparent dime-sized disc that covers the front of the eye; among the most sensitive parts of the body; sometimes called the window of the eye. The cornea and the air–tear film interface, along with the lens, focus light on the retina.

CORNEA AND EXTERNAL DISEASE A subspecialty of ophthalmology that focuses on diseases of the ocular surface.

CORNEAL EPITHELIUM The most superficial cells covering the corneal surface, several cell layers thick.

CORNEAL NEUROPATHIC PAIN, CORNEAL NEUROPATHY, CORNEAL NEURALGIA (also called ocular neuropathic pain; informally called ocular neuropathy) A diagnosis of exclusion given when no cause can be found for ocular surface pain.

CORTICOSTEROID Topical drops used for reducing and eliminating inflammation; a nonspecific therapy.

CRUSTING Dry foreign substance found near the roots of the lashes or along the lid margin; usually a sign of infectious anterior blepharitis.

CYCLOSPORINE An immunosuppressant drug produced by a fungus, sometimes used to inhibit organ transplant rejection. Used in topical medications and thought to reduce inflammation in patients with Dry Eye.

CYSTIC Ballooning out.

DACRYOCYSTITIS An infection of the tear sac that lies between the inner corner of the eyelids and the nose.

DAUGHTER CELLS The generation of cells produced by stem cells or progenitor cells.

DECONGESTANT A medication, often found in over-the-counter as well as prescription drugs, that breaks up congestion in the sinuses or chest by reducing swelling.

DELAYED TEAR CLEARANCE Improper drainage of tears. Often accompanied by aqueous tear deficiency and sometimes caused by a clogged tear duct, which can cause inflammation of the eye surface.

DERMATITIS (also called eczema) Inflammation of the upper layers of the skin, causing itching, redness, swelling, and scaling.

DERMATOCHALASIS Loosening of the eyelid skin tissues.

DESTABILIZED TEAR FILM, UNSTABLE TEAR FILM Tear film that breaks up too quickly.

DIABETES A serious but common disorder in which the pancreas produces insufficient or no insulin; often involves eye problems, which can include Dry Eye.

DIAGNOSIS OF EXCLUSION A diagnosis given when all other possible diseases have been ruled out. May lead to misdiagnosis if diseases are occult (hidden) or test results are false negative.

DIFFUSE A symptom felt regionally, that is, more than focally, but not necessarily globally.

DILATE To widen or spread apart.

DISTAL Situated closer to the terminal end. Distal periductal fibrosis develops between the orifice and the first acinus, near the terminal end of the gland.

DISTICHIASIS An extra row of lashes sometimes emanating from a Meibomian gland orifice.

DIURETIC A substance or drug that causes the body to eliminate water, increasing urine output. May cause aqueous tear deficiency.

DROOPY EYELID, see **ptosis.**

DROPOUT, MEIBOMIAN GLAND DROPOUT One or more of a Meibomian gland's acinar-ductular units has atrophied. Illuminated with meibography, there is an empty space where the acinar-ductular unit should be.

DRY EYE, DRY EYE SYNDROME A disease characterized by faulty production of tears resulting in damage to the surface of the eye and at times painful eyes.

DUCT The central structure of a Meibomian gland through which meibum travels to the orifice at the lid margin. Its interior space is called the lumen. See **lumen.**

DUCTAL INTEGRITY (lumen integrity) A noncompromised duct with a patent lumen that allows Meibomian gland secretions to flow freely and without resistance; confirmed or established with intraductal Meibomian gland probing.

DUCTULE The small duct that connects one or more acini to the central duct of the Meibomian gland.

ECTROPION The condition in which the eyelid turns away from the eyeball and fails to cover the eye properly, leaving the ocular surface exposed.

ECZEMA, see **dermatitis.**

EDEMA The accumulation of excessive water in cells, tissues, or body cavities.

ENDOTHELIUM The single layer of cells lining the inner cornea that keeps the cornea from swelling by removing excess water.

ENTROPION The condition in which the eyelid turns inward; often associated with eyelashes rubbing against the eye (trichiasis).

EPISCLERA A layer of loose fibroelastic tissue underlying and attached to the Tenon's capsule.

EPISCLERITIS Inflammation of the episclera; may indicate systemic diseases, such as gout.

EPITHELIUM The layers of cells that make up the covering of most of the surfaces of the body, including the eyes.

ESSENTIAL NUTRIENTS Nutrients, including vitamin C, omega-3, and omega-6 fatty acids, that the body does not produce on its own and must come from a food or supplement source.

ESTROGEN Any of several hormones secreted by the ovaries and placenta, which stimulate the female secondary sex characteristics.

ETIOLOGY The cause of a disease or abnormal condition.

EVAPORATION The rate at which tears are converted into vapor after they are secreted and distributed onto the surface of the eye.

EVAPORATIVE DRY EYE A form of Dry Eye characterized by abnormal tear film lipid; results in rapid evaporation of tear film.

EXFOLIATING Removing outer epithelial layer of eyelid margin cells.

EXOCRINE A gland that secretes its contents through a duct to reach its destination.

EXPRESS To press on the lids with the aim of forcing meibum or other sequestered material out of a Meibomian gland; can be performed diagnostically or therapeutically.

EXPRESSIBLE A Meibomian gland that secretes meibum when pressure is applied to the lid.

FALSE NEGATIVE A test result wherein the test indicates no disease when disease exists.

FALSE POSITIVE A test result wherein the test indicates a disease exists when there is no disease.

FATTY ACIDS Chemicals that are the building blocks of fat in food and in the human body.

FIBROSIS, FIBROTIC TISSUE Scar tissue; fibrous connective tissue that replaces healthy tissue in the setting of inflammation or injury. Fibrotic, vascularized tissue develops around the Meibomian gland duct wall and invades the duct wall epithelium.

FIBROVASCULAR Having both fibrotic and vascular tissue.

FILAMENT Small strands of degenerated epithelial cells and mucus attached to the ocular surface at one end.

FILAMENTARY KERATITIS A disorder wherein stringy filaments of mucus and degenerated epithelial cells are found attached to the cornea, creating pain, redness, and fluctuating vision.

FISSURE See **lid fissure width.**

FLAXSEED OIL A vegetable oil high in omega-3 fatty acids; seems to help reduce Dry Eye.

FLOPPY EYELID SYNDROME A disorder characterized by lax or flaccid upper eyelids.

FLUORESCEIN An orange-red compound that exhibits intense yet harmless fluorescence (an emission of electromagnetic radiation); used in ophthalmology to reveal corneal lesions and to test for delayed tear clearance.

FLUORESCEIN CLEARANCE TEST Using fluorescein dye for the delayed tear clearance test. See also **delayed tear clearance.**

FOCAL A symptom felt in a specific spot.

FOLLICULITIS Infection at the base of the lashes.

FOREIGN-BODY SENSATION The feeling that an object—a speck of dust, an eyelash, a wood sliver—has lodged in the eye, causing irritation or pain.

FORNICEAL Pertaining to the conjunctival fornix.

FORNIX, CONJUNCTIVAL The loose pouch formed at the junction of the bulbar and palpebral conjunctiva. Because the fornix is lax, it allows the eyeball to move in the eye socket.

FRICTIONAL STRESS Occurs with Dry Eye and MGD; the physical force of the lining of the lids rubbing against the surface tissues of the eye.

GERD (gastroesophageal reflux disease) A common, chronic digestive disease; acidified contents of the stomach refluxes into the esophagus.

GIANT PAPILLARY CONJUNCTIVITIS (GPC) A disorder affecting people who wear contact lenses. Features "giant papillae," or bumps of swollen tissue, with a central dilated vessel on the lining of the upper eyelid, making contact lens wear difficult or impossible.

GLAND A cell or group of cells, or an organ, that selectively removes material from the blood, concentrates or alters it as necessary, and secretes it for further use by the body or eliminates it from the body.

GLAUCOMA A blinding disease caused by elevated intraocular pressure that usually results from inadequate functioning of the eye's internal fluid-drainage structures.

GLOBAL A symptom felt across the entire eyeball.

GOBLET EPITHELIAL CELL A conjunctival cell that produces mucin, which enables tear film to adhere to the eye surface.

GRAFT-VERSUS-HOST DISEASE Incompatibility reaction against the host after bone marrow transplant. This reaction may cause severe Dry Eye and may need aggressive treatment.

GRAVES' DISEASE A condition caused by excessive thyroid hormone; sometimes characterized by an enlarged thyroid gland, protrusion of the eyeballs, rapid heartbeat, and nervousness. If the eyes protrude or the lids retract, the ocular surface may become desiccated and irritated.

GRAY LINE Where the posterior and anterior lamella of the eyelid tissue meet, visible on the eyelid margin.

HERPES SIMPLEX A common virus that affects the skin, mucous membranes, nervous system, and eyes.

HISTAMINE a compound released by white blood cells as part of the body's immune system response.

HOLOCRINE A gland whose cells mature, disintegrate, and become the secreted material.

HORDEOLUM Acute blockage of a Meibomian gland with secondary inflammation, characterized by acute pain and eyelid tenderness.

HORMONE REPLACEMENT THERAPY (HRT) Treatment with natural or synthetic hormones.

HYDROPHOBIC Has properties that repel moisture.

HYPEROSMOLAR A liquid that contains a high concentration of solutes.

IATROGENIC COMORBIDITIES Comorbidities caused by medical intervention.

INCOMPLETE BLINKING (also called partial blinking) Blinking with the eyelids not completely closing before opening again; may reduce the amount of secreted meibum and build up pressure on the acini of the Meibomian glands.

INFERIOR Situated below.

INFLAMMATORY MEDIATOR A chemical produced by the body that causes an inflammatory response.

INTRADUCTAL Inside the ductal space.

INTRADUCTAL MEIBOMIAN GLAND PROBE, PROBING, see **Maskin® Probe** and **Maskin® Probing.**

JOJOBA ANESTHETIC OINTMENT Topical anesthetic refrigerated ointment used to prepare the lids, lid margins, and Meibomian glands for Maskin probing, containing 8% lidocaine and 25% jojoba oil in a proprietary formula.

KERATITIS Inflammation of the cornea.

KERATOCONJUNCTIVITIS SICCA Inflammation of the cornea and conjunctiva from insufficient aqueous tears.

KERATOCONUS A degenerative disease of the cornea that causes it to gradually thin and bulge into a conelike shape.

LACRIMAL APPARATUS The tear production and drainage system consisting of tear glands, lacrimal puncta, tear drainage ducts, collection sac within the nose, and duct from the sac to the internal lining of the nose.

LACRIMAL CANALICULUS One of the tear drainage ducts leading from the lacrimal puncta to the collection sac inside the nose.

LACRIMAL CARUNCLE The ball of tissue found in the inner corner of each eye, which helps to channel tear film into the lacrimal puncta.

LACRIMAL FUNCTIONAL UNIT The integrated tear secretory system whereby tear gland secretion and blinking are stimulated by the sensory nerves on the surface of the cornea through a subconscious neurologic pathway within the brain stem.

LACRIMAL GLAND A gland behind the conjunctival fornix in the upper outer corner of the eye, which produces watery tears.

LACRIMAL PUNCTA (singular is punctum) The openings or portals at the nasal end of the eyelid closest to the nose, where tears enter the lacrimal drainage system. See **lacrimal apparatus.**

LACRIMAL SYSTEM, NASOLACRIMAL APPARATUS A complex of glands that produce aqueous (water) tears and excretory ducts, which allows "old" or "dirty" tears to drain from the eyes into the nose. See also **lacrimal functional unit** and **lacrimal apparatus.**

LAGOPHTHALMOS A condition in which the eyelids do not close completely. Nocturnal lagophthalmos occurs when the eyelids do not close completely during sleep. Blink lagophthalmos occurs when the eyelids do not close completely during blinks.

LAMELLA Layers of the eyelid. See **anterior lamella** and **posterior lamella.**

LASIK (laser in situ keratomileusis) A common refractive procedure used to correct nearsightedness, farsightedness, and astigmatism; the nerve endings are cut or ablated to reconfigure the cornea. Because the corneal nerves are cut, they become desensitized, leading to a reduced blink rate.

LATERAL CANTHAL CROWDING A cluster of comorbidities affecting the lateral canthus, or outer corner of the eye, and may include in variable severity dermatochalasis, entropion, trichiasis, and conjunctivochalasis, leading to altered blink patterns. Prevents normal spreading of tear film. Causes local microtrauma and inflammation.

LAVAGE Washing or clearing by rinsing with a solution.

LENS (also called crystalline lens) The internal optical component of the eye, responsible for adjusting focus; elastic and transparent. Located behind the iris.

LEVATOR MUSCLE The primary retractor muscle in the upper lid. See also **retractor muscles.**

LID FISSURE WIDTH The vertical distance between the upper and lower lid margins at rest after a blink. If increased, can lead to ocular surface desiccation and discomfort. May have association with blink lagophthalmos.

LID LAXITY A condition in which the lower lid does not properly hug or cover the eyeball. Usually age related, and closely associated with ectropion.

LID MARGIN The smooth, flat edge of the eyelid between the skin and palpebral conjunctiva; about 2 millimeters wide (about 1.5 millimeters in children). The lid margins of the upper and lower lid meet during a blink.

LID WIPER The region of the lining of upper lid that is responsible for spreading tears during blinks.

LIMBUS In healthy tissue the limbus is found at the junction of the bulbar conjunctiva and the cornea and is notable for containing corneal stem cells.

LIPID LAYER The oily, outer layer of the tear film, made up of waxy meibum produced by the Meibomian glands.

LIQUIDITY How readily a substance can flow.

LISSAMINE GREEN TEST A standard dye test given to Dry Eye patients to determine whether the epithelial cells are degenerating.

LUMEN The central cavity or interior space of a duct, tube, or orifice.

LUPUS ERYTHEMATOSUS An autoimmune disorder in which the body's immune system attacks tissues and organ systems throughout the body, causing inflammation. The skin is often involved; a red, blotchy, butterfly-shaped rash on the cheeks and bridge of the nose is common.

LYSOZYME An antibacterial agent found in tears, which in a matter of minutes inactivates bacteria on the surface of the eye.

MAP-DOT-FINGERPRINT DYSTROPHY A condition in which an irregular corneal surface can lead to Dry Eye when the overlying tear film becomes unstable. Also known as anterior basement membrane dystrophy and Cogan's dystrophy.

MASKIN® MICROTUBE A specially configured and dimensioned hollow, non-sharp, stainless-steel tube that is inserted through the Meibomian gland orifice and into the duct after probing; used to deliver a therapeutic medicament (medication) or biologic to the intraductal space; also used to lavage and rinse the intraductal space.

MASKIN® PROBE A specially configured and dimensioned nonsharp, stainless-steel device for insertion through the Meibomian gland orifice into the duct.

MASKIN® PROBING The method (or protocol) of inserting a Maskin Probe into a Meibomian gland orifice and duct to release periductal fibrotic tissue, equilibrate intraductal pressure, restore ductal integrity and functional Meibomian glands, and diagnose or confirm lumen patency.

MASKING SCENTS Chemicals used to cover up undesirable scents.

MAST CELL A type of cell found in connective tissue (mucous membranes, lung tissue, conjunctiva, nose), which contains numerous basophilic granules and releases substances such as heparin and histamine in response to injury or inflammation of bodily tissue. Often associated with allergies.

MEIBOCYTES The daughter cells produced by progenitor cells in the acini. As they travel toward the ductule, the meibocyte material breaks down and turns into the oil, known as meibum, secreted by Meibomian glands.

MEIBOMIAN GLAND A holocrine, exocrine sebaceous gland in the eyelid that produces oil known as meibum for the lipid layer of tear film.

MEIBOMIAN GLAND CLASSIFICATION FORM (MCF) A form used to record the characteristics of the entire population of Meibomian glands in each lid, including the number of diagnostically expressible glands and presence or absence of lid tenderness.

MEIBOMIAN GLAND DYSFUNCTION Abnormally functioning Meibomian glands, most often due to circumferential ductal constriction as well as external duct wall invasion by periductal fibrotic and/or fibrovascular tissue. Results in lid pain and tenderness and an abnormal tear film. Alternatively, the patient may be asymptomatic while the disease progresses. The most common cause of Dry Eye.

MEIBOMIAN GLAND PROBE, PROBING, see **Maskin® Probe, Maskin® Probing.**

MEIBUM A complex mix of lipids, consisting of wax and sterol esters, hydrocarbons, triglycerides, free sterols, free fatty acids, and polar lipids; secreted by the Meibomian glands.

MEIBUM SECRETING UNIT When functionally classifying Meibomian glands, the entire population of glands in a lid are considered as a single entity.

MICROBIOME The collection of microorganisms, such as bacteria, fungi, and parasites, that live on or in the human body.

MOISTURE CHAMBER GLASSES or GOGGLES Special eye protectors engineered to minimize evaporation of tears in Dry Eye sufferers.

MUCIN A glycoprotein, mucuslike substance produced by the goblet cells of the epithelial layer of the conjunctiva.

MUCIN LAYER The layer of the tear film that lies closest to the surface of the eye. Stabilizes the tear film and helps to spread tears across the cornea. Combines in varying degrees with the aqueous layer of tear film to create a muco-aqueous layer. Becomes denser closer to the ocular surface epithelium.

MUCOCUTANEOUS JUNCTION The site along the lid margin where keratinized skin of the eyelid and mucosal tissue of the conjunctiva meet. Also called the Line of Marx.

MUCUS An opaque discharge of mucins.

NANOMETER One billionth of a meter.

NASAL, NASALLY Closer to the nose, on the same side of the eye as the nose. The inner corner of the eye is the nasal side of the eye.

NEURODEGENERATIVE DISORDER Diseases that result in the destruction of brain cells or the peripheral nervous system, such as Parkinson's disease and multiple sclerosis.

NEUROPATHIC PAIN Neuropathic pain is pain generated by altered or damaged nerves; believed to be either peripheral, emanating from nerves on the ocular surface, or central, emanating from within the brain. Although the patient experiences ocular symptoms, there is no detectable external stimulus causing the pain.

NOCICEPTIVE PAIN Pain caused by mechanical, thermal, or chemical injury. You feel nociceptive pain when you stub your toe, burn your finger, or splash soap in your eye.

NONEDEMATOUS Tissue that is not inflamed or swollen (has no edema).

NONOBVIOUS MGD (NOMGD) Minimal to no signs of MGD visible at the slit lamp, except reduced numbers of expressible glands.

NONREFRACTIVE CORNEA AND EXTERNAL DISEASES Diseases of the ocular surface excluding those concerned with refraction, the eyes' ability to focus.

NON-SJÖGREN'S AQUEOUS TEAR DEFICIENCY, see **primary acquired lacrimal gland disease.**

NOXIOUS AGENT Poisonous or harmful substance.

NSAID Nonsteroidal anti-inflammatory drug.

OCCULT DISEASE A disease that is not immediately apparent or is not discovered during an exam and not revealed by tests.

OCULAR CICATRICIAL PEMPHIGOID A chronic autoimmune disease that features scarring of the conjunctiva and at times other mucosal tissues in the nose, throat, esophagus, urethra, vagina, and anus. The scarring can lead to obstruction of the lacrimal or Meibomian glands and destruction of the goblet cells of the conjunctiva, resulting in tear instability and Dry Eye.

OCULAR NEUROPATHIC PAIN (also informally called ocular neuropathy) A diagnosis of exclusion given when no cause can be found for ocular surface pain. See also **corneal neuropathic pain, corneal neuropathy, corneal neuralgia.**

OCULAR SURFACE DISEASE INDEX (OSDI) Developed by a pharmaceutical company, a survey often administered to Dry Eye patients, which assesses how often patients experience common Dry Eye symptoms, how often symptoms affect common tasks, and if certain environments trigger symptoms. The survey neglects to ask about the severity of symptoms and about lid heaviness.

OMEGA-3 FATTY ACID Any of various polyunsaturated fatty acids found primarily in fish, fish oils, vegetables, and vegetable oils (including flaxseed oil). These fatty acids are thought to improve meibum secretion.

OPHTHALMOLOGIST A medical doctor who specializes in care of the eyes, who diagnoses and treats eye diseases and disorders as well as associated systemic medical diseases, performs eye surgery as necessary, prescribes medications, and conducts examinations to determine the quality of vision and the need for corrective glasses.

OPHTHALMOLOGY The study of the eye; the branch of medicine and surgery that specializes in the diagnosis and treatment of disorders of the eye.

OPTICIAN A technician who fills prescriptions for ophthalmic lenses and dispenses eyeglasses.

OPTOMETRIST A specialist trained to examine the eyes, check for and treat diseases of the eye, and prescribe, supply, and adjust glasses or contact lenses. In some states allowed to perform intraductal Meibomian gland probing. A graduate of optometry school.

OPTOMETRY The practice of assessing vision, diagnosing eye diseases and disorders, and nonsurgically treating general eye problems, as well as establishing whether glasses or contact lenses are needed.

ORBICULARIS MUSCLE The main protractor muscle in the upper eyelid; closes the upper eyelid. See also **protractor muscles.**

ORBIT, see **socket.**

ORIFICE METAPLASIA Visible threadlike keratin within the orifice.

PALLIATIVE Treatment that reduces symptoms but does not treat the disease.

PALPEBRAL CONJUNCTIVA The conjunctiva that covers the inner lining of the eyelid.

PARTIAL BLINKING See **incomplete blinking.**

PARTIAL DISTAL OBSTRUCTION (PDO) A classification assigned to a lid with obstructive MGD based on the predominant condition of the glands. Glands may have visible threadlike obstruction within the orifice (orifice metaplasia) and/or mildly constricting occult periductal fibrosis. There are five or more expressible glands. There is no lid tenderness because obstruction is partial and does not cause elevated intraductal pressure.

PARTIAL DISTAL OBSTRUCTION–NONFUNCTIONAL (PDO-NF) A classification assigned to a lid with obstructive MGD based on the predominant condition of the glands. Glands may have visible threadlike obstruction within the orifice (orifice metaplasia) and/or mildly constricting occult periductal fibrosis. There are four or fewer expressible glands. There is no lid tenderness because obstruction is partial and meibum is not being produced, as though the glands were dormant. Seen in cases of binge eating.

PARTICULATE MATTER Tiny particles suspended in air or liquid.

PATENT, PATENCY Fully open, lacking obstruction.

PATHOGENS Microorganisms that can cause disease.

PATHOPHYSIOLOGY The study of disease and how it develops and progresses.

PEPTIDES Amino acids that make up proteins.

PERIDUCTAL Surrounding a duct.

PERIGLANDULAR Surrounding one or more glands.

PHOTOPHOBIA A sensitivity to bright lights.

PINGUECULA A benign, yellowish degenerative growth that can form on the conjunctiva of the eye. Often causes no symptoms but can also cause severe pain if inflamed (pingueculitis).

PINK EYE, see **conjunctivitis.**

PLICA SEMILUNARIS A loose fold in the palpebral conjunctiva adjacent to the lacrimal caruncle, which allows the eyeball to move around in the eye socket and helps to channel tear film into the lacrimal punctum.

POLARITY, POLAR MOLECULE Having one end positively charged and the other end negatively charged; a molecule charged this way.

POSTERIOR Situated in the back.

POSTERIOR BLEPHARITIS Inflammation of the rear part of the eyelid, including the lid margin and Meibomian glands. The term is often used instead of Meibomian gland dysfunction. See also **blepharitis** and **Meibomian gland dysfunction.**

POSTERIOR LAMELLA The inner layer of the eyelid; includes the tarsal plate (dense connective tissue that forms and supports the lid) and the Meibomian glands.

PRECORNEAL TEAR FILM The portion of tear film that covers the cornea.

PRESERVATIVE A substance, such as benzalkonium chloride, that is added to artificial tears and other eye drops, inhibiting microbial contamination for a longer shelf life. Can damage surface epithelium, leading to and exacerbating pain and irritation.

PRESERVATIVE-FREE EYE DROP An eye drop or artificial tear that does not contain any preservatives, to increase tolerance for the eye.

PRIMARY ACQUIRED LACRIMAL GLAND DISEASE (also called non-Sjögren's aqueous tear deficiency) The most common cause of aqueous tear deficiency, involving the lacrimal glands failing to produce sufficient aqueous tears.

PROBE, PROBING, see **Maskin® Probe, Maskin® Probing.**

PROBE FINDINGS FORM A form used to record the results of probing each individual Meibomian gland.

PROGENITOR CELLS Produced by stem cells, which themselves produce daughter cells with one or more specific functions. Progenitor cells do not reproduce themselves indefinitely.

PROTRACTOR MUSCLES Muscles that close the eyelids. See also **orbicularis muscle, retractor muscles,** and **levator muscle.**

PROXIMAL Situated away from the terminal end. Proximal periductal fibrosis develops deeper within in the lid and farther away from the orifice (the terminal end of the gland).

PROXIMATE CAUSE The primary cause; the cause immediately precipitating a condition.

PSEUDO SLK A disease that presents with the same signs and symptoms as SLK (superior limbic keratoconjunctivitis) but is actually due to aqueous tear deficiency (ATD) and therefore resolves when ATD is accurately diagnosed and effectively treated. See **superior limbic keratoconjunctivitis.**

PSYCHOSOMATIC A physical illness caused by a mental or emotional condition such as stress.

PTERYGIUM A raised, wedge-shaped growth of the conjunctiva onto the cornea.

PTOSIS (also called droopy eyelid) A sagging of the eyelid that may occur as a result of disease, injury, birth defect, eye surgery, or age.

PUNCTAL OCCLUSION Closing the punctum to retain tear film on the ocular surface and prevent it from draining out.

PUNCTUM (plural is puncta) A small opening or portal at the inner corner of the eye that permits tears to drain into the nose. Each eye has two, an upper and a lower punctum.

PUPIL The black "dot" at the center of the iris; actually a hole through which light travels to the retina.

P-VALUE Short for "probability value"; a value that indicates if data is of statistical significance. Data with a p-value less than or equal to 0.05 is considered statistically significant.

RECURRENT EROSION SYNDROME A periodic breakdown of the corneal epithelium in which the upper lids pull a thin layer of cells off the cornea; typically causes acute sharp pain upon opening the eyes when awakening.

REFLEX TEARING Tearing that happens in response to an external stimulus like a foreign body or a foreign body sensation; tearing that happens when the eyes feel dry.

REFRACTIVE SURGERY One of the surgical procedures—LASIK, LASEK, PRK, and epi-LASIK—used to correct refractive eye problems, such as nearsightedness, farsightedness, and astigmatism.

REFRACTORY A term describing a disease that does not respond as expected to treatment and the disease persists.

RETINA Processes the light projected through the cornea and the lens; comparable to film in a camera.

RETINOIDS Vitamin A compounds.

RETRACTOR MUSCLES Muscles in the upper and lower eyelids that open the eyelids and hold them open. Lower lid retractors open the lids and hold them in place during a downward gaze. See also **levator muscle, protractor muscles,** and **orbicularis muscle.**

RHEUMATOID ARTHRITIS An autoimmune disorder that affects joints of the fingers, wrists, toes, and other body joints, making them swollen, stiff, painful, and sometimes deformed. Often seen in conjunction with Sjögren's syndrome, thus, the lacrimal and salivary glands may also be affected.

ROSACEA A chronic skin condition characterized by sebaceous gland inflammation, most recognizable when involving the nose and cheeks with blood vessel dilation. Can be associated with ocular surface and Meibomian periglandular inflammation. Often accompanied by delayed tear clearance. Can lead to blood vessel invasion of the peripheral cornea often in the setting of delayed tear clearance. May be difficult to diagnose in darkly pigmented individuals.

ROSE BENGAL TEST An evaluation using rose bengal, a red vital dye, to assess the health of the conjunctival epithelial cells, specifically which cells are inadequately coated with mucin.

SALZMANN'S NODULAR DEGENERATION A noninflammatory, slowly progressive, degenerative condition of the surface of the cornea.

SAPONIFICATION (also called frothy tears) Tear film becomes soaplike and bubbly due to the liberation of free acids from meibum by microbial enzymes; causes burning, irritation, and inflammation. Patients may complain that it feels like they have soap in their eyes.

SCARRING, SCAR TISSUE Fibrous connective tissue that replaces healthy tissue in the setting of inflammation or injury.

SCHIRMER'S TEST A method of assessing the volume of aqueous tear production, using a filter paper wetting strip. See also serial **Schirmer's test.**

SCLERA The dense white outer wall of the eye.

SCLERAL LENS A contact lens that rests on the sclera, clear of the cornea and limbus, allowing a diseased or damaged cornea to stay moist and protected.

SEBACEOUS GLAND An oil-secreting gland. Meibomian glands are a type of sebaceous gland.

SEBORRHEIC MEIBOMIAN GLAND DISEASE A type of Meibomian gland dysfunction with excess lipid secretion.

SECONDARY ACQUIRED LACRIMAL GLAND DISEASES Aqueous tear deficiency caused by various disorders, including graft-versus-host disease and HIV/AIDS, which can affect the functioning of the lacrimal glands.

SECONDARY BLEPHAROSPASM Spasm of the eyelids from an identifiable cause, such as tear or ocular surface problems, for example, ATD, MGD, allergy, conjunctivochalasis, and distichiasis or trichiasis; dehydration; stimulants; or electrolyte imbalance. The eyelid spasm may further increase irritation, causing a cycle of more forceful spasms. Can occur simultaneously with benign essential blepharospasm (BEB). See **blepharospasm, benign essential blepharospasm.**

SECRETAGOGUE A hormone or other agent that stimulates moisture-producing glands, including salivary glands and lacrimal glands; usually administered orally.

SELF-LIMITING BLEEDING Stops on its own without applying pressure.

SERIAL SCHIRMER'S TEST A method of immediately repeating a Schirmer's test to evaluate the volume of aqueous tears and avoid potentially false negative test results from a single Schirmer's test.

SEVENTH CRANIAL NERVE One of twelve cranial nerves, it controls facial muscles and therefore facial expressions.

SHEARING FORCES Forces that push in different directions.

SJÖGREN'S SYNDROME A condition in which the secretory glands, most commonly the lacrimal gland of the eyes and salivary glands of the mouth, are gradually destroyed by autoimmune inflammation, leading to excessively dry eyes and mouth. May occur in conjunction with other autoimmune disorders, such as rheumatoid arthritis or systemic lupus erythematosus.

SLIT LAMP A type of biomicroscope used to examine the surface of the eye.

SOCKET (also called orbit) The bony structure formed by the brow, the cheek-bone, and the bridge of the nose, which holds and protects the eyeball.

SOLUTE A substance dissolved in liquid.

SQUAMOUS METAPLASIA In the context of a Meibomian gland, a change in the shape, characteristics, and function of acinar cells, becoming flat and nonsecretory.

SQUAMOUS NEOPLASIA A type of cancer found on the surface of the eye.

STANDARD PATIENT EVALUATION OF EYE DRYNESS (SPEED™) QUESTION-NAIRE A questionnaire often used to assess the frequency and severity of Dry Eye and MGD symptoms: "dryness, grittiness, or scratchiness," "soreness or irritation," burning or watering," and "eye fatigue." The questionnaire groups symptoms together, which can distort results, and it neglects to ask about lid heaviness.

STEM CELL DEFICIENCY A lack of stem cells.

STEM CELLS Found throughout the body, cells that produce daughter cells and have the potential to differentiate into specialized cells. Meibomian gland stem cells are thought to be found in the external duct wall epithelium at the junction of the central duct and the acinar-ductular unit. Stem cells can reproduce indefinitely.

STENOTIC Narrowed.

STEVENS-JOHNSON SYNDROME A very rare but severe inflammatory eruption of the skin and mucous membranes, similar to a burn; may occur in children and young adults following an infection or as a reaction to drugs.

STROMA The layer of cornea under the epithelium that accounts for 90 percent of the corneal thickness and is optically clear under normal conditions to allow the passage of light to reach the retina.

SUBCLINICAL A condition that is has not progressed to the degree that it causes symptoms. See **asymptomatic.**

SUPERFICIAL The outermost layer.

SUPERIOR Situated above.

SUPERIOR LIMBIC KERATOCONJUNCTIVITIS Inflammation of the superior (top) part of the eye, including the conjunctiva and upper part of the cornea (the superior limbus); can occur concomitantly with Dry Eye or in association with thyroid conditions.

SYMBLEPHARON Fibrotic adhesion of the palpebral conjunctiva to the bulbar conjunctiva.

SYMPTOM ASSESSMENT IN DRY EYE (SANDE) Developed at Harvard Medical School in 2007, a questionnaire often used to diagnose Dry Eye that asks only about the frequency and severity of symptoms on a 100-point visual analog scale (VAS), but does not ask which symptoms are present.

TEAR BREAKUP TIME (TBUT) The time it takes for the tear film to destabilize on the surface of the eye.

TEAR CLEARANCE (also called tear turnover) The rate at which tears are cleared from the surface of the eye.

TEAR CLEARANCE TEST, see **fluorescein clearance test.**

TEAR DRAINAGE SYSTEM Part of the nasolacrimal apparatus; includes the punctum, lacrimal canaliculus, lacrimal sac, and nasolacrimal duct.

TEAR FILM The moist substance that covers the exposed surface of the eye all the time; about 3 microns thick.

TEAR MENISCUS The thin strip of tear film adjacent to the lid margins where most exposed tear volume pools. Aqueous tear deficiency is suggested by an inadequate or missing tear meniscus.

TELANGIECTASIA Abnormal blood vessel growth.

TEMPORAL, TEMPORALLY Closer to the temple, on the same side of the eye as the temple. The outer corner of the eye is the temporal side of the eye.

TENDER, TENDERNESS A sensation of pain from tissue when pressure is applied.

TENON'S CAPSULE A layer of connective tissue between the bulbar conjunctiva and episclera and attached to both.

TETRACAINE An anesthetic drop used to numb the eyes.

TORTUOSITY Twisting and turning.

TOXICITY The condition of being poisonous or injurious; also the degree to which a substance is toxic.

TRANSILLUMINATION Lighting tissue from behind.

TRANSILLUMINATOR A flashlight-like device that shines light through the lids, used to illuminate the gross outlines of the Meibomian glands within the eyelids.

TRICHIASIS A disease in which the eyelashes become misdirected, growing inward toward the surface of the eye instead of outward and thus irritate or abrade the ocular surface. Can cause discomfort and possibly corneal ulceration and perforation.

ULTRAVIOLET (UV) LIGHT Electromagnetic radiation beyond the spectrum of light visible by humans; UV light can be harmful to the ocular surface.

VASCULAR, VASCULARIZED TISSUE Tissue that contains blood vessels. Vascularized fibrotic tissue develops around the Meibomian gland duct wall and invades the duct wall epithelium.

VASOCONSTRICTOR A drug that constricts blood vessels in the eyes, thus eliminating redness.

VISCOSITY The consistency of a liquid measured by its degree of thickness, stickiness, and fluidity.

VISUAL ACUITY A measure of one's ability to see clearly.

VISUAL ANALOG SCALE A standardized measurement tool for recording patients' subjective evaluations of the severity of their symptoms. Patients make a handwritten vertical mark on a horizontal line that has 0 on the left, representing no pain, and 10 (sometimes 100) on the right, representing the worst pain they have ever experienced.

VITAL DYE STAINING Using water-soluble stains on living (vital) tissue as part of an ocular examination.

WHOLE GLAND ATROPHY (WGA) The status of an individual gland. Viewed with infrared meibography or transillumination, there is a complete lack of organized glandular tissue; the orifice may be still visible at the lid margin.

WRAPAROUND GLASSES Glasses that have wide sides preventing free flow of air across the ocular surface.

BIBLIOGRAPHY

CHAPTER 1. MEIBOMIAN GLAND DYSFUNCTION: THE MOST COMMON FACTOR IN DRY EYE

Andrews, John, et al., "The Impact of Digital Devices on Meibomian Gland Structure and Function." Poster presented at the annual meeting of the American Academy of Optometry, October 23–27, 2019, Orlando, FL.

"The Epidemiology of Dry Eye Disease: Report of the Epidemiology Subcommittee of the International Dry Eye WorkShop (2007)," *Ocular Surface,* April 2007, 93–107.

Lemp, Michael A., et al., "Distribution of Aqueous-Deficient and Evaporative Dry Eye in a Clinic-Based Patient Cohort: A Retrospective Study," *Cornea,* May 2012, 427–428.

Maskin, Steve L., and Erin L. Greenberg, "Meibomian Gland Dysfunction, Dry Eye Disease, and Unhappy Cataract Surgery Patients," *Cataract & Refractive Surgery Today,* October 2018, 18–21.

Maskin, Steven L., and Scheffer C. G. Tseng, "Clonal Growth and Differentiation of Rabbit Meibomian Gland Epithelium in Serum-Free Culture: Differential Modulation by EGF and FGF," *Investigative Ophthalmology & Visual Science* 33 (1992), 205–217.

———, "Culture of Rabbit Meibomian Gland Using Collagen Gel," *Investigative Ophthalmology & Visual Science* 32 (1991), 214–223.

Restasis®, "Full Prescribing Information." Accessed January 4, 2019, https://www.allergan.com/assets/pdf/restasis_pi.pdf.

CHAPTER 2. THE EYE

Beers, Mark H., et al. (eds.), *The Merck Manual of Medical Information*. New York: Pocket Books, 2003, passim.

Clayman, Charles B., *The American Medical Association Encyclopedia of Medicine*. New York: Random House, 1989, passim.

Culhane, Shamus, *Animation from Script to Screen*. New York: St. Martin's Press, 1988, 165.

Dartt, Darelene A., and Mark Duncan Willcox, "Complexity of the Tear Film: Importance in Homeostasis and Dysfunction During Disease," *Experimental Eye Research*, December 2013, 1–3.

Foster, Brian J., and W. Barry Lee, "The Tear Film: Anatomy, Structure and Function," in Holland, Mannis, and Lee (eds.), *Ocular Surface Disease: Cornea, Conjunctiva, and Tear Film*. London: Elsevier Saunders, 2013, 17–21.

Foulks, Gary N., and Anthony J. Bron, "Meibomian Gland Dysfunction: A Clinical Scheme for Description, Diagnosis, Classification, and Grading," *The Ocular Surface*, July 2003, 107–111.

Glaser, Dee, et al., "Epidemiologic Analysis of Change in Eyelash Characteristics with Increasing Age in a Population of Healthy Women," *Dermatologic Surgery*, November 2014, 1208–1213.

Goldman, Lee, and Andrew I. Schaefer, *Goldman-Cecil Medicine*, 25th ed. Philadelphia: Elsevier, 2016, passim.

Hamrah, Pedram, and Afsun Sahin, "Limbus and Corneal Epithelium," in Holland, Mannis, and Lee (eds.), *Ocular Surface Disease: Cornea, Conjunctiva, and Tear Film*. London: Elsevier Saunders, 2013, 29–33.

Harvey, Thomas M., et al., "Conjunctival Anatomy and Physiology," in Holland, Mannis, and Lee (eds.), *Ocular Surface Disease: Cornea, Conjunctiva, and Tear Film*. London: Elsevier Saunders, 2013, 23–27.

Knop, Erich, et al., "The International Workshop on Meibomian Gland Dysfunction: Report of the Subcommittee on Anatomy, Physiology, and Pathophysiology of the Meibomian Gland," *Investigative Ophthalmology & Visual Science*, March 2011, 1938–1978.

Lawrenson, John G., "Anterior Eye," in Efron (ed.), *Contact Lens Practice*, 3rd ed. Philadelphia: Elsevier, 2018, 10–27.

Lin, Lily K., "Eyelid Anatomy and Function," in Holland, Mannis, and Lee (eds.), *Ocular Surface Disease: Cornea, Conjunctiva, and Tear Film*. London: Elsevier Saunders, 2013, 11–15.

Maskin, Steven L., *Reversing Dry Eye Syndrome: Practical Ways to Improve Your Comfort, Vision, and Appearance*. New Haven, CT: Yale University Press, 2007, passim.

Wang, Michael T. M., and Jennifer P. Craig, "Investigating the Effect of Eye Cosmetics on the Tear Film: Current Insights," *Clinical Optometry*, April 2018, 33–40.

CHAPTER 3. THE MEIBOMIAN GLAND

Arita, Reiko, et al., "Increased Tear Fluid Production as a Compensatory Response to Meibomian Gland Loss: A Multicenter Cross-sectional Study," *Ophthalmology* vol. 122, 5 (2015): 925–933.

Bründl, Maximilian, et al., "Characterization of the Innervation of the Meibomian Glands in Humans, Rats and Mice," *Annals of Anatomy = Anatomischer Anzeiger: Official Organ of the Anatomische Gesellschaft*, vol. 233 (2021).

Goto, E., and Scheffer C. Tseng, "Differentiation of Lipid Tear Deficiency Dry Eye by Kinetic Analysis of Tear Interference Images," *Archives of Ophthalmology*, February 2003, 173–180.

Hwang, Hyeonha, et al., "Image-Based Quantitative Analysis of Tear Film Lipid Layer Thickness for Meibomian Gland Evaluation," *Biomedical Engineering Online*, November 23, 2017, https://biomedical-engineering-online.biomedcentral.com/articles/10.1186/s12938-017-0426-8.

Knop, Erich, et al., "The International Workshop on Meibomian Gland Dysfunction: Report of the Subcommittee on Anatomy, Physiology, and Pathophysiology of the Meibomian Gland," *Investigative Ophthalmology & Visual Science*, March 2011, 1938–1978.

Maskin, Steve L., and Whitney R. Testa, "Growth of Meibomian Gland Tissue After Intraductal Meibomian Gland Probing in Patients with Obstructive Meibomian Gland Dysfunction," *British Journal of Ophthalmology,* January 2018, cover, 59–68.

Meibom, Heinrich, *De Vasis Palpebrarum Novis Epistola.* Helmstadt, Germany: Henningi Mulleri, 1666, cover, 17. Accessed December 15, 2020, https://archive.org/details/b31623839.

Olami, Y., et al., "Turnover and Migration of Meibomian Gland Cells in Rats' Eyelids," *Ophthalmic Research,* May–June 2001, 170–175.

Parfitt, Geraint J., et al., "Renewal of the Holocrine Meibomian Glands by Label-Retaining, Unipotent Epithelial Progenitors," *Stem Cell Report,* September 2016, 399–410.

Renker, L. W., et al., "Meibomian Gland (MG) Acinar Regeneration from Atrophy in a *Fgfr2* Conditional Knockout Mouse Model," *Investigative Ophthalmology & Visual Science* 60 (2019), 1412.

Suzuki, Tomo, et al., "Meibomian Gland Physiology in Pre- and Postmenopausal Women," *Investigative Ophthalmology & Visual Science,* February 2017, 763–771.

Wang, Michael T. M., et al., "Impact of Blinking on Ocular Surface and Tear Film Parameters," *Ocular Surface,* October 2018, 424–429.

Xie, Hya-Tao, et al., "Biomarkers for Progenitor and Differentiated Epithelial Cells in the Human Meibomian Gland," *Stem Cells Translational Medicine,* December 2018, 887–892.

CHAPTER 4. MEIBOMIAN GLAND DYSFUNCTION EXPLORED

Blackie, Caroline A., et al., "Nonobvious Obstructive Meibomian Gland Dysfunction," *Cornea,* December 2010, 1333–1345.

Bron, Anthony J., et al., "A Solute Gradient in the Tear Meniscus. I. A Hypothesis to Explain Marx's Line," *The Ocular Surface,* April 2011, 70–91.

———, "A Solute Gradient in the Tear Meniscus. II. Implications for Lid Margin Disease, Including Meibomian Gland Dysfunction," *The Ocular Surface*, April 2011, 92–97.

Butovich, Igor A., Juan C. Arciniega, and Jadwiga C. Wojtowicz, "Meibomian Lipid Films and the Impact of Temperature," *Investigative Ophthalmology & Visual Science*, November 2010, 5508–5518.

Cher, Ivan, "Meibomian Margin Dimples: Clinical Indicants of Reactive Pathogenic Processes," in Lass (ed.), *Advances in Corneal Research*. New York: Plenum Press, 1997, 27–35.

"Dry Eye Redefined: TFOS Dews II Report," website of the Tear Film and Ocular Surface Society. Accessed December 2, 2020, https://www.tfosdewsreport.org/.

The Editors of Encyclopaedia Britannica, "Keratin Biology," in *Encyclopaedia Britannica*. Accessed May 30, 2019, https://www.britannica.com/science/keratin.

Foulks, Gary N., and Anthony J. Bron, "Meibomian Gland Dysfunction: A Clinical Scheme for Description, Diagnosis, Classification, and Grading," *The Ocular Surface*, July 2003, 107–126.

Hwan, Ho Sik, et al., "Meibocyte Differentiation and Renewal: Insights into Novel Mechanisms of Meibomian Gland Dysfunction (MGD)," *Experimental Eye Research*, October 2017, 37–45.

Hykin, Philip G., and Anthony J. Bron, "Age-Related Morphological Changes in Lid Margin and Meibomian Gland Anatomy," *Cornea*, July 1992, 334–342.

Jester, James V., Geraint J. Parfitt, and Donald J. Brown, "Meibomian Gland Dysfunction: Hyperkeratinization or Atrophy?," *BMC Ophthalmology*, December 2015.

Knop, Erich, et al., "The International Workshop on Meibomian Gland Dysfunction: Report of the Subcommittee on Anatomy, Physiology, and Pathophysiology of the Meibomian Gland," *Investigative Ophthalmology & Visual Science*, March 2011, 1938–1978.

Knop, Erich, M. Ludescher, and Nadja Knop, "Keratinisation Status and Cytokeratins of the Human Meibomian Gland Epithelium," *Acta Ophthalmologic* 87, September 1, 2009, https://doi.org/10.1111/j.1755-3768.2009.2232.x.

Liu, Jingbo, Hosam Sheha, and Scheffer C. G. Tseng, "Pathogenic Role of Demodex Mites in Blepharitis," *Current Opinion in Allergy and Clinical Immunology*, October 2010, 505–510.

Maskin, Steven L., "Intraductal Meibomian Gland Probing Relieves Symptoms of Obstructive Meibomian Gland Dysfunction," *Cornea*, October 2010, 1145–1152.

Maskin, Steven L., and Sreevardhan Alluri, "Expressible Meibomian Glands Have Occult Fixed Obstructions: Findings from Meibomian Gland Probing to Restore Intraductal Integrity," *Cornea*, July 2019, 880–887.

———, "Meibography Guided Intraductal Meibomian Gland Probing Using Real-Time Infrared Video Feed," *British Journal of Ophthalmology*, December 2020, cover, 1676–1682.

———, "Real Time Infrared Video Meibography Feed Shows Intraductal Meibomian Gland Probing Confirms Presence of Duct and Restores Intraductal Integrity in Setting of Whole Gland Atrophy." Poster presented at the American Academy of Optometry, October 2019, Orlando, FL.

Parfitt, Geraint J., et al., "Absence of Ductal Hyper-Keratinization in Mouse Age-Related Meibomian Gland Dysfunction (ARMGD)," *Aging*, November 2013, 825–834.

Rastogi, Vaibhav, et al., "Abdominal Physical Signs and Medical Eponyms: Movements and Compression," *Clinical Medicine & Research*, December 2018, 76–82.

Suhalim, J. L., et al., "Effect of Desiccating Stress on Mouse Meibomian Gland Function," *The Ocular Surface*, January 2014, 59–68.

Syed, Zeba A., and Francis C. Sutula, "Dynamic Intraductal Meibomian Probing: A Modified Approach to the Treatment of Obstructive Meibomian Gland Dysfunction," *Ophthalmic Plastic and Reconstructive Surgery*, July–August 2017, 307–309.

CHAPTER 5. COMORBIDITIES AND COFACTORS

Alsuhaibani, Adel, et al., "Floppy Eyelid Syndrome," EyeWiki of the American Academy of Ophthalmology, January 6, 2020, https://eyewiki.org/Floppy_Eyelid_Syndrome.

Asproudis, Ioannis, et al., "Irritable Bowel Syndrome Might Be Associated with Dry Eye Disease," *Annals of Gastroenterology,* October–December 2016, 487–491.

Barba Gallardo, Luis Fernando, et al., "Extended Low Oxygen Transmissibility Contact Lens Use Induces Alterations in the Concentration of Proinflammatory Cytokines, Enzymes and Electrolytes in Tear Fluid," *Experimental and Therapeutic Medicine,* May 2018, 4291–4297.

Barta, Zsolt, et al., "Evaluation of Objective Signs and Subjective Symptoms of Dry Eye Disease in Patients with Inflammatory Bowel Disease," *BioMed Research International,* January 8, 2019, https://doi.org/10.1155/2019/8310583.

Beard, Crowell, "Wendell L. Hughes, MD," *Transactions of the American Ophthalmological Society* 92 (1994), 16–18.

Bert, Benjamin B., "How to Manage Conjunctivochalasis," *Review of Ophthalmology,* September 12, 2017, https://www.reviewof ophthalmology.com/article/how-to-manage-conjunctivochalasis.

Bron, Anthony J., et al., "A Solute Gradient in the Tear Meniscus. I. A Hypothesis to Explain Marx's Line," *The Ocular Surface,* April 2011, 70–91.

———, "A Solute Gradient in the Tear Meniscus. II. Implications for Lid Margin Disease, Including Meibomian Gland Dysfunction," *The Ocular Surface,* April 2011, 92–97.

Burkat, Cat Nguyen, et al., "Blepharospasm," EyeWiki of the American Academy of Ophthalmology, October 22, 2019. Accessed August 16, 2021, https://eyewiki.org/Blepharospasm.

Caffery, Barbara E., "Influence of Diet on Tear Function," *Optometry and Vision Science: Official Publication of the American Academy of Optometry* 68, no. 1 (1991), 58–72.

Chaudhary, Omar R., "Can Toenail Fungus Cause a Fungal Infection in the Eye?," website of American Academy of Ophthalmology, EyeSmart®, May 6, 2019, https://www.aao.org/eye-health/ask-oph thalmologist-q/can-toenail-fungus-cause-fungal-infection-in-eye.

"Cleaning Supplies and Household Chemicals," website of American Lung Association. Accessed July 23, 2019, https://www.lung .org/our-initiatives/healthy-air/indoor/indoor-air-pollutants /cleaning-supplies-household-chem.html.

Cole, Gary W., "Atopic Dermatitis Symptoms, Causes, vs. Eczema, Remedies, and Treatment," Medicinenet.com. Accessed October 31, 2019, https://www.medicinenet.com/atopic_dermatitis/article .htm.

Doshi-Velez, Finale, Yaorong Ge, and Isaac Kohane, "Comorbidity Clusters in Autism Spectrum Disorders: An Electronic Health Record Time-Series Analysis," *Pediatrics* 133, no. 1 (2014), e54–e63.

Efron, Nathan, "Contact Lens Wear Is Intrinsically Inflammatory," *Clinical and Experimental Optometry*, January 2017, 3–19.

Efron, Nathan, Munira Al-Dossari, and Nicola Pritchard, "In Vivo Confocal Microscopy of the Bulbar Conjunctiva," *Clinical & Experimental Ophthalmology*, May 2009, 335–344.

Efron, Nathan, and Philip B. Morgan, "Rethinking Contact Lens Associated Keratitis," *Clinical and Experimental Optometry*, September 2006, 280–298.

Gomes, José Alvaro P., et al., "TFOS DEWS II Iatrogenic Report," *The Ocular Surface* 15, no. 3 (2017), 511–538.

"High Blood Pressure," website of NIH, National Heart, Lung and Blood Institute. Accessed July 18, 2019, https://www.nhlbi.nih .gov/health-topics/high-blood-pressure.

Huang, Yukan, Hosam Sheha, and Scheffer C. G. Tseng, "Conjunctivochalasis Interferes with Tear Flow from Fornix to Tear Meniscus," *Ophthalmology*, August 2013, 1681–1687.

Ibraheem, Waheed A., et al., "Tear Film Functions and Intraocular Pressure Changes in Pregnancy," *African Journal of Reproductive Health,* December 2015, 118–122.

Jalbert, Isabelle, "Diet, Nutraceuticals and the Tear Film," *Experimental Eye Research* 117 (2013), 138–146.

Kan, Emrah, et al., "Presence of Dry Eye in Patients with Hashimoto's Thyroiditis," *Journal of Ophthalmology* 2014 (2014), https://doi.org/10.1155/2014/754923.

Karpecki, Paul M., and Diana L. Shechtman, "This Is NOT Dry Eye: Conjunctival Chalasis Is a Painful Condition That Produces Symptoms Similar to Dry Eye—But Don't Confuse the Two," *Review of Optometry,* February 2009.

Koçer, Emel, et al., "Dry Eye Related to Commonly Used New Antidepressants," *Journal of Clinical Psychopharmacology,* August 2015, 411–413.

Kramer, Elise, "Scleral Lenses—A Practice Builder," *Contact Lens Spectrum,* August 1, 2019.

Larrazabal, Luis Ignacio (contribs. and eds.), "Conjunctivochalasis," EyeWiki of the American Academy of Ophthalmology, November 15, 2019, https://eyewiki.org/Conjunctivochalasis.

Maki, Kara L., and David S. Ross, "Exchange of Tears Under a Contact Lens Is Driven by Distortions of the Contact Lens," *Integrative and Comparative Biology,* December 2014, 1043–1050.

Maskin, Steven L., "Effect of Ocular Surface Reconstruction by Using Amniotic Membrane Transplant for Symptomatic Conjunctivochalasis on Fluorescein Clearance Test Results," *Cornea,* July 2008, 644–649.

Maskin, Steven L., and Sreevardhan Alluri, "Intraductal Meibomian Gland Probing: Background, Patient Selection, Procedure, and Perspectives," *Clinical Ophthalmology,* July 10, 2019, 1203–1223.

Master, Jordan Scott, et al., "Vernal Keratoconjunctivitis," EyeWiki of the American Academy of Ophthalmology, March 7, 2020, https://eyewiki.org/Vernal_Keratoconjunctivitis.

Meller, Daniel, et al., "Amniotic Membrane Transplantation for Symptomatic Conjunctivochalasis Refractory to Medical Treatments," *Cornea,* November 2000, 796–803.

Mimura, Tatsuya, et al., "Changes of Conjunctivochalasis with Age in a Hospital-Based Study," *American Journal of Ophthalmology,* January 2009, 171–177.e1, https://doi.org/10.1016/j.ajo.2008.07.010.

Moen, Bente E., et al., "Can Air Pollution Affect Tear Film Stability? A Cross-Sectional Study in the Aftermath of an Explosion Accident," *BMC Public Health,* April 14, 2011, 235.

Moy, Allison, Nancy A. McNamara, and Meng C. Lin, "Effects of Isotretinoin on Meibomian Glands," *Optometry and Vision Science: Official Publication of the American Academy of Optometry,* September 2015, 925–930.

Mukamal, Reena, "Facts About Tears," website of American Academy of Ophthalmology, EyeSmart®, December 21, 2016, https://www.aao.org/eye-health/tips-prevention/facts-about-tears.

Neff, Kristiana D., "Conjunctivochalasis," in Holland, Mannis, and Lee (eds.), *Ocular Surface Disease: Cornea, Conjunctiva, and Tear Film.* London: Elsevier Saunders, 2013, 161–166.

Ohtomo, Kazuyoshi, et al., "Quantitative Analysis of Changes to Meibomian Gland Morphology Due to S-1 Chemotherapy," *Translational Vision Science & Technology,* December 2018, 37.

Papas, Eric B., "The Significance of Oxygen During Contact Lens Wear," *Contact Lens & Anterior Eye: The Journal of the British Contact Lens Association,* December 2014, 394–404.

"Parkinsons Overview," website of WebMD. Accessed March 26, 2020, https://www.webmd.com/parkinsons-disease/default.htm.

Periman, Laura M., and Leslie E. O'Dell, "When Beauty Doesn't Blink," *Ophthalmology Management,* August 1, 2016, https://www.ophthalmologymanagement.com/issues/2016/august-2016/when-beauty-doesn-8217;t-blink.

Pray, W. Steven, and Gabriel E. Pray, "Nonprescription Products for Minor Eye Condition," *U.S. Pharmacist,* April 20, 2011, https://www.uspharmacist.com/article/nonprescription-products-for-minor-eye-conditions.

Richards, Shawn C., and Richard S. Davidson, "Superior Limbic Keratoconjunctivitis," in Holland, Mannis, and Lee (eds.), *Ocular Surface Disease: Cornea, Conjunctiva, and Tear Film.* London: Elsevier Saunders, 2013, 167–169.

Samra, Khawla Abu, "The Eye and Visual System in Pregnancy, What to Expect? An In-Depth Review," *Oman Journal of Ophthalmology,* May 2013, 87–91.

Schuster, Alexander Karl-Georg, et al., "Eye Pain and Dry Eye in Patients with Fibromyalgia," *Pain Medicine,* December 1, 2018, 2528–2535.

Shamsheer, R. P., and Cynthia Arunachalam, "A Clinical Study of Meibomian Gland Dysfunction in Patients with Diabetes," *Middle East African Journal of Ophthalmology,* October–December 2015, 462–466.

Silpa-Archa, Sukhum, Joan J. Lee, and C. Stephen Foster, "Ocular Manifestations in Systemic Lupus Erythematosus," *The British Journal of Ophthalmology,* January 2016, 135–141.

Stone, John H., et al., "Recommendations for the Nomenclature of IgG4-Related Disease and Its Individual Organ System Manifestations," *Arthritis and Rheumatism,* October 2012, 3061–3067.

Sullivan, David A., et al., "Meibomian Gland Dysfunction in Primary and Secondary Sjögren Syndrome," *Ophthalmic Research* 59, no. 4 (2018), 193–205.

Szczotka-Flynn, Loretta B., Eric Pearlman, and Mahmoud Ghannoum, "Microbial Contamination of Contact Lenses, Lens Care Solutions, and Their Accessories: A Literature Review," *Eye & Contact Lens,* March 2010, 116–129.

Tamer Cengaver, Huseyin Oksuz, and Sadik Sogut, "Androgen Status of the Nonautoimmune Dry Eye Subtypes," *Ophthalmic Research* 38, no. 5 (2006), 280–286.

Varikooty, Jalaiah, "What Is Lid Wiper Epitheliopathy? Epidemiology, Associated Conditions, and How to Grade/Assess This Condition," *Contact Lens Spectrum,* November 1, 2015, https://www.clspectrum.com/issues/2015/november-2015/what-is-lid-wiper-epitheliopathy.

Wang, Michael T., and Jennifer P. Craig, "Investigating the Effect of Eye Cosmetics on the Tear Film: Current Insights," *Clinical Optometry,* April 3, 2018, 33–40.

Wong, John, et al., "Non-Hormonal Systemic Medications and Dry Eye," *The Ocular Surface,* October 2011, 212–226.

Ziemanski, Jillian F., et al., "Relation Between Dietary Essential Fatty Acid Intake and Dry Eye Disease and Meibomian Gland Dysfunction in Postmenopausal Women," *American Journal of Ophthalmology,* May 2018, 29–40.

CHAPTER 6. SYMPTOMS: LIVING WITH PAIN

Akpek, Esen K., et al., "Dry Eye Syndrome Preferred Practice Pattern®," *Ophthalmology,* January 2019, 286–334.

Arita, Reiko, et al., "Increased Tear Fluid Production as a Compensatory Response to Meibomian Gland Loss: A Multicenter Cross-sectional Study," *Ophthalmology* vol. 122,5 (2015): 925–933.

Asbell, Penny A., and Scott Spiegel, "Ophthalmologist Perceptions Regarding Treatment of Moderate to Severe Dry Eye: Results of a Physician Survey," *Transactions of the American Ophthalmological Society,* December 2009, 205–213.

Bleichrodt, Han, and Magnus Johannesson, "Standard Gamble, Time Trade-Off and Rating Scale: Experimental Results on the Ranking Properties of QALYs," *Journal of Health Economics,* April 1997, 155–175.

Buchholz, Patricia, et al., "Utility Assessment to Measure the Impact of Dry Eye Disease," *The Ocular Surface,* July 2006, 155–161.

Chalmers, Robin L., et al., "The Agreement Between Self-Assessment and Clinician Assessment of Dry Eye Severity," *Cornea,* October 2005, 804–810.

"Dizziness, Lightheadedness and Nausea or Vomiting," *Web MD Symptoms Checker.* Accessed August 13, 2019, https://symptom checker.webmd.com/multiple-symptoms?symptoms=dizziness %7Clightheadedness%7Cnausea-or-vomiting&symptomids=81 %7C141%7C156&locations=2%7C2%7C22.

Ducharlet, Kathryn, et al., "Patient-Reported Outcome Measures and Their Utility in the Management of Patients with Advanced Chronic Kidney Disease," *Nephrology*, August 2019, 814–818.

Enoch, Jamie, et al., "Evaluating Whether Sight Is the Most Valued Sense," *JAMA Ophthalmology*, October 3, 2019, 1317–1320.

Farrand, Kimberly F., et al., "Prevalence of Diagnosed Dry Eye Disease in the United States Among Adults Aged 18 Years and Older," *American Journal of Ophthalmology*, October 2017, 90–98.

Ghose, Tia, "Pediatricians: No More than 2 Hours Screen Time Daily for Kids," *Scientific American Health*, October 28, 2013.

Hamrah, Pedram, and Afsun Sahin, "Limbus and Corneal Epithelium," in Holland, Mannis, and Lee (eds.), *Ocular Surface Disease: Cornea, Conjunctiva, and Tear Film*. London: Elsevier Saunders, 2013, 29–33.

"Hip Fractures Among Older Adults," website of Centers for Disease Control and Prevention. Accessed August 21, 2019, https://www .cdc.gov/homeandrecreationalsafety/falls/adulthipfx.html.

King-Smith, P. E., et al., "The Thickness of the Human Precorneal Tear Film: Evidence from Reflection Spectra," *Investigative Ophthalmology & Visual Science*, October 2000, 3348–3359.

McDonald, Marguerite, et al., "Economic and Humanistic Burden of Dry Eye Disease in Europe, North America, and Asia: A Systematic Literature Review," *The Ocular Surface*, April 2016, 144–167.

McMonnies, Charles W., "The Potential Role of Neuropathic Mechanisms in Dry Eye Syndromes," *Journal of Optometry*, January–March 2017, 5–13.

"Medscape Physician Compensation Report: 2011 Results, Amount of Time Spent with Each Patient," *Medscape.* Accessed October

23, 2019, https://www.medscape.com/features/slideshow/compen sation/2011/#:~:text=Anesthesiologists%2C%20neurologists %2C%20and%20radiologists%20spend,9%2D12%20minutes %20per%20encounter.

Miller, Scott, "Kidney Stones vs. Childbirth: Which Is More Painful?" Accessed August 12, 2018, https://www.scottdmillermd.com /kidney-stones-vs-childbirth-painful/.

Mundi, Simran, et al., "Similar Mortality Rates in Hip Fracture Patients Over the Past 31 Years," *Acta Orthopaedica,* February 2014, 54–59.

"Ocular Surface Disease Index© (OSDI©)," Allergan an AbbVie Company. Accessed March 27, 2020, https://static1.squarespace.com /static/5a7915b649fc2b945a095fa3/t/5aadf828562fa7d5c70a 4be0/1521350696433/OSDI.pdf.

Schaumberg, Debra A., et al., "Development and Validation of a Short Global Dry Eye Symptom Index." *The Ocular Surface,* January 2007, 50–57.

Schiffman, Rhett M., et al., "Utility Assessment Among Patients with Dry Eye Disease," *Ophthalmology,* July 2003, 1412–1419.

Smith, Yolanda, "What Is the Difference Between Nociceptive and Neuropathic Pain?," News-Medical.Net, August 23, 2018, https:// www.news-medical.net/health/What-is-the-Difference-Between -Nociceptive-and-Neuropathic-Pain.aspx.

"Standardized Patient Evaluation of Eye Dryness (SPEED™) Questionnaire," TearScience Inc., 2011, https://eyewiki.aao.org/File:Official _SPEED_Questionnaire_copy.png.

"Symptoms," website of Not A Dry Eye Foundation. Accessed December 7, 2018, https://www.notadryeye.org/all-about-dry-eye-syn drome/symptoms-of-dry-eye-syndrome-and-related-conditions/.

Tichenor, Anna A., et al., "Tear Film and Meibomian Gland Characteristics in Adolescents," *Cornea,* December 2019, 1475–1482.

Wan, K. H., L. J. Chen, and A. L. Young, "Depression and Anxiety in Dry Eye Disease: A Systematic Review and Meta-Analysis," *Eye,* December 2016, 1558–1567.

Whelan, David, "Clayton Christensen: The Survivor," *Forbes*, February 23, 2011.

Xue, Wenwen, Xian Xu, and Haidong Zou, "A Rating Scale Is a Proper Method to Evaluate Changes in Quality of Life Due to Dry Eye Symptoms," *International Ophthalmology*, March 2019, 563–569.

Yu, Junhua, Carl V. Asche, and Carol J. Fairchild, "The Economic Burden of Dry Eye Disease in the United States: A Decision Tree Analysis," *Cornea*, April 2011, 379–387.

Zhang, Xingru, et al., "Bulbar Conjunctival Thickness Measurements with Optical Coherence Tomography in Healthy Chinese Subjects," *Investigative Ophthalmology & Visual Science*, July 2013, 4705–4709.

CHAPTER 7. THE LAST DAY OF MY LIFE

Maskin, Steven L., email message to Natalia A. Warren, August 17, 2011.

Restasis®, "Full Prescribing Information." Accessed January 4, 2019, https://www.allergan.com/assets/pdf/restasis_pi.pdf.

CHAPTER 8. SEVEN PRINCIPLES OF MEIBOMIAN GLANDS AND MEIBOMIAN GLAND DYSFUNCTION

Brissette, Ashley R., et al., "The Utility of a Normal Tear Osmolarity Test in Patients Presenting with Dry Eye Disease Like Symptoms: A Prospective Analysis," *Contact Lens & Anterior Eye: The Journal of the British Contact Lens Association*, April 2019, 185–189.

Ding, Juan, Yang Liu, and David A. Sullivan, "Effects of Insulin and High Glucose on Human Meibomian Gland Epithelial Cells," *Investigative Ophthalmology & Visual Science*, December 2015, 7814–7820.

Ma, Xiao, and Yan Lu, "Bilateral Tear Film Alterations in Patients with Unilateral Quiescent Herpes Simplex Keratitis," *Acta Ophthalmologica*, September 2017, 629–633.

Maskin, Steven L., and Whitney R. Testa, "Infrared Video Meibography of Lower Lid Meibomian Glands Shows Easily Distorted Glands: Implications for Longitudinal Assessment of Atrophy or Growth Using Lower Lid Meibography," *Cornea,* October 2018, 1279–1286.

Mukamal Reena, "Facts About Tears," website of American Academy of Ophthalmology, EyeSmart®, December 21, 2016, https://www.aao.org/eye-health/tips-prevention/facts-about-tears.

Nitoda, Eirini, et al., "Tear Film Osmolarity in Subjects with Acute Allergic Rhinoconjunctivitis," *In vivo,* March–April 2018, 403–408.

Parfitt, Geraint J., et al., "Absence of Ductal Hyper-Keratinization in Mouse Age-Related Meibomian Gland Dysfunction (ARMGD)," *Aging,* November 2013, 825–834.

Vorvick, Linda J., et al. (reviewers), "Exercise and Immunity," MedlinePlus, January 14, 2018, https://medlineplus.gov/ency/article/007165.htm.

CHAPTER 9. THE DIAGNOSIS

Arita, Reiko, et al., "Increased Tear Fluid Production as a Compensatory Response to Meibomian Gland Loss: A Multicenter Cross-sectional Study," *Ophthalmology* vol. 122,5 (2015): 925–933.

Baenninger, Philipp B., et al., "Variability of Tear Osmolarity Measurements with a Point-of-Care System in Healthy Subjects—Systematic Review," *Cornea,* July 2018, 938–945.

Blackie, Caroline A., and Donald R. Korb, "A Novel Lid Seal Evaluation: The Korb-Blackie Light Test," *Eye Contact Lens,* March 2015, 98–100.

Bunya, Vatinee Y., et al., "Variability of Tear Osmolarity in Patients with Dry Eye," *JAMA Ophthalmology,* June 2015, 662–667.

Compañ, Vicente, et al., "Oxygen Diffusion and Edema with Modern Scleral Rigid Gas Permeable Contact Lenses," *Investigative Ophthalmology & Visual Science,* September 4, 2014, 6421–6429.

Galor, Anat, et al., "Neuropathic Pain and Dry Eye," *The Ocular Surface,* January 2018, 31–44.

"InflammaDry," website of Quidel. Accessed February 2, 2020, https://www.quidel.com/immunoassays/inflammadry.

Maskin, Steven L., *Reversing Dry Eye Syndrome: Practical Ways to Improve Your Comfort, Vision, and Appearance.* New Haven, CT: Yale University Press, 2007, 140.

McMonnies, Charles W., "The Potential Role of Neuropathic Mechanisms in Dry Eye Syndromes," *Journal of Optometry,* January–March 2017, 5–13.

Stiles, J., et al., "The Efficacy of 0.5% Proparacaine Stored at Room Temperature," *Veterinary Ophthalmology,* September 2001, 205–207.

TearLab®. Accessed August 8, 2020, https://www.tearlab.com/.

CHAPTER 10. TREATING MEIBOMIAN GLAND DYSFUNCTION AND COMORBIDITIES

Beery, Brooke, "FDA Approves Bausch + Lomb Alaway Antihistamine Eyedrops," *Optometry Times,* September 25, 2020, https://www.optometrytimes.com/view/fda-approves-bausch-lomb-alaway-antihistamine-eyedrops.

Borchman, Douglas, "The Optimum Temperature for the Heat Therapy for Meibomian Gland Dysfunction," *The Ocular Surface,* April 2019, 360–364.

Bron, Anthony J., et al., "A Solute Gradient in the Tear Meniscus. I. A Hypothesis to Explain Marx's Line," *The Ocular Surface,* April 2011, 70–91.

Cher, Ivan, "Meibomian Margin Dimples: Clinical Indicants of Reactive Pathogenic Processes," in Lass (ed.), *Advances in Corneal Research.* New York: Plenum Press, 1997, 27–35.

"CyclASol®," website of Novalique. Accessed September 8, 2020, https://www.novaliq.com/products/cyclasol/.

Dell, Steven J., "Intense Pulsed Light for Evaporative Dry Eye Disease," *Clinical Ophthalmology*, June 20, 2017, 1167–1173.

"Depression: FDA-Approved Medications May Help," website of the U.S. Food & Drug Administration. Accessed June 11, 2020, https://www.fda.gov/consumers/consumer-updates/depression-fda-approved-medications-may-help.

Dogan, Cezmi, et al., "Effect of Scleral Lens Use on Conjunctival Microbiota," *Contact Lens & Anterior Eye: The Journal of the British Contact Lens Association*, April 2020, 189–191.

"Dry Eye," website of Lubris BioPharma. Accessed September 8, 2020, http://lubris.net/dry-eye/.

Dry Eye Assessment and Management Study Research Group, et al., "n-3 Fatty Acid Supplementation for the Treatment of Dry Eye Disease," *The New England Journal of Medicine*, May 3, 2018, 1681–1690.

"EyeLipid Mobilizer," website of Eyedetec. Accessed September 8, 2020, https://www.eyedetec.com/#eyedetec-solution.

Foulks, Gary N., et al., "Topical Azithromycin and Oral Doxycycline Therapy of Meibomian Gland Dysfunction: A Comparative Clinical and Spectroscopic Pilot Study," *Cornea*, January 2013, 44–53.

Hara, Shuya, et al., "Evaluation of Tear Stability After Surgery for Conjunctivochalasis," *Optometry and Vision Science: Official Publication of the American Academy of Optometry*, September 2011, 1112–1118.

Huang, Xiaodan, et al., "Clinical Results of Intraductal Meibomian Gland Probing Combined with Intense Pulsed Light in Treating Patients with Refractory Obstructive Meibomian Gland Dysfunction: A Randomized Controlled Trial," *BMC Ophthalmology*, October 28, 2019.

"iTear® 100," website of Olympic Ophthalmics. Accessed September 8, 2020, http://www.olympicophthalmics.com/devices/iTEAR100/.

Jehangir, Naz, et al., "Comprehensive Review of the Literature on Existing Punctal Plugs for the Management of Dry Eye Disease," *Journal of Ophthalmology*, March 7, 2016.

Kim, Ho-Yun, et al., "Clinical Efficacy of Combined Topical 0.05% Cyclosporine A and 0.1% Sodium Hyaluronate in the Dry Eyes with Meibomian Gland Dysfunction," *International Journal of Ophthalmology,* April 18, 2018, 593–600.

Korb, Donald R., and Caroline A. Blackie, "Meibomian Gland Therapeutic Expression: Quantifying the Applied Pressure and the Limitation of Resulting Pain," *Eye & Contact Lens,* September 2011, 298–301.

Liu, Jingbo, Hosam Sheha, and Scheffer C. G. Tseng, "Pathogenic Role of Demodex Mites in Blepharitis," *Current Opinion in Allergy and Clinical Immunology,* October 2010, 505–510.

Liu, S., et al., "Analysis of Factors Leading to Lid Wiper Epitheliopathy," *European Review for Medical and Pharmacological Sciences,* February 2020, 1593–1601.

LYRICA®, "Full Prescribing Information." Accessed June 11, 2020, http://labeling.pfizer.com/showlabeling.aspx?id=56.

Macedo-de-Araújo, Rute Juliana, Eef van der Worp, and José Manuel González-Méijome, "In Vivo Assessment of the Anterior Scleral Contour Assisted by Automatic Profilometry and Changes in Conjunctival Shape After Miniscleral Contact Lens Fitting," *Journal of Optometry,* April–June 2019, 131–140.

Marcet, Marcus M., et al., "Safety and Efficacy of Lacrimal Drainage System Plugs for Dry Eye Syndrome: A Report by the American Academy of Ophthalmology," *Ophthalmology,* August 2015, 1681–1687.

Maskin, Steven L., "Effect of Ocular Surface Reconstruction by Using Amniotic Membrane Transplant for Symptomatic Conjunctivochalasis on Fluorescein Clearance Test Results," *Cornea,* July 2008, 644–649.

———, "Regression of Limbal Epithelial Dysplasia with Topical Interferon," *Archives of Ophthalmology,* September 1994, 1145–1146.

———, *Reversing Dry Eye Syndrome: Practical Ways to Improve Your Comfort, Vision, and Appearance.* New Haven, CT: Yale University Press, 2007, passim.

Maskin, Steven L., and Whitney R. Testa, "Growth of Meibomian Gland Tissue After Intraductal Meibomian Gland Probing in Patients with Obstructive Meibomian Gland Dysfunction," *British Journal of Ophthalmology,* January 2018, cover, 59–68.

McMonnies, Charles W., "The Potential Role of Neuropathic Mechanisms in Dry Eye Syndromes," *Journal of Optometry,* January–March 2017, 5–13.

Neurontin®-Gabapentin, "Full Prescribing Information." Accessed June 11, 2020, http://labeling.pfizer.com/ShowLabeling.aspx?id =630#S5.6.

"NuLids FAQs," website of NuSight Medical. Accessed September 8, 2020, https://www.nusightmedical.com/faq/.

"OC-01 (Varenicline) Nasal Spray for Treatment of the Signs and Symptoms of Dry Eye Disease," website of Oyster Point Pharma, Inc. Accessed February 20, 2020, https://oysterpointrx.com/pipe line/oc-01/.

Oleñik, Andrea, et al., "A Randomized, Double-Masked Study to Evaluate the Effect of Omega-3 Fatty Acids Supplementation in Meibomian Gland Dysfunction," *Clinical Interventions in Aging,* August 29, 2013, 1133–1138.

Opitz, Dominick L., and Jennifer S. Harthan, "Review of Azithromycin Ophthalmic 1% Solution (AzaSite®) for the Treatment of Ocular Infections," *Ophthalmology and Eye Diseases,* February 23, 2012, 1–14.

Periman, Laura M., and Leslie E. O'Dell, "When Beauty Doesn't Blink," *Ophthalmology Management,* August 1, 2016, https://www .ophthalmologymanagement.com/issues/2016/august-2016 /when-beauty-doesn-8217;t-blink.

Restasis®, "Full Prescribing Information." Accessed January 4, 2019, https://www.allergan.com/assets/pdf/restasis_pi.pdf.

Salem, Doaa Abdel-Badie, et al., "Evaluation of the Efficacy of Oral Ivermectin in Comparison with Ivermectin-Metronidazole Combined Therapy in the Treatment of Ocular and Skin Lesions of

Demodex Folliculorum," *International Journal of Infectious Diseases (IJID): Official Publication of the International Society for Infectious Disease,* May 2013, e343–e347.

Schornack, Muriel M., and Cherie B. Nau, "Changes in Optical Density of Postlens Fluid Reservoir During 2 Hours of Scleral Lens Wear," *Eye & Contact Lens,* November 2018, S344–S349.

Sheppard, John D., Jr., et al. "Long-term Supplementation with n-6 and n-3 PUFAs Improves Moderate-to-Severe Keratoconjunctivitis Sicca: A Randomized Double-Blind Clinical Trial," *Cornea,* October 2013, 1297–1304.

Sherman, Suzanne W., Christina Cherny, and Leejee H. Suh, "Epithelial Inclusion Cyst of the Bulbar Conjunctiva Secondary to Scleral Lens Impingement Managed with a MicroVault," *Eye & Contact Lens,* November 2020, e56-e58.

Tauber, Joseph, "A 6-Week, Prospective, Randomized, Single-Masked Study of Lifitegrast Ophthalmic Solution 5% Versus Thermal Pulsation Procedure for Treatment of Inflammatory Meibomian Gland Dysfunction," *Cornea,* April 2020, 403–407.

Tauber, Joseph, et al., "Comparison of the iLUX and the LipiFlow for the Treatment of Meibomian Gland Dysfunction and Symptoms: A Randomized Clinical Trial," *Clinical Ophthalmology,* February 12, 2020, 405–418.

"TP-03," website of Tarsus Pharmaceuticals. Accessed September 8, 2020, https://www.tarsusrx.com/tp03.

Website of Azura Ophthalmics. Accessed September 8, 2020, https://azuraophthalmics.com/pipeline.

Website of Eye Eco Inc. Accessed December 10, 2020, https://www.eyeeco.com.

Website of TearCare®. Accessed December 10, 2020, https://www.tearcare.com/.

Website of TearScience® Inc. Accessed January 22, 2020, https://dryeyeandmgd.com/product-safety-info/.

Xiidra®, "Full Prescribing Information," website of Novartis US. Accessed December 10, 2020, https://www.novartis.us/sites/www.novartis.us/files/xiidra.pdf.

CHAPTER 11. INTRADUCTAL MEIBOMIAN GLAND
PROBING: THE MASKIN® PROBE AND PROTOCOL

Cárdenas Díaz, Taimi, et al., "Efficacy of Intraductal Probing in the Dysfunction of the Meibomian Glands," *Revista Cubana de Oftalmología*, [S.l.], v. 30, n. 2, 2017. Available in: http://www.revoftalmologia.sld.cu/index.php/oftalmologia/article/view/496.

Cher, Ivan, "Meibomian Margin Dimples: Clinical Indicants of Reactive Pathogenic Processes," in Lass (ed.), *Advances in Corneal Research*. New York: Plenum Press, 1997, 27–35.

Dongju, Qin, Liu Hui, and Xu Jianjiang, "Clinical Research on Intraductal Meibomian Gland Probing in the Treatment of Patients with Meibomian Gland Dysfunction," *Chinese Journal of Optometry, Ophthalmology, and Visual Science* 16, no. 10 (2014), 615–621.

Fermon, S., Hindi I. Zaga, and Alvarez D. Melloni, "Sondaje intraductal de las glándulas de Meibomio para el tratamiento de blefaritis posterior severa" [Intraductal Meibomian gland probing for the treatment of blepharitis], *Archivos de la Sociedad Española de Oftalmologí*, February 2015, 76–80.

Huang, X., et al., "Clinical Results of Intraductal Meibomian Gland Probing Combined with Intense Pulsed Light in Treating Patients with Refractory Obstructive Meibomian Gland Dysfunction: A Randomized Controlled Trial," *BMC Ophthalmology*, October 28, 2019.

Incekalan, T. K., et al., "Effectiveness of Intraductal Meibomian Gland Probing in Addition to the Conventional Treatment in Patients with Obstructive Meibomian Gland Dysfunction," *Ocular Immunology and Inflammation*, September 2019, 1345–1351.

Kheirkhah, Ahmad, et al., "A Randomized, Sham-Controlled Trial of Intraductal Meibomian Gland Probing with or Without Topical Antibiotic/Steroid for Obstructive Meibomian Gland Dysfunction," *The Ocular Surface*, October 2020, 852–856.

Ma, Xiao, and Yan Lu, "Efficacy of Intraductal Meibomian Gland Probing on Tear Function in Patients with Obstructive Meibomian Gland Dysfunction," *Cornea,* June 2016, 725–730.

Maskin, Steven L., "Effect of Ocular Surface Reconstruction by Using Amniotic Membrane Transplant for Symptomatic Conjunctivochalasis on Fluorescein Clearance Test Results," *Cornea,* July 2008, 644–649.

———, "Fantastic Voyage into the Meibomian Gland: Results of Intraductal Probing (MGP) and Successful Treatment of Meibomian Gland Dysfunction (MGD) from Within." Virtual presentation for the Japanese Dry Eye Research Society, 2011, Tokyo.

———, "Intraductal Meibomian Gland Probing: A Paradigm Shift for the Successful Treatment of Obstructive Meibomian Gland Dysfunction," in Tsubota (ed.), *Diagnosis and Treatment of MGD.* Tokyo: Kanehara, September 2016, chap. 17, 130–167.

———, "Intraductal Meibomian Gland Probing for Meibomian Gland Dysfunction Using VAS Testing." Poster presented at the annual meeting of the American Academy of Ophthalmology, October 2010, Chicago.

———, "Intraductal Meibomian Gland Probing for Meibomian Gland Dysfunction Using VAS Testing." Poster presented at the World Cornea Congress VI, April 2010, Boston.

———, "Intraductal Meibomian Gland Probing Relieves Symptoms of Obstructive Meibomian Gland Dysfunction." Abstract published in *Investigative Ophthalmology & Visual Science,* April 2009, 4636.

———, "Intraductal Meibomian Gland Probing Relieves Symptoms of Obstructive Meibomian Gland Dysfunction," *Cornea,* October 2010, 1145–1152.

———, "Intraductal Meibomian Gland Probing Relieves Symptoms of Obstructive Meibomian Gland Dysfunction." Poster presented at the annual meeting of the Association for Research in Vision and Ophthalmology, May 2009, Fort Lauderdale, FL.

———, "Meibomian Gland Probing (MGP): Safely Providing Outflow Patency with Positive Physical Proof: Concepts, Literature Review and Results." Presented at a course on New Treatments for Meibomian Gland Dysfunction at the annual meeting of the American Academy of Ophthalmology, October 2018, Chicago.

———, "Meibomian Gland Probing (MGP): Safely Providing Patency with Positive Physical Proof: Literature Review, Concepts and Results." Presented at a course on New Treatments for Meibomian Gland Dysfunction at the annual meeting of the American Academy of Ophthalmology, November 2017, New Orleans, LA.

———, "Meibomian Gland Probing (MGP): Safely Providing Patency to Glands Using Verifiable Physical Proof: Background, Technique and Results." Presented at a course on New Treatments for Meibomian Gland Dysfunction at the annual meeting of the American Academy of Ophthalmology, October 2016, Chicago.

———, "Meibomian Gland Probing (MGP): Safely Providing Patency to Glands Using Verifiable Physical Proof: Background, Technique and Results." Presented at a course on New Treatments for Meibomian Gland Dysfunction at the annual meeting of the American Academy of Ophthalmology, November 2015, Las Vegas, NV.

———, "Regression of Limbal Epithelial Dysplasia with Topical Interferon," *Archives of Ophthalmology,* September 1994, 1145–1146 (also selected for publication in the Chinese and Spanish editions).

———, "Results of Intraductal Meibomian Gland Probing (MGP) for Symptoms of Inflammatory Meibomian Gland Dysfunction (MGD) Excluding Lid Tenderness." Poster presented at the annual meeting of the American Society of Cornea and Refractive Surgery, April 2010, Boston.

———, *Reversing Dry Eye Syndrome: Practical Ways to Improve Your Comfort, Vision, and Appearance.* New Haven, CT: Yale University Press, 2007.

———, "Treatment of Obstructive Meibomian Gland Dysfunction Using Intraductal Probing: Emerging Importance of Restoring Ductal Integrity." Presented at a course on New Treatments for

Meibomian Gland Dysfunction at the annual meeting of the American Academy of Ophthalmology, October 2019, San Francisco.

Maskin, Steven L., and Sreevardhan Alluri, "An Alternative Hypothesis of Atrophic Meibomian Gland Dysfunction Using Stem Cell Concept." Abstract published in *Investigative Ophthalmology & Visual Science,* June 2020, 343.

———, "An Alternative Hypothesis of Atrophic Meibomian Gland Dysfunction Using Stem Cell Concept." Poster presented at the annual meeting of the Association for Research in Vision and Ophthalmology, virtual meeting, March 2020.

———, "Expressible Meibomian Glands Have Occult Fixed Obstructions: Findings from Meibomian Gland Probing to Restore Intraductal Integrity," *Cornea,* July 2019, 880–887.

———, "Infrared Video Meibography Feed Reveals Meibomian Gland Probing Restores and Confirms Central Duct Integrity in Areas of Whole Gland Atrophy." Paper presented at the World Cornea Congress VIII, virtual meeting, March 2020.

———, "Intraductal Meibomian Gland Probing: Background, Patient Selection, Procedure, and Perspectives," *Clinical Ophthalmology,* July 10, 2019, 1203–1223.

———, "Intraductal Meibomian Gland Probing (MGP) Leads to Ductal Epithelial Proliferation with Increased Duct Wall Thickness." Abstract published in *Investigative Ophthalmology & Visual Science,* June 2020, 96.

———, "Intraductal Meibomian Gland Probing (MGP) Leads to Ductal Epithelial Proliferation with Increased Duct Wall Thickness." Poster presented at the annual meeting of the Association for Research in Vision and Ophthalmology, virtual meeting, March 2020.

———, "Meibography Guided Intraductal Meibomian Gland Probing Using Real-Time Infrared Video Feed," *British Journal of Ophthalmology,* December 2020, cover, 1676–1682.

————, "Real Time Infrared Video Feed Enables Visualization of Intraductal Meibomian Gland Probing." Poster presented at the World Cornea Congress VIII, virtual meeting, March 2020.

————, "Real Time Infrared Video Meibography Feed Shows Intraductal Meibomian Gland Probing Confirms Presence of Duct and Restores Intraductal Integrity in Setting of Whole Gland Atrophy." Poster presented at the American Academy of Optometry, October 2019, Orlando, FL.

————, "Visualization of Intraductal Meibomian Gland Probing Using Real Time Infrared Video Feed." Poster presented at the American Academy of Optometry, October 2019, Orlando, FL.

Maskin, Steven L., et al., "Loteprednol Etabonate 0.5% (Lotemax) Versus Vehicle in the Management of Patients with KCS and at Least Moderate Inflammation." Abstract published in *Investigative Ophthalmology & Visual Science,* May 2003, 686.

————, "Loteprednol Etabonate 0.5% (Lotemax) Versus Vehicle in the Management of Patients with KCS and at Least Moderate Inflammation." Poster presented at the meeting of the Association for Research in Vision and Ophthalmology, May 2003, Fort Lauderdale, FL.

Maskin, Steven L., and Whitney Hethorn, "Meibomian Gland Probing for Lid Tenderness and Non-Functioning Meibomian Glands in Meibomian Gland Dysfunction." Poster presented at the annual meeting of the American Academy of Ophthalmology, November 2015, Las Vegas, NV.

Maskin, Steven L., and Kelly Kantor, "Intraductal Meibomian Gland Probing to Restore Functionality for Obstructive Meibomian Gland Dysfunction." Poster presented at the annual meeting of the American Academy of Ophthalmology, October 2011, Orlando, FL.

————, "Intraductal Meibomian Gland Probing with Adjunctive Intraductal Microtube Steroid Injection (MGPs) for Meibomian Gland Dysfunction (MGD)." Abstract published in *Investigative Ophthalmology & Visual Science,* April 2011, 3817.

———, "Intraductal Meibomian Gland Probing with Adjunctive Intraductal Microtube Steroid Injection (MGPs) for Meibomian Gland Dysfunction (MGD)." Poster presented at the annual meeting of the Association for Research in Vision and Ophthalmology, May 2011, Fort Lauderdale, FL.

Maskin, Steven L., and Jody Leppla, "Meibomian Gland Probing Findings Suggest Fibrotic Obstruction Is a Major Cause of Obstructive Meibomian Gland Dysfunction (O-MGD)." Abstract published in *Investigative Ophthalmology & Visual Science*, March 2012, 605.

———, "Meibomian Gland Probing Findings Suggest Fibrotic Obstruction Is a Major Cause of Obstructive Meibomian Gland Dysfunction (O-MGD)." Poster presented at the annual meeting of the Association for Research in Vision and Ophthalmology, May 2012, Fort Lauderdale, FL.

Maskin, Steven L., and Whitney R. Testa, "Growth of Meibomian Gland Tissue After Intraductal Meibomian Gland Probing in Patients with Obstructive Meibomian Gland Dysfunction," *British Journal of Ophthalmology*, January 2018, cover, 59–68.

———, "Infrared Video Meibography of Lower Lid Meibomian Glands Shows Easily Distorted Glands: Implications for Longitudinal Assessment of Atrophy or Growth Using Lower Lid Meibography," *Cornea*, October 2018, 1279–1286.

———, "Regrowth of Meibomian Gland Tissue After Intraductal Meibomian Gland Probing in Patients with Obstructive Meibomian Gland Dysfunction (O-MGD)." Abstract published in *Investigative Ophthalmology & Visual Science*, June 2017, 4392.

———, "Regrowth of Meibomian Gland Tissue After Intraductal Meibomian Gland Probing in Patients with Obstructive Meibomian Gland Dysfunction (O-MGD)." Poster presented at the annual meeting of the Association for Research in Vision and Ophthalmology, May 2017, Baltimore, MD. Selected by ARVO Annual Program Committee as 2017 Hot Topic.

Maskin, Steven L., and Scheffer C. G. Tseng, "Clonal Growth and Differentiation of Rabbit Meibomian Gland Epithelium in Serum-

Free Culture," *Investigative Ophthalmology & Visual Science,* January 1992, 205–217.

———, "Culture of Rabbit Meibomian Gland Using Collagen Gel," *Investigative Ophthalmology & Visual Science,* January 1991, 214–223.

Maskin, Steven L., and Courtney Warsinski, "Long Term Safety and Retreatment Data After Intraductal Meibomian Gland Probing for Obstructive Meibomian Gland Dysfunction." Abstract published in *Investigative Ophthalmology & Visual Science,* April 2010, 6283.

———, "Long Term Safety and Retreatment Data After Intraductal Meibomian Gland Probing for Obstructive Meibomian Gland Dysfunction." Poster presented at the annual meeting of the Association for Research in Vision and Ophthalmology, May 2010, Fort Lauderdale, FL.

Meller, Daniel, et al., "Amniotic Membrane Transplantation for Symptomatic Conjunctivochalasis Refractory to Medical Treatment," *Cornea,* November 2000, 796–803.

Nakayama, Naohiko, et al., "Analysis of Meibum Before and After Intraductal Meibomian Gland Probing in Eyes with Obstructive Meibomian Gland Dysfunction," *Cornea,* October 2015, 1206–1208.

Nirupama, D., et al., "Meibomian Gland Probing in Patients with Meibomian Gland Dysfunction," *Indian Journal of Clinical and Experimental Ophthalmology* 5, no. 1 (2019), 78–81.

Pflugfelder, Stephen C., et al., "A Randomized, Double-Masked, Placebo-Controlled, Multicenter Comparison of Loteprednol Etabonate Ophthalmic Suspension, 0.5%, and Placebo for Treatment of Keratoconjunctivitis Sicca in Patients with Delayed Tear Clearance," *American Journal of Ophthalmology,* September 2004, 444–457.

Pires R. T. F., et al., "Amniotic Membrane Transplantation for Symptomatic Bullous Keratopathy," *Archives of Ophthalmology,* October 1999, 1291–1297.

Prozornaia, L. P., and V. V. Brzhevskiǐ, "Efficacy of Physiotherapy and Hygienic Procedures in Treatment of Adults and Children with

Chronic Blepharitis and Dry Eye Syndrome," *Vestnik oftalmologii,* May–June 2013, 68–70, 72–73.

Sarman, Zuleyha Sik, et al., "Effectiveness of Intraductal Meibomian Gland Probing for Obstructive Meibomian Gland Dysfunction," *Cornea,* June 2016, 721–724.

Syed, Zeba A., and Francis C. Sutula, "Dynamic Intraductal Meibomian Probing: A Modified Approach to the Treatment of Obstructive Meibomian Gland Dysfunction," *Ophthalmic Plastic and Reconstructive Surgery,* July/August 2017, 307–309.

Tseng, Scheffer C. G., et al., "Classification of Conjunctival Surgeries for Corneal Disease Based on Stem Cell Concept," in Sugar and Soong (eds.), *Ophthalmology Clinics of North America,* vol. 3, no. 4. Philadelphia: Saunders, December 1990, 595–610.

Wladis, Edward J., "Intraductal Meibomian Gland Probing in the Management of Ocular Rosacea," *Ophthalmic Plastic and Reconstructive Surgery,* November–December 2012, 416–418.

CHAPTER 12. GUIDELINES FOR MANAGING YOUR LIFE WITH MEIBOMIAN GLAND DYSFUNCTION

Jester, James V., et al., "Meibomian Gland Dysfunction. II. The Role of Keratinization in a Rabbit Model of MGD," *Investigative Ophthalmology & Visual Science,* May 1989, 936–945.

Trope, G. E., and A. G. Rumley, "Catecholamine Concentrations in Tears," *Experimental Eye Research,* September 1984, 247–250.

INDEX

Tables and figures are indicated by *t* and *fig* respectively following the page number.

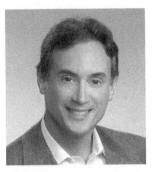

STEVEN L. MASKIN, MD, is a board-certified ophthalmologist who specializes in solving difficult Dry Eye, Meibomian gland dysfunction (MGD), and ocular surface disorders. He treats patients from across the globe at the Dry Eye and Cornea Treatment Center in Tampa, Florida. He is the founder of MGDinnovations (mgdi .com), a translational bio-tech company focused on Meibomian gland dysfunction.

Dr. Maskin was the first researcher to confirm the presence of periductal fibrosis, the tissue that constricts Meibomian glands, is the inventor of intraductal Meibomian gland probing, the therapy that targets fibrosis, and holds six US patents related to the treatment of Meibomian gland dysfunction. In 1994, he published a peer-reviewed scientific paper describing his discovery of a cure for ocular surface squamous neoplasia (cancer), using interferon alpha-2b, that is now widely used.

He has published over 22 scientific papers on MGD, Meibomian gland probing, and other ophthalmic topics and is the author of *Reversing Dry Eye Syndrome: Practical Ways to Improve Your, Comfort, Vision, and Appearance* (Yale University Press, 2007).

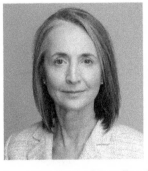

NATALIA A. WARREN, MBA, MHA, has been Dr. Maskin's patient since 2011. Prior to her Dry Eye diagnosis, she enjoyed a successful career as an award-winning executive in strategy, product management, and conference production at global technology and entertainment companies. She is the cofounder of Not A Dry Eye Foundation, the first non-profit patient-founded organization dedicated to raising awareness of Dry Eye Syndrome, where she chairs the Board of Directors, volunteers as a patient advocate, and oversees independent patient-centered research projects on Dry Eye, MGD, and related comorbidities. She lives in Orlando, Florida with her family.